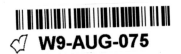

NURSING
THEORIES

The Base for
Professional Nursing Practice

JULIA B. GEORGE, EDITOR
The Nursing Theories Conference Group

NURSING THEORIES

The Base for Professional Nursing Practice

SECOND EDITION

PRENTICE-HALL, INC., Englewood Cliffs, New Jersey 07632

Library of Congress Cataloging in Publication Data
Main entry under title:

Nursing theories.

Includes bibliographies and index.
1. Nursing—Philosophy—Congresses. I. George,
Julia B. II. Nursing Theories Conference Group.
[DNLM: 1. Philosophy, Nursing. WY 86 N9755]
RT84.5.N89 1985   610.73'01   84-17919
ISBN   0-13-627407-2

Printed in the United States of America

10   9   8   7   6   5   4   3   2   1

Editorial/production supervision: Paul Spencer
Interior design: Eleanor Henshaw Hiatt
Cover design: Ben Santora
Manufacturing buyer: John Hall

ISBN   0-13-627407-2   01

Prentice-Hall International, Inc., *London*
Prentice-Hall of Australia Pty. Limited, *Sydney*
Editora Prentice-Hall do Brasil, Ltda., *Rio de Janeiro*
Prentice-Hall Canada Inc., *Toronto*
Prentice-Hall of India Private Limited, *New Delhi*
Prentice-Hall of Japan, Inc., *Tokyo*
Prentice-Hall of Southeast Asia Pte. Ltd., *Singapore*
Whitehall Books Limited, *Wellington, New Zealand*

CONTRIBUTING AUTHORS

Janice Ryan Belcher, R.N., M.S., Psychiatric Clinical Nurse Specialist, Kettering Medical Center, Kettering, Ohio.

Agnes M. Bennett, R.N., M.S., Assistant Professor, Department of Nursing, Miami University, Oxford, Ohio.

Mary Disbrow Crane, R.N.C., M.S., Family and Community Health Clinical Specialist, Potomac, Maryland.

Joanne R. Cross, R.N., M.S.N., M.S. Counseling, Assistant Professor, School of Nursing, Wright State University, Dayton, Ohio.

Suzanne M. Falco, R.N., Ph.D., Associate Professor, School of Nursing, The University of Wisconsin-Milwaukee, Milwaukee, Wisconsin.

Lois J. Brittain Fish, R.N., M.S.N., Instructor, School of Nursing, Wright State University, Dayton, Ohio.

Peggy Coldwell Foster, R.N., M.S.N., Staff Nurse, Bethesda Hospitals, Bethesda, Maryland, and Instructor, Childbirth Education Association, Cincinnati, Ohio.

Chiyoko Yamamoto Furukawa, R.N., M.S., Assistant Professor, College of Nursing, University of New Mexico, Albuquerque, New Mexico.

Julia Gallagher Galbreath, R.N., C.S., M.S., Adjunct Assistant Professor, Wright State University, Dayton, Ohio, and Certified Clinical Nurse Specialist, Piqua Memorial Hospital, Piqua, Ohio.

Julia B. George, R.N., Ph.D., Associate Professor and Chairperson, Parent and Child Health Nursing Graduate Program, College of Nursing and Health, University of Cincinnati, Cincinnati, Ohio.

Christina R. Hogarth, R.N., M.S., Director of Nursing, Dartmouth Center, Dayton, Ohio.

Joan K. Howe, R.N., M.S., Lecturer in Nursing, Lima Technical College, Lima, Ohio.

Nancy P. Janssens, R.N., M.S., Assistant Professor, School of Nursing, Wright State University, Dayton, Ohio.

Mary Kathryn Leonard, R.N., M.S., Ph.D. Candidate, Vice-President for Nursing, Herbert J. Thomas Memorial Hospital, South Charleston, West Virginia.

Marie L. Lobo, R.N., Ph.D., Associate Professor, Director, Chairperson Nursing Care of Children, Frances Payne Bolton School of Nursing, Case Western Reserve University, Rainbow Babies and Children's Hospital, Cleveland, Ohio.

Charlotte Paul, R.N., Ph.D., Associate Professor, School of Nursing and Psychology, Edinboro State College, Edinboro, Pennsylvania.

Susan G. Praeger, R.N., Ed.D., Assistant Professor, School of Nursing, Wright State University, Dayton, Ohio.

Joan S. Reeves, R.N., M.S.N., Assistant Professor, College of Nursing, University of Illinois, Chicago, Illinois.

Marjorie Stanton, R.N., Ed.D., Chairperson, Division of Nursing, D'Youville College, Buffalo, New York.

Gertrude Torres, R.N., Ed.D., Dean of Academic Affairs, D'Youville College, Buffalo, New York.

CONTENTS

PREFACE

As an emerging profession, nursing continues to be deeply involved in identifying its own unique knowledge base. In identifying this base of knowledge, various concepts, models, and theories specific to nursing are being recognized, defined, and developed. Although these concepts, models, and theories have been published in a variety of journals and books, there is a need for them to be gathered in one volume and applied to nursing practice through the nursing process.

This book is designed to consider the ideas of sixteen nursing theorists and relate the work of each to the nursing process of assessing, diagnosing, planning, implementing, and evaluating. It must be recognized that the book serves as a secondary source in relation to the statements and purposes of the individuals whose writings are discussed. It is intended for use as a tool for the thoughtful and considered application of nursing concepts and theories to nursing practice.

There are essentially three areas of focus. First, Chapters 1 and 2 present the place of concepts and theories in nursing and discuss the nursing process. These chapters provide a common base for the next fifteen chapters and should be read first.

Next, Chapters 3 through 17 present the major components of

the work of Florence Nightingale, Hildegard E. Peplau, Virginia Henderson, Ernestine Wiedenbach, Lydia E. Hall, Dorothea E. Orem, Faye G. Abdellah, Ida Jean Orlando, Myra Estrin Levine, Dorothy E. Johnson, Martha E. Rogers, Imogene M. King, Betty Neuman, Josephine E. Paterson and Loretta T. Zderad, and Sister Callista Roy. Each chapter presents one theorist (or pair of theorists). Although an effort has been made to present the information chronologically, these fifteen chapters may be read in any order. Each chapter gives the historical setting of the nursing theorist and the specific components that she identified as meaningful to nursing. This material is drawn from the work of each theorist. The components are then interpreted and discussed by the chapter author(s) in relation to the four basic concepts: (1) The human or individual, (2) health, (3) society/environment, and (4) nursing and to the use of these concepts in the nursing process. In addition, the work of each theorist is discussed in relation to the characteristics of a theory. This discussion is not to be considered a comprehensive critique of the work but rather an effort to give one view of the strengths and weaknesses of the work and to stimulate the reader's thought processes about the characteristics of a theory and those of the particular work. The terms *theory, model, conceptual framework,* and *conceptual model* are not used consistently in the nursing literature. Thus the work being presented may meet the characteristics of a theory as described in this book and still not be generally accepted as a theory.

Finally, Chapter 18 is an aid to the reader for using several or all of these theories in the nursing process in a given situation. This last chapter gives some examples of application of the components as a guide and stimulus to the reader's utilization of theory and the nursing process for professional nursing practice. Chapter 18 will be most meaningful if it is read after becoming familiar with the contents of Chapters 1 through 17. A glossary is also provided for quick reference to some common terms and to terms specific to the work of particular theorists.

Some of the theorists, as appropriate to their times, used *she* to refer to the nurse and *he* to refer to the recipient of care. In some chapters, it would have been awkward to change the theorist's use of such words. In these situations, we have indicated that the use is that of the original author. In like manner, we have tried to reflect the original author's use of the terms *patient* and *client.*

The Nursing Theories Conference Group was formed out of a concern for the need for materials to help students of nursing understand and use nursing theories in nursing practice. The original group of ten nursing faculty began discussion in 1975. The need for a text that included the elements of nursing theories and their application to practice soon became apparent and resulted in the publication of the first edition of this book. As the theories to be included have expanded, the group has gradually evolved to include the twenty authors who have contributed to this second edition. They will continue their efforts to enhance the development of theory-based professional nursing practice.

A special "thank you" is due the staff at Prentice-Hall for their help and encouragement during the process of developing the first and second editions of this book. They have been patient, understanding, and supportive. In particular, Dudley Kay was helpful in the development of the second edition.

Suggestions and comments from users of this text are requested and welcomed.

Julia B. George

1

THE PLACE OF CONCEPTS
AND THEORIES WITHIN NURSING

Gertrude Torres

Basic to any professional discipline is the development of a body of knowledge that can be applied to its practice. Such knowledge is often expressed in terms of concepts and theories, especially in the area of the behavioral or social sciences. Thus, nursing as a young, evolving profession is beginning to develop a body of knowledge in terms of the concepts and theories that support its practice.

DEFINITION OF TERMS

The use and meanings of the terms *concept* and *theory* within nursing and other disciplines are often conflicting. This confusion can be caused by differences of opinion. However, such confusion is more likely to be caused by the frequent use of these terms in a broad non-defined sense, leaving the listeners or readers uncertain as to the purpose of the presentation and encouraging them to focus on details or specifics rather than on concepts.

In 1920, Lavinia Dock and I. M. Stewart, in discussing the education of nursing for the future, stated that the *concept* of public health and the normal healthy individual should be taught before the care of the sick individual. Although they did not define what was meant by *concept,* one can conjecture that the term was used because they apparently viewed public health as a concept.[1]

In 1933, the New York League of Nursing Education prepared a *concept* of nursing that defined nursing as "using skillfully scientific methods in adapting prescribed therapy and preventive treatment to the specific physical and psychic needs of the individual."[2] A year later in the *American Journal of Nursing,* Effie Taylor spoke of the prevailing concept of nursing as practical, having real depths through love, sympathy, knowledge, and culture.[3] In 1969, Faye Abdellah proposed that nursing theories are the basis for nursing sciences. Among those she identified as being pioneers in the development of nursing theories were Ida Jean Orlando, Ernestine Wiedenbach, and Hildegard Peplau.[4]

The use of the word *concept* is not a new phenomenon; it is one that has been part of nursing's historical background. This is also probably true in other disciplines within and outside the health care fields. Nursing has used the word *concept* for over fifty years without its having a specific meaning and probably continue to do so for several more decades.

The main purpose of this chapter is to present the various approaches to the meanings of the words *concept* and *theory* and to identify each definition that is functional and should be applied in reading this book.

Concepts are basically vehicles of thought that involve images.[5] They are abstract notions and are similar in definition to ideas.[6] Impressions received by sensing our environment evolve into concepts.[7] Chinn and Jacobs define a concept as "a complex mental formulation of an object, property or event that is derived from individual perception and experience."[8] Individuals vary in the specific images or notions they perceive in relation to a given concept. In nursing, the most significant concepts that influence and determine its practice include: (1) the human or individual, (2) society/environment, (3) health, and (4) nursing (see Figure 1–1). Among these four concepts, the core of the practice of nursing is the individual. It is from the client or patient that the other nursing concepts arise. Without any of these concepts, nursing cannot evolve either as a science or as a professional practice field. For example, the concepts of nursing and the individual may have little relationship unless one recognizes some aspect of health, such as its promotion or restora-

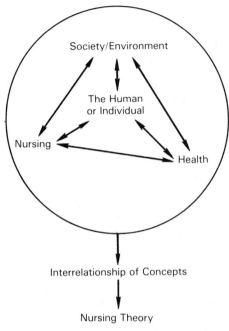

Interrelationship of Concepts

↓

Nursing Theory

Figure 1-1. Concepts essential to practice.

tion, as part of a mutual concern. Also, to attempt to envision the individual without a society is impossible.

Since concepts create images abstract in nature, these concepts tend to have different meanings and can lead to different interpretations. Concepts are strongly influenced by previous learning experiences. Thus, the concept of the individual creates an almost endless supply of notions and ideas. For example, it creates images related to woman, soldier, client/patient, daughter, father, son, and so forth. This kind of word association also leads to identifying related concepts so that increased clarification can occur. In communicating, nurses often use concepts followed by some explanation or description in order to increase the clarity of the message. Misinterpretation, which can lead to misunderstanding, is caused by lack of clarification in the meaning of words representing concepts. It is not essential to agree on the meaning of a particular term, but it is important to describe it sufficiently so that the image one attempts to project becomes more explicit. Undefined concepts tend to be too generalized in nature to assist in understanding specifics of our unique experience, and defined concepts do not necessarily indicate a plan for implementation. For this reason, the use of concepts alone without theories is of little assistance in influencing nursing practice.

If nursing accepts the idea that concepts are the elements used to develop theories—theories that form the basis for nursing practice—the profession must then have a thorough understanding of the meaning of the word *theory*.

Within nursing and many disciplines the meaning of the word *theory* varies. This variety of interpretations is a method of searching and exploring for truths and clarity. Although the lack of precise definition may lead some to a state of confusion and frustration, it allows the option of developing a definition of *theory* that is functional for nursing practice. As the nursing profession matures, sophistication in the understanding and utilizing of nursing theories will probably increase.[9]

In order to give some clarity to the word *theory* so that it can be functional throughout this book, a review of some of the literature is necessary. The word evolves from the Greek word *theoria* signifying a "vision." Based on this sensory nature, the development of theories should be viewed as rational and intellectual and leading to the disclosure of truth. Involved in this intellectual process is comparing, experimenting, and uncovering relationships.[10] This approach to the meaning of theory makes most individuals in nursing potential theory builders. Thus, it is important that nursing recognize that anyone who is capable of speaking is a potential theorist. Nursing practitioners frequently claim to have visions or truths about beliefs that strongly influence their actions. Although this interpretation is helpful in allowing the profession to believe that anyone is capable of theorizing as an intellectual human being, it is of little true value in the development of a sound body of knowledge based on research derived from theory. Theories need to do more than foster intellectual visions of how nurses might practice.

Theories are also viewed as a set of interrelated concepts that give a systematic view of a phenomenon that is explanatory and predictive in nature.[11] Ideally, nursing theories should be viewed as an interrelationship of these basic concepts and should be used to systematically explain approaches to nursing care and to predict outcomes. The extent of predictability depends on the amount of research available and on the theorist's skill in studying existing knowledge and in linking concepts and theories to form new theories. Nurses previously used only intuition, habit, or tradition as the basis for making nursing decisions. For example, in caring for a person with a particular need/problem, using a particular nursing theory should give strong clues as to the outcomes of nursing care. If we relate this to the use of a particular drug, given the correct data about the person and the drug, we can expect certain results to occur from the administration of that drug. Thus, the outcome has the element of prediction. In nursing we should view a theory as a way of relating concepts through the use of definitions that assist in developing significant interrelationships to describe or classify approaches to practice (see Figure 1-1). Classification is used to relate facts and to generalize about them. This will assist in explaining events.[12] From this approach we can develop the important predictive ingredients of a theory and can view nursing theories as a way of assisting and explaining approaches to practice.

In other fields, especially the biological sciences, there are laws as well as theories. Laws are truly *predictable* and can be utilized with assurance because they provide a sound body of knowledge in which to function. For example, in chemistry, if one correctly places a salt and an acid in the same vehicle, one can predict the results. Laws compose the basis of the most mature sciences. On the other hand, since nursing is a behavioral *and* a new science, its knowledge is based primarily on theories that have not yet been validated and are not predictable. In the future, the predictability of nursing theories will become more reliable as concepts are better defined and as the research from which theories develop grows.

Theories are a way of combining concepts for the purpose of deriving hypotheses about practice. In reviewing theories, it is important to understand their basic characteristics. These are reviewed below.

BASIC CHARACTERISTICS
OF A THEORY

1. **Theories can interrelate concepts in such a way as to create a different way of looking at a particular phenomenon.** Theories are constructed from concepts, which are abstract ideas or mental images that represent reality. A theory is only a theory if more than one major concept is identified and defined, and if explicit or clearly stated relationships are projected between these concepts. The definitions of the concepts should provide a clear mental picture of the events or experiences that the theory is designed to explain, and

should clarify how these experiences fit together to describe, explain, and predict reality. Theory provides a way of viewing our everyday experiences in a way that is not always evident based on our limited experience, and it also provides a way of looking at possible goals that might not otherwise occur to us.

For example, a theory might identify the two concepts "need" and "nursing." The concept of need may be described in terms of actual experiences that a person might encounter that interfere with an optimal health state. The concept of nursing may be defined in terms of actions that can be taken to reach an optimal health state such as touch, listening, or teaching. The theory, in turn, may connect the two concepts of need and nursing in such a way that nursing actions can be deliberately viewed as meeting needs, and in so doing reach a goal of optimal health. Without the theory, we may not perceive the relationship between a need and a nursing action, but the theory should provide a unique way of viewing nursing actions as meeting a particular goal: a specific relationship.

With the theory we begin to look more closely at a need and relate our nursing actions more directly to that need, rather than simply doing what we think we should be doing in a situation because someone says that is what we should do. For example, we can approach a typical care giving situation by providing information because we have been taught that a young mother must be given information about how to feed her infant. If we have a theory on which to base our nursing practice that relates the abstract ideas of "need" and "nursing action," and these concepts are defined in the theory so that our experiences with this young mother are consistent with the theory, then we can begin to look for evidence that she *needs* this information and can provide the type of information that is viewed as consistent with her need. If the theory includes a concept of family or society, then we would also integrate our notions about families or societies into our view of this situation.

2. Theories must be logical in nature. Logic involves orderly reasoning. Interrelationships must be sequential and must follow principles of reasoning. Theories must have clearly defined concepts, and the concepts and their relationships must be consistent; that is, there must not be any apparent contradictions between the definitions of the concepts, the relationships within the theory, and the goals of the theory. Theories all have basic underlying assumptions that must be consistent with the goals and the relationships of the theory. For example, a theory might be based on the underlying assumption that humans are basically good in nature. Then all the concepts and the relationships must be consistent with this basic assumption. Therefore, if the theory defines human beings as basically good, but then goes on to describe relationships that focus on sick or unhealthy goals or outcomes, the theory lacks logical consistency. Such a theory would be logical only if it describes, explains, and predicts the natural and healthy outcomes as well as the hazards that threaten these naturally healthy or good outcomes or goals.

3. Theories should be relatively simple yet generalizable. A theory that is thought of as a "good" theory is stated in the most simple terms possible, but at the same time it includes a wide range of possible experiences in nursing practice. The concept of motion is a relatively simple term in that it can be applied to a wide range of experiences, such as or including blood flow, muscles, objects (air, automobiles, etc.), and even ideas. Likewise, the concept of time can be simply defined in relation to the moon or sun cycles, but it can also be generalized to include how people perceive its passage as slow or fast. If a theory relates the relatively simple concepts of time and motion, then it is said to be simple yet generalizable to a wide range of specific events and experiences in the real world. Such theories that are both simple and generalizable may be referred to as *parsimonious*.

4. Theories can be the bases for hypotheses that can be tested. If a particular theory cannot be tested, it offers little as a base of knowledge. The definitions of the concepts in the theory should suggest precise experiences that can be observed or measured in some way. A broad concept such as need might have many possible real-world experiences that can be measured either directly or indirectly. For example, an imbalance of electrolytes might imply a direct observation of need for electrolyte substances that would restore balance in the physiological system. An indirect measurement might be indicated for something more abstract such as attachment or adaptation. If the concepts of the theory cannot be measured, observed, or demonstrated in some way, then the theory cannot be tested empirically. On the other hand, if the theory suggests some means of measuring or observing the abstract concepts that form the relationships, then research can be designed that tests the precision of the theory in predicting relationships, and the theory grows in meaning and significance.

5. Theories contribute to and assist in increasing the general body of knowledge within the discipline through the research implemented to validate them. Theories that are not tested empirically (through measurement or observation of real-world events) contribute little to the body of knowledge of a discipline. If the theory stimulates research, then this research and the theory on which it is based will contribute to the present body of knowledge of the discipline. Since all research raises additional questions for investigation, the research and the theory on which it is based lead to the development of other scientific theories from which new hypotheses can be drawn. Thus theories, if sound, assist in developing nursing hypotheses that can be used to develop new theories.

6. Theories can be utilized by the practitioners to guide and improve their practice. One of the most significant characteristics of a theory is its usefulness to the practitioner. A theory should provide an indication of the goal that is to be attained if the relationships of the theory are accurate in reality. If the goal of the theory is high-level wellness, and the relationships of the theory are accurate in reality, then if the practitioner provides for the conditions and realities implied in the theory, the goal of high-level wellness should be attained. Although theories are not principles or rules for practice but rather serve to stimulate further testing of reality, they can provide guidelines that can be used in the ongoing process of improvement of nursing practice. As the theories of nursing are tested with research and are shown to be reliable, the profession will continue to grow and develop new and evolving approaches to its practice.[13]

7. Theories must be consistent with other validated theories, laws, and principles but will leave open unanswered questions that need to be investigated. Unless nursing theories build upon scientific findings that have been validated, much confusion will occur. The logic of theory is based on the underlying laws, previously validated knowledge, and humanitarian values that are generally accepted as "good" and "right." Theory within nursing must be consistent with previously established knowledge; however, the tentative nature of theory continues to raise questions that challenge aspects of that knowledge that have not yet been challenged. For example, most previous research has demonstrated that adaptation is a response that leads to an improved state of health. However, the question still persists as to whether this is always the case or under what conditions adaptation best exists. Nursing theory will build on and support previously developed knowledge about adaptation but will leave open the possibility of new knowledge that has not yet been explored about adaptation.

THEORETICAL APPROACH TO NURSING PRACTICE

By examining the following situation, one can identify how a theoretical approach can be utilized in nursing practice.

Situation.   Mrs. Mary Dolphin is nine months pregnant and is expecting her first child within a week. She is visiting her obstetrician for an examination. The office nurse has been requested to do health teaching either during the office visits or in Mrs. Dolphin's home. Mrs. Dolphin is an executive career woman of Irish descent who has been married for one year. Mr. Dolphin is in governmental service and travels a great deal, frequently leaving Mrs. Dolphin alone. During the entire pregnancy, Mrs. Dolphin has been cooperative and enthusiastic. No complications or unusual problems (other than morning sickness, which lasted for six weeks during her first trimester) have occurred during the pregnancy.

In reviewing the above situation, many theories, especially those related to the sciences, can be identified that would show the need of special knowledge in order to practice professional nursing. The following kinds of theories reflect only a sample.

KINDS OF THEORIES

Stress Theories

The nurse needs to assess Mrs. Dolphin's previous ability to deal with stress. Theories that give clues as to how individuals deal physiologically and psychologically with stress will assist the nurse in understanding how people can be expected to react. Stress theories will also enable the nurse to differentiate between typical and atypical reactions to stress, thus leading to more appropriate nursing diagnoses.

Developmental Theories

Theories relating to the development of each member of the family will give the nurse an appropriate knowledge base on which to assess specific developmental levels and tasks for each member of the family. For example, during Mrs. Dolphin's pregnancy it is important for the nurse to teach her what is the "normal" physical, intellectual, and emotional development of the newborn and the infant, as well as the "normal" development of the pregnant family.

Family Theories

The structure and function of the family unit and the interrelationships of a family group are reflected in theories relating to the family. Although the office nurse may not have seen Mr. Dolphin, the nurse is able to assess Mrs. Dolphin's relationship with her husband as perceived by Mrs. Dolphin and the impact that a new child may have on the family relationships. Theories concerning family structure and needs will assist the professional nurse in health teaching and nursing diagnoses.

Interactive Theories

The professional nurse must have a sound base of theoretical knowledge about interactions since the base of health teaching relates to the nurse's ability to interact with Mrs. Dolphin and Mrs. Dolphin's ability to interact with others.

Adaptation Theories

Mrs. Dolphin needs to be assessed in terms of her ability to adapt to both her pregnancy and the birth of a child. The nurse needs to be able to explain and hypothesize physical and emotional changes in Mrs. Dolphin.

Other Theories

Other theories can also be identified that will offer the nurse insight into both assessing and planning care. For example, *role* theories will assist in explaining both the role of the nurse and Mrs.

Dolphin's role as a mother. *Change* theories will offer insight into the expected behaviors that evolve when significant change occurs within an environment. *Nursing* theories that explain phenomena and guide the nurse in giving care would be instrumental as guidelines to care. Also, involved in the care of Mrs. Dolphin is a variety of scientific knowledge related to physiology, such as fetal nourishment, labor, and delivery.

In caring for Mrs. Dolphin, the nurse needs a breadth of knowledge. The greater the nurse's sophistication and expertise in theories, the greater the potential for the utilization of appropriate approaches to care. A strong theoretical knowledge base assists the nurse in providing quality nursing care.

Figure 1–2 gives us a visual reference point by which to identify how various theories assist the nurse in the care of Mrs. Dolphin. Other theories can be identified that would enhance the knowledge base upon which to provide care for Mrs. Dolphin. A beginning student in nursing should review theories that are foundational to nursing.

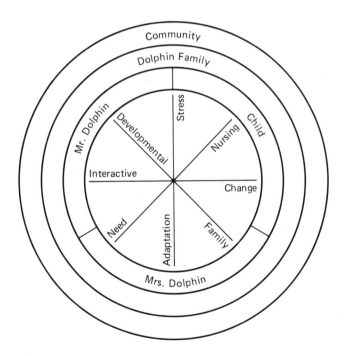

Figure 1–2. Theories—Base of knowledge.

SUMMARY

Concepts represent abstract notions and ideas that, when interrelated, provide the foundation of a theory. Theories may be viewed as visions giving intellectual insight into phenomena, but for maximum significance and impact they should be explanatory and predictive in nature so as to guide professional practice. Nursing theories need to be viewed in the context of how they describe or classify approaches to practice by interrelating the four concepts of (1) the human or individual, (2) society/environment, (3) health, and (4) nursing. Nursing research, through testing hypotheses derived from theories and through assisting in the development of more predictive theories, will thus build a body of nursing science.

Within any given nursing situation, a variety of theories can be identified that will give the professional nurse a strong base of knowledge on which to practice and explain the approach to nursing care. The main function of this text is to demonstrate how nursing theories provide this knowledge base for professional nursing practice and ultimately for improving health care.

NOTES

1. Lavinia L. Dock and I. M. Stewart, A Short History of Nursing, 4th ed. (New York: G. P. Putnam's Sons, 1920), p. 249.
2. New York League of Nursing Education, "A Concept of Nursing," The American Journal of Nursing, 33 (June 1933), 565.
3. Effie J. Taylor, "Of What Is the Nature of Nursing?" The American Journal of Nursing, 34 (May 1934), 476.
4. Faye G. Abdellah, "The Nature of Nursing Science," Nursing Research, 18, no. 5 (September-October 1969), 390.
5. Rom Harre, "The Formal Analysis of Concepts," Analysis of Concept Learning, eds. Herbert Klausmerer and Chester Harris (New York: Academic Press, Inc., 1966), pp. 3–4.
6. Webster's New Collegiate Dictionary (Springfield, Mass.: G. & C. Merriam Company, 1974), p. 233.
7. A. Toffler, "The Psychology of the Future," Learning for Tomorrow—The Role of the Future in Education (New York: Vintage Books, 1974), p. 12.
8. P. L. Chinn and M. K. Jacobs, Theory and Nursing: Systematic Approach (St. Louis: The C. V. Mosby Company, 1983), p. 200.
9. Ibid.

10.   P. H. Phenix, "Educational Theory and Inspiration," *Educational Theory*, 13, no. 1 (January 1963), 1–2.
11.   F. N. Kerlinger, *Foundations of Behavorial Research* (New York: Holt, Rinehart and Winston, 1965), p. 11.
12.   G. Beauchamp, *Curriculum Theory*, 2nd ed. (Wilmette, Ill.: Kagg Press, 1968), pp. 23–24.
13.   Chinn and Jacobs, *Theory and Nursing*.

2

AN OVERVIEW
OF THE NURSING PROCESS

Marjorie Stanton, Charlotte Paul, and Joan S. Reeves

This chapter is based on the assumption that professional nursing practice is interpersonal in nature. Recognizing the importance and effect of the nurse's relationship with the client/patient, professional nurses use this knowledge in proceeding through each phase of the nursing process.

It is also assumed that professional nurses view human beings as holistic, thereby acknowledging that mind and body are not separate but function as a whole. People respond as whole beings. What happens in one part of the mind or body affects the person as a whole entity.

Given these two assumptions, it would be impossible for a nurse to view a client/patient as "the hysterectomy in room 201" or "the paranoid in bed 2." The woman who has experienced a hysterectomy may have physiological, spiritual, and psychological health problems, i.e., physiological and psychological adjustments due to induced menopause, and spiritual adjustments if her life style includes a religious orientation related to a life of childbearing. Or the person with symptoms of paranoia may refuse to eat, causing physiological changes related to malnutrition. These two assumptions, that nursing is interpersonal in nature and that professional nurses view human beings as holistic, give guidance and direction to the use of the nursing process.

The nursing process is the underlying scheme that provides order and direction to nursing care. It is the essence of professional nursing practice. It is the "tool" and methodology of the nursing profession and, as such, helps nurses in arriving at decisions and in predicting and evaluating consequences. The nursing process can be defined as a deliberate intellectual activity whereby the practice of nursing is approached in an orderly, systematic manner. Each of these terms for defining the process can be further delineated as follows:*

Deliberate: Careful, thoughtful, intentional.

Intellectual: Rational, knowledgeable, reasonable, conceptual.

Activity: The state or condition of functioning, initiating, changing, behaving.

Orderly: A methodical, efficient, logical arrangement.

Systematic: Purposeful, pertaining to classification.

Students of nursing using the nursing process are learning to behave as professional nurses in practice behave. Since the nursing process is the essence and tool (methodology) of professional nursing practice, students must become familiar with and adept at using the nursing process as their basis for practice. The nursing process also provides a means for evaluating the quality of nursing care given by nurses and assures their accountability and responsibility to the client/patient. In order to use the nursing process effectively, nurses need to understand and apply appropriate concepts and theories from nursing, from the biological, physical, and behavioral sciences, and from the humanities, in order to provide a rationale for decision making, judgments, interpersonal relationships, and actions. These concepts and theories provide the framework for nursing care.

FIVE PHASES

Most authors agree that four phases, or components, are considered necessary to the nursing process: assessment, nursing diagnosis or identification of problem, intervention or implementation, and evalua-

---

*This list is based on definitions found in the *American Heritage Dictionary*, 1975.

tion.[1,2,3,4] However, some authors do not mention the nursing diagnosis as such, and some consider the nursing care plan separately. In this book, because nursing diagnosis is considered an essential component of the nursing process and planning is included as an integral part of it, we will consider five different phases or components, as listed below:

1. Assessment.
2. Nursing diagnosis.
3. Planning.
4. Implementation.
5. Evaluation.

Although this listing suggests a forward movement of the process through each discrete phase, this does not always occur in the actual process. Assessment must always begin the process, and it always leads to a nursing diagnosis. The assessment phase includes collection and analysis of data. The nursing diagnosis is derived from assessment. However, during the planning, implementation, and evaluation phases, *reassessment* can lead to immediate changes in each of these three stages. Reassessment, the further collection and analysis of data, is a continuous, ongoing process; and it is not to be confused with evaluation, which measures outcomes. Reassessment may also lead to a change in diagnosis, which could lead to a change in planning, implementation, and evaluation as the process continues (see Figure 2–1).

Assessment

Assessment is the first phase in the nursing process. It consists of the systematic and orderly collection and analysis of data pertaining to and about the health status of the client/patient for the purpose of making the nursing diagnosis. It always leads to a nursing diagnosis. Thus insufficient or incorrect assessment could lead to an incorrect nursing diagnosis, which could mean inappropriate planning, implementation, and evaluation. Therefore, the importance of accurate assessment cannot be overemphasized. It is vital to the process and is the basis for all other stages in the process. Although assessment is the first phase, it may also occur as reassessment during any other phase of the process when new data are obtained.[5]

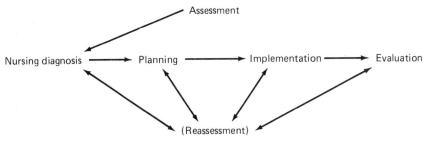
Figure 2-1. The nursing process.

The exception is the diagnosis phase during which no data are collected.

The systematic and orderly collection of data is essential in order for the nurse to know if sufficient data have been collected, and it also serves to provide a method of quick retrieval of information relative to the client/patient for auditing professional practice and for doing nursing research. Several authors have provided guidelines for the systematic collection of data.[6,7,8,9] The American Nurses' Association's (ANA) *Standards of Nursing Practice* also provides information.[10] A holistic view during the assessment phase ensures that the biological, psychological, social, and spiritual spheres of the individual are considered. Any assessment guidelines should include the following:

Biographical data.

A health history including family and social history.

Subjective and objective data about the current health status, including reasons for contact with health care professional and medical diagnosis if the client/patient has a medical problem.

By using these guidelines, the data collected are classified into discrete areas that can be compared, contrasted for relationships, and clustered during the analysis of the data.

The biographical data are generally provided during an interview with the client or the person responsible for the client.[11] Such data are necessary to appropriately identify the client as an individual and may provide clues to the client's health status. For example, the age of clients gives an indication of their growth and developmental status.

A health history is "the client's story of past and present events

17

which may affect current and future health status."[12] The history is obtained through interviewing the client and/or the individual responsible for the client, i.e., parent, and by reviewing previous health records of the client if available. Clients may, if able, fill out part of the biographical data and health history forms. Interviewing the client is essential for discerning clues and cues and for beginning the establishment of a therapeutic relationship.

The currrent health status of the client is also ascertained through interviewing the client or person responsible for the client (subjective data) and through examination and observation of the client to obtain data that can be seen or measured objectively (objective data). For example, a client's description of pain is considered to be subjective data, whereas vital signs are an example of an objective measurement of physiological data.[13] When possible, objective data should be obtained to verify subjective data. For example, the client complains of abdominal pain (subjective data), which the nurse verifies by observation of the position of the client and palpation of the abdomen for tenderness and/or rigidity (objective data).

Situation.   Mrs. James has come to the outpatient department medical clinic because "I just don't feel well." Her medical diagnosis is general malaise. An excerpt of the assessment data collected by the nurse for Mrs. James might look like Table 2-1.

Table 2-1
Assessment of Mrs. James

Bio Data	Health History	Subjective Data	Objective Data
Client—Mrs. James Age 45 Housewife Husband Philip, age 46 electrical helper Daughters Ann, age 18 Jean, age 15	Italian/Spanish heritage. Mother of Mrs. James had diabetes in older years. "All family are overweight." Shops at local fast-food market. Usually shops daily. Mrs. James responsible for cooking. Family does not have regular mealtimes.	"Fingernails break easily." Favorite foods are pizza, pasta with butter, french fries, biscuits with gravy. Drinks are coffee and Tab. Dislikes milk, meats, and vegetables.	Height—5'2" Weight—180 lb Skin pale, dry to touch. Hair lifeless and dry to touch. Nails are ragged and broken.

After the data are collected, analysis of the data takes place. This is the professional nurse's responsibility and *must* occur in order to make a nursing diagnosis. The nurse examines the data to identify, compare, and contrast the relationship of one piece of data to another. The data collected are also compared to societal norms to identify an actual or potential health problem. For example, a four-year-old who is unable to walk does not meet the developmental standards for four-year-olds, and this is an example of an actual health problem.

It is during the analysis stage of assessment that the nurse uses her/his knowledge of various theories and concepts to cluster the collected data. Clustering the data is the grouping of data pieces that fit together and show relationships. Nursing diagnoses are derived from clusters of data that show relationships, make sense, and lead to a logical conclusion. The clustering of data in Table 2–2 indicates that the client may have a potential health problem in relation to diabetes based on age, family history of diabetes, and obesity problem.

When analyzing the data related to age, the nurse needs to know what is expected of people during each stage of development. Abraham Maslow's hierarchy of needs,[14] E. H. Erikson's eight stages of man,[15] and other sources in the literature are useful references to consider in looking at the data.

Identification of gaps in the data should occur during the analysis stage in order to ensure that all important information has been supplied and that the nursing diagnosis is based on actual data and not on inaccurate assumptions. For example, assessing a young child without talking to the mother or to the person responsible for the child will immediately tell the nurse that there are gaps in the data. An analysis of the data should also give clues as to the kinds of patterns developing. In the case of Mrs. James, there is a pattern of poor eating habits, poor selection of foods, and little understanding of diet for good health. These patterns may be handed down from generation to generation.

Table 2–2
Comparison and Relationship of Data
for Mrs. James

Biographical Data	Health History	Current Health Status
45 years old	Mother had adult onset diabetes.	Height—5′2″ Weight –180 lb

Nursing Diagnosis

Nursing diagnosis, the second phase of the nursing process, is recognized in the ANA definition of nursing as "the diagnosis and treatment of human responses to actual or potential health problems.[16] Nursing diagnosis may be defined here as the identification of the human responses and resource limitations of the client for the general purpose of identifying and directing nursing care. The diagnostic statement identifies the client's actual or potential health problem, deficit, or concern, which can be affected by nursing actions. Models for these diagnostic statements have been provided in the reports of the National Nursing Diagnosis Conferences and by Campbell and Gordon.[17] For most clients, there will be more than one nursing diagnosis.

These diagnostic statements are derived from the nurse's inferences, based on the assessed and validated data coupled with nursing, scientific, and humanistic concepts and theories. As one proceeds through the analysis of data, certain patterns develop, and the utilization of relevant concepts and theories is appropriate. Nursing diagnoses are formulated after conclusions or decisions have been reached based on analysis of the data. Each nursing diagnosis can be considered a client-related behavioral statement that identifies the area for the focus of nursing action. A diagnosis may deal with an actual (present-oriented) or a potential (future-oriented) health problem.

After the nursing diagnoses are identified, they should be ranked in order of priority. This ranking should take into consideration both the client's and the nurse's opinions. Those areas that have the greatest impact on the client and/or family should receive particular attention. The nurse also determines priorities based on past nursing experience and on scientific knowledge of the needs and functions of human beings. Therefore, a continuum of priorities of nursing diagnoses is developed, based on the degree of threat to the level of wellness of the client.

The nursing diagnosis can be considered a decisive statement concerning the client's nursing needs. It is important to remember that diagnoses are based on the client's concerns as well as on actual or potential problems that may be symptoms of physiological disorders or of behavioral, psychosocial, and/or spiritual problems.

Situation. Mrs. James's medical diagnosis has been altered to: adult onset diabetes mellitus. She asks the nurse if this means she will need to make any changes in how she lives. She says she remembers her mother "took some kind of shots."

For Mrs. James, an actual health problem can be identified as a lack of information regarding diabetes management. This is based on data about her height, weight, personal and family nutrition patterns, and the status of her integumentary system. In this case, the nursing diagnosis could be: "Inadequate information relating to diabetes management: lack of information regarding cause, effect, and therapeutic action associated with diabetes management (more specific nutritional needs)."[18] This statement indicates the client has inadequate information, as determined from assessed validated data.

The nursing diagnosis also states the categories where lack of information is pertinent. This assists the nurse in developing a plan of action. Another way to state the diagnosis would be: "Alterations in nutrition (eating and drinking)." This statement identifies the need to investigate the client's eating habits, her motivation to change, and her knowledge of nutritional needs.

Other nursing diagnoses for Mrs. James may deal with potential problems that can be identified through assessment and/or reassessment. These problems are related to significant risk factors, factors that can be modified to reduce the impact of the illness. In this case, a nursing diagnosis could be: "Inadequate knowledge relating diabetic skin care: lack of information regarding special skin care, peripheral circulation and the healing process."[19] This nursing diagnosis establishes the potential problem and identifies the categories where lack of knowledge can create problems to assist the nurse in developing the plan for care. Another way to state this diagnosis could be: "Potential for alterations in skin integrity." This diagnosis implies the need to evaluate the knowledge base of the client about special skin care and the healing process in persons with diabetes. These diagnoses, the needs, and the problem categories they represent are presented in Table 2-3.

Planning

Planning is the third phase of the nursing process. The plan for providing nursing care can be described as the determination of what can be done to assist the client, and involves the mutual setting of goals and objectives, judging priorities, and designing methods to resolve actual or potential problems.[20]

Table 2-3

Classification of Nursing Diagnoses

Nursing Diagnosis Statement	Type of Need	Problem Category Actual (present)	Potential (future)
I.			
Inadequate information relating to diabetes management: lack of information regarding cause, effect, and therapeutic action associated with diabetes management (more specific nutritional needs).	Biopsycho-social	Lack of information regarding diabetes management	
OR			
Alterations in nutrition (eating and drinking).	Biological	Lack of knowledge pertaining to nutrition, eating habits; lack of motivation to change	
II.			
Inadequate knowledge relating to diabetic skin care: lack of information regarding special skin care, peripheral circulation, and the healing process.	Biopsycho-social		Lack of knowledge regarding the need for special skin care
OR			
Potential for alterations in skin integrity.	Biological		Implies the need to evaluate knowledge base of client regarding special skin care and healing process in diabetics

The first stage in the planning is setting goals and objectives. These goals and objectives are derived from the nursing diagnoses and are established for each nursing diagnosis listed.

In preparing to write the plan, the client and his/her family should be consulted before formulating the goals and objectives. The goals and objectives should be realistic and attainable, supportive of the client's needs, and mutually acceptable. It is important to consider the need for objectives that can be defined and stated concisely in an "act-of-being" phrase. This phrase should contain a performer (the client), a performance (action), and a change in behavior to be accomplished (objectives). The expected end behavior needs to be identified and be placed in the proper time frame, and can be utilized as a means for evaluation.

Goals are stated in broad terms in order to identify effective criteria for evaluating nursing action. These goals can pertain to rehabilitation, prevention of complications associated with stressors, and/or the ability of the client to adapt to these stressors. Other goals may deal with the achievement of the highest potential for wholeness of the system. A sample of a goal statement would be, "Mrs. James will have an adequate understanding of the basic food groups and their relationship to recommended daily allowance (RDA) requirements within one month."

From the goals, objectives are determined that need to be stated in observable behavioral terms. Objectives should define the conditions under which the expected end behaviors are to occur and should specify the performance level and specific behaviors that will be accepted as being evidence of meeting the desired outcomes. The behaviors in question refer to psychological, physiological, social, and intellectual activities and other observable responses. Objectives related to the above goal for Mrs. James could be:

1. Identify the basic four food groups from a chart.
2. Prepare a shopping list to include at least two necessary foods from each group by the end of Week I.
3. Prepare family menus for three days using the basic four food groups as a guide by Week II.
4. Make substitutions in family menus for three days using the basic four food groups chart as guide by Week III.
5. Evaluate eating patterns of family for one week using the basic four food groups chart as guide and identify at least two problem areas to discuss with nurse by Week IV.

Desired behavioral outcomes (objectives) should be stated in a manner that everyone is able to understand without having to seek clarification. Robert Mager in his book on preparing objectives indicates that a meaningfully stated outcome would be one that communicates to the staff the intent of the individual who stated it.[21]

"The statement which communicates best will be one which describes the terminal behavior of the learner well enough to prevent misinterpretation."[22]

Time is another consideration when specifying desired outcomes. The time limits should be precise for evaluation purposes but should not be so rigid that changes cannot readily be made based on reassessment of the priorities and necessary outcomes. It is important to remember to state the desired outcomes in terms of client behaviors rather than nurse behaviors, in keeping with the ANA *Standards of Nursing Practice.*[23]

The second stage in nursing care planning is the identification of nursing actions for each nursing diagnosis, based on carefully thought out scientific rationale. The nursing action specifies what kind of nursing care is to be done to effectively meet the client's problem. Nursing actions should be precisely spelled out. These actions are part of the scheme for providing good nursing care.

Nursing actions can be said to be hypotheses established for testing if they contribute to the solution of the problem. It is up to the nurse in conjunction with the client and/or family to select appropriate actions to produce the desired results. In selecting these nursing actions, it is important to analyze the options available and to determine the probability of success in reaching the objective. Sometimes compromises must be made in order to provide the best care for the client, and the nurse needs to be aware of this when specifying nursing actions.

The nursing care plan deals with actual as well as potential problems. Nursing actions are based on scientific principles and theories of nursing and need to be specific. The plan serves as a means for resolving the problems and for meeting established goals in an orderly fashion. Also, it provides a means for organization, giving direction and meaning to the nursing action used in helping the client and/or family to resolve the health problems. A plan of action is essential in that it aids in the efficient utilization of time, thus saving time and energy by providing essential data for those individuals responsible for giving care.

Since the client's condition is continuously changing, the written nursing care plan needs to reflect these changes. Therefore, planning becomes a continuous process based on evaluation and reassessment and is the most efficient way of keeping all individuals involved in the client's care informed of modifications in the plan of nursing care.

Implementation

After planning, implementation is the next or fourth phase of the nursing process. Implementation refers to the action or actions initiated to accomplish the defined goals and objectives. Implementation is often considered as the actual giving of nursing care. It is putting the plan into action. Other terms used to describe this part of the process are *action* or *intervention.* According to *The Random House Dictionary,* the two words *implementation* and *intervention* are not synonymous.[24] The definition of implementation is "to put into effect according to or by means of a definite plan or procedures." Intervention is defined as "interposition or interference of one state in the affairs of another, a coming between." Therefore the term *implementation* seems more appropriate to describe this phase of the process if nursing actions are to follow from stated goals and objectives.

Since the nursing process is interpersonal in nature, it must take place between the nurse and the client. The client may be a person, a group, a family, or even a community. The beliefs that the nurse and the client have about human beings, nurses, and clients, and about interactions between nurses and clients will affect the types of actions that both consider appropriate. If human beings are considered unique, then nursing actions should reflect this uniqueness. Therefore, the philosophy of nursing that a nurse develops will affect the nursing actions that he/she uses in meeting the needs of clients. Helen Yura and Mary Walsh in their book *The Nursing Process* indicate that the implementation phase of the nursing process draws heavily on the intellectual, interpersonal, and technical skills of the nurse.[25] Even though the focus is on action, the action is intellectual, interpersonal, and technical in nature.

The implementation phase begins when the nurse considers various alternative actions and selects those most suitable to achieve the planned goals and objectives. Just as goals and objectives have priorities in the plan, actions may also have priorities. Nursing actions may be carried out by the nurse who developed the nursing care plan or by other nurses or nursing assistants. Nursing actions may also be carried out by the client and/or family. To carry out a nursing action, the nurse refers to the written plan for specific information. Many nursing actions fall into the broad categories of counseling, teaching, providing physical care, carrying out delegated medical therapy, coordination of resources, referral to other sources of help, and therapeutic communication (verbal and nonverbal).

Based on the goals and objectives for Mrs. James, as discussed on page 23, there are several nursing actions that could be implemented. For example, under objective 1 (identify the basic four food groups from a chart), the following actions could be considered:

1. Establish an agreed upon time when Mrs. James and her family could meet with the nurse in their home during the next week.
2. Establish base-line knowledge about Mrs. James's and the family members' understanding of basic food groups.
3. Bring chart and booklets containing information about the four basic food groups to Mrs. James's home.
4. Teach family about using the four basic food groups for good nutrition (base teaching on information gained from base-line knowledge).
5. Focus on the value of the food groups for each family member based on age, height, weight, and activity.
6. Request a return demonstration in which Mrs. James and other family members will identify foods by placing the food in a food group and will state why each food group is important.

In Campbell's study of nursing diagnoses and nursing actions, seven categories of nursing actions were developed. These are: assertive, hygienic, rehabilitative, supportive, preventive, observational, and educative.[26] Campbell also points out that almost all nursing actions are initiated by nurses without medical direction. Nurses can initiate and carry out all activities that fall within the nursing domain. In the hospital setting, nurses are also asked to assist physicians in carrying out medical prescriptions. Therefore, nurses need to be clear about their dependent and independent functions.

For every nursing action, the client responds as a total person or as a whole. The concept of *holism*, which states that a person is more than the sum of that person's parts, means that the nurse may be treating a person's leg, but the person will respond as a whole person.[27] The concept is useful in thinking about the consequences of any nursing actions. For example, the simple action of turning the patient every two hours will have a variety of consequences. Some of these consequences should or could be: (1) increased circulation, (2) improved muscle tone, (3) improved breathing, (4) less flatus (gas) in the intestinal tract, (5) prevention of pressure sores, (6) increased or decreased pain, (7) opportunity for communication with care giver, (8) increased ability to socialize with patient in next bed, and (9) increased or decreased ability to reach articles at bedside. There may be other consequences that could not have been predicted, such as an opportunity to express values or beliefs. Therefore, in planning nursing actions, it is important to consider the cluster of consequences of both positive and negative value that can be expected to occur with and following each action.[28] Utilizing this knowledge will help the nurse in selecting the most appropriate actions. Even though not all consequences are predictable for a specific client, it is possible to develop a general knowledge of expected consequences. Knowledge of consequences is an important aspect of the implementation phase of the nursing process. The implementation phase is completed when the nursing actions are finished and results are recorded.

Evaluation

Evaluation is the fifth and final phase of the nursing process. It may be defined as the appraisal of the client's behavioral changes due to the action of the nurse.[29] Although evaluation is considered to be the final phase, it frequently does not end the process. As mentioned earlier in this chapter, evaluation may lead to reassessment, which in turn may result in the nursing process beginning all over again. The main questions to ask in evaluation are: Were the goals and objectives met? Were there identifiable changes in the client/patient behavior? If so, why? If not, why not? Were the consequences of nursing actions predicted? These questions help the nurse to determine which problems have been solved and which problems need to be reassessed and replanned. Unsolved problems cannot be assumed to reflect faulty data collection or inadequate data collection; rather each part of the nursing process may need to be evaluated to determine the cause of ineffective actions.

The key to appropriately evaluating nurse/client actions lies in the planning phase of the process. When objectives are described in behavioral terms with clearly stated expected outcomes, it is easy to determine whether or not the nurse/client actions were successful. These objectives become the criteria for evaluating nurse/client actions. Just as goals should be mutually set with a client/patient, whenever possible, it is also important for the nurse and client to mutually establish the objectives (criteria for evaluation).

According to Dolores Little and Doris Carnevali, evaluation consists of three sequential steps:[30]

1. Selecting criteria (objectives) that will guide the nurse's observation to specified areas of the client's anticipated behavioral changes related to the diagnosis and goals.
2. Collecting specific evidence (data) after goals have been set and client-nurse activities have taken place.
3. Comparing the evidence collected to the criteria and baseline data (if available); then making judgments about the nature of the behavioral change (such as direction, stability, achievement).

Step 1 has been briefly discussed in relation to the planning phase of the process. In addition to stating the desired behavior change, it is also important for the nurse to decide how the change will be measured and when it will be measured.

Step 2 involves the collection of evidence (data). Although data are collected in both assessment and evaluation, the data collection during evaluation is utilized differently from data collected during assessment. In assessment, data are collected for the purpose of making a nursing diagnosis. In evaluation, data are collected as evidence to determine whether the goals and objectives were met. This is an important difference to note in using the nursing process.

Step 3 in evaluation is the one that often is the most difficult because it is easy to use different measurements in making judgments. For example, if a nurse observed that a client "ate well," would this mean the same thing to the client or to another nurse? "Ate well" could be interpreted to mean that the client was able to chew, swallow, and digest the food with no difficulty, or it could refer to the amount and kind of food consumed. Therefore, in evaluation it is not only important to determine the criteria (objectives) but also to determine the exact way(s) in which evidence will be gathered and interpreted to ascertain whether the criteria were met.

In the third step, base-line data refer to information that should be collected in the assessment of the client. To observe a change and to measure a change, the nurse must know the current status of the client or the base from which the change will take place. An example of base-line data could be the weight of the client on initial contact.

In the situation regarding Mrs. James, objectives can be mutually set in measurable terms. Using Little and Carnevali's Step 1, it would be possible to select criteria for measuring the first objective (identify the basic four food groups from a chart). The criteria set could include eighteen out of twenty foods correctly identified. If at the end of Week 1, Mrs. James could identify nineteen foods correctly by food groups, then objective 1 would be evaluated as "accomplished." Specific evidence could then be collected (Step 2) and compared to the criteria (Step 3). Base-line data could be obtained so that change in knowledge about food groups could be measured.

Under objective 2 (prepare a shopping list to include at least two foods from each group by the end of Week 1), the criteria established could be:

1. The shopping list will include all foods essential for preparing three meals per day for seven days.
2. Two foods from each food group would be included on the shopping list.

In looking at the shopping list, the nurse may discover that no red meats were included, therefore creating a limited use of one food group. (Mrs. James revealed that her husband did not believe in eating red meat.) This information would then be included as reassessment data, and the nurse would collect information about foods containing protein that the family could eat. By evaluating the family eating patterns (objective 5), the nurse would have information to enable him/her to help Mrs. James in choosing high protein foods, thereby meeting objective 2.

When objectives have not been met, reassessment should occur and the process will begin again. If the evaluation shows that the nurse/client objectives have been met, the nursing process is complete at that particular point in time.

Evaluation that is based on behavioral changes is called *outcome evaluation*. There are two other types of evaluation that may also be considered: (1) structure and (2) process. *Structure evaluation* relates to such things as appropriate equipment to assess the client or carry out the plan. For example, if the scales were inaccurate, then correct base-line data could not be obtained. Structure evaluation may also relate to the organization within which the nurse works. If the nurse is unable to carry out the nursing process appropriately due to agency time limitation, this must be considered as part of the evaluation.

Process evaluation, which focuses on the activities of the nurse, can be done during each phase of the nursing process, or it may be carried out at the end of the process. The following are examples of process evaluation questions that could be used in evaluating each phase of the process:

Assessment:

1. Was historical data that might be related to health problems collected?
2. Was a physical examination carried out and the results recorded?
3. Was the analysis logical? Did it make use of data collected? Were significant findings mentioned in the analysis?

Diagnosis:

1. Was the diagnosis based on the analysis?
2. Is the diagnosis a logical conclusion from the data collected?

Planning:

1. Are goals and objectives stated?
2. Does the plan rationally follow from the diagnosis?
3. Were goals and objectives mutually established with the client?

Implementation:

1. What activities did the nurse carry out?
2. What activities did the client carry out?
3. Were the activities consistent with the objectives?

Evaluation:

1. Were the goals and objectives accomplished?
2. What evaluation methods were utilized?

The nurse and the client are responsible for carrying out outcome evaluation. Structure and process evaluations are typically carried out by the nurse and/or others in nursing administration within an agency.

SUMMARY

In summary, the nursing process is the "tool" or methodology of professional nursing that helps nurses arrive at decisions and helps them predict and evaluate consequences. To use the nursing process successfully, a nurse needs to apply concepts and theories from nursing; from biological, physical, and behavioral sciences; and from the humanities, in order to provide a rationale for decision making, judgments, interpersonal relationships, and actions. The five components considered necessary to the nursing process are: assessment, nursing diagnosis, planning, implementation, and evaluation.

It is expected that students learning about the use of the nursing process will need to use many references and resources to augment their knowledge and skills as they proceed through their nursing program.

NOTES

1. Helen Yura and Mary B. Walsh, *The Nursing Process: Assessing, Planning, Implementing, Evaluating,* 2nd ed. (New York: Appleton-Century-Crofts, 1973), p. 69.
2. Fay Louise Bower, *The Process of Planning Nursing Care—A Model for Practice* (St. Louis, Mo.: The C. V. Mosby Company, 1977), p. 11.
3. Pamela Holsclaw Mitchell, *Concepts Basic to Nursing* (New York: McGraw-Hill Book Company, 1973), p. 71.
4. Ann Marriner, *The Nursing Process: A Scientific Approach to Nursing Care* (St. Louis, Mo.: The C. V. Mosby Company, 1975), p. 1.
5. Bower, *The Process of Planning,* pp. 10–11.
6. Judith Bloom Walter, Geraldine P. Pardee, and Doris M. Malbo, *Dynamics of Problem-Oriented Approaches: Patient Care and Documentation* (Philadelphia: J. B. Lippincott Company, 1976), pp. 32–39.
7. Bower, *The Process of Planning,* pp. 11–13, 48–70.
8. Donna S. Zimmerman and Carol Gohrke, "The Goal-Directed Nursing Approach: It Does Work," *The Nursing Process: A Scientific Ap-*

proach, Ann Marriner, compiler (St. Louis, Mo.: The C. V. Mosby Company, 1975), p. 150.

9. Lucille Lewis, *Planning Patient Care* (Dubuque, Iowa: William C. Brown Company, Publishers, 1976), Chapter 3.

10. Congress for Nursing Practice, *Standards of Nursing Practice* (Kansas City, Mo.: American Nurses' Association, 1973).

11. Elizabeth Anne Mahoney, Laurie Verdisco, and Lillie Shortridge, *How to Collect and Record a Health History* (Philadelphia: J. B. Lippincott Company, 1976), pp. 9-52.

12. Ibid., p. 5.

13. Dolores Little and Doris Carnevali, *Nursing Care Planning,* 2nd ed. (Philadelphia: J. B. Lippincott Company, 1976), p. 12.

14. Abraham Maslow, *Motivation and Personality* (New York: Harper & Row, Publishers, Inc., 1954).

15. E. H. Erikson, *Childhood and Society* (New York: W. W. Norton & Co., Inc., 1963), pp. 247-74.

16. American Nurses' Association, *Nursing: A Social Policy Statement* (Kansas City, Mo.: American Nurses' Association, 1980), p. 3.

17. Kristine M. Gebbie, ed., *Summary of the Second National Conference: Classification of Nursing Diagnoses* (St. Louis, Mo.: Clearinghouse, 1976); Kristine M. Gebbie and Mary Ann Lavin, *Classification of Nursing Diagnoses* (St. Louis, Mo.: The C. V. Mosby Company, 1975); Marjory Gordon, *Manual of Nursing Diagnosis* (New York: McGraw-Hill Book Company, 1982); idem, *Nursing Diagnosis: Process and Application* (New York: McGraw-Hill Book Company, 1982); Mi Ja Kim and Derry Ann Moritz, eds., *Classification of Nursing Diagnoses* (New York: McGraw-Hill Book Company, 1982); and Claire Campbell, *Nursing Diagnosis and Intervention in Nursing Practice* (New York: John Wiley & Sons, Inc., 1980).

18. Campbell, *Nursing Diagnosis,* p. 849.

19. Ibid., p. 829.

20. Gertrude Torres and Marjorie Stanton, *Curriculum Process in Nursing: A Guide to Curriculum Development* (Englewood Cliffs, N. J.: Prentice-Hall, Inc., 1982), pp. 128-29.

21. Robert Mager, *Preparing Instructional Objectives* (Palo Alto, Calif.: Fearon Publishers, Inc., 1962), p. 12.

22. Ibid., p. 11.

23. Congress for Nursing Practice, *Standards of Nursing Practice* (Kansas City, Mo., 1973).

24. *The Random House Dictionary of the English Language* (New York: Random House, Inc., 1966).

25. Yura and Walsh, *The Nursing Process,* p. 108.

26. Campbell, *Nursing Diagnosis,* pp. 21-22.

27. Jan Christiaan Smuts, *Toward a Better World* (New York: World Book Company, distributed by Duell, Sloan and Pearce, 1944), pp. 123–33.
28. Marjorie L. Byrne and Lida F. Thompson, *Key Concepts for the Study and Practice of Nursing* (St. Louis, Mo.: The C. V. Mosby Company, 1972), pp. 67–75.
29. Ibid., Chapter 6.
30. Little and Carnevali, *Nursing Care Planning,* p. 230.

3

FLORENCE NIGHTINGALE

Gertrude Torres

Florence Nightingale (1820–1910) was born to English parents while they were on a trip to Florence, Italy. Her greatest achievement was the establishment of the concept of formal preparation for the practice of nursing; thus, the profession of nursing started with her commitment to the care of the sick.

Miss Nightingale's fame spread rapidly after she and a group of devoted women cared for the sick during the Crimean War. She was a proficient bedside nurse with a great concern for the soldiers. An account of her nightly rounds with her lamp ("The Lady with the Lamp") was given special attention by Henry Wadsworth Longfellow.

Organized nursing began in the mid-1800s with the leadership of Florence Nightingale. Before her era, nursing care was done by paupers and drunkards, persons unfit for any other type of work. Hospitals were places where the poor frequently suffered more from the environment than from the disease that brought them there. Surgery without anesthesia, little or no sanitation, and filth within hospitals were prevalent everywhere.

Nightingale's beliefs about nursing form the basic foundation on which nursing care is practiced today. Her religious convictions and military nursing experience during the Crimean War had a strong influence on her approach and beliefs about the care of the sick. Her writing ability, which is well demonstrated in her *Notes on Nursing*,[1] can be attributed to her education, which was achieved mainly through her father's tutoring. She traveled extensively and had the ability to deal in government and politics. Many have called her a genius. Thus, in understanding her theoretical approach to professional nursing, the reader needs to keep in mind her unique characteristics in relation to the place of a woman of the mid-nineteenth century.

Nightingale did not specifically approach her writings in the context of today's terminology, that of concepts and theories. Yet these writings about nursing care can be interpreted to reflect the present emphasis on a theoretical approach to the nursing process. There may be the temptation to see her ideas as "old-fashioned" or "out-of-date." This must be avoided since many of her sound ideas about nursing are still not being universally carried out in contemporary practice.

NIGHTINGALE'S ENVIRONMENTAL THEORY OF NURSING

The core concept that is most reflective of Nightingale's writings is that of environment. Although she tends to emphasize the physical more than the psychological or social environment, this needs to be viewed in the context of her time and her activities as a nurse leader in a war-torn environment. It is understandable that she, having witnessed in the early 1850s the filth, vermin, and death within an enormous barracks hospital, would focus so heavily on improving the environment to assist soldiers to merely survive. Through such an emphasis, the death rate went from a staggering 42 per 100 to a low of 22 per 1000. This success gave her a strong data base on which to view nursing in her own unique way.

The environment is viewed as all the external conditions and influences affecting the life and development of an organism and capable of preventing, suppressing, or contributing to disease or death.[2] Nightingale's writing speaks of providing such things as ventilation, clean air and water, cleanliness, and warmth, so the reparative process that nature has instituted will not be hindered. Assisting patients toward the retention of their vital powers by meeting their needs is viewed as a goal of nursing. The flavor of her beliefs is expressed when she speaks of the environmental elements that disturb health, such as dirt, dampness, chills, drafts, smells, and darkness.[3]

Medical practice is not viewed as a curative process but as having the function of assisting nature. Thus, nursing is also a noncurative practice in which the patient is put in the best condition for nature to act. This condition was seen by her as enhanced by providing an environment conducive to health promotion.

At this point it is helpful to think of a patient who has had surgery, such as an appendectomy, and relate what Nightingale proposes. Medicine is seen as functioning to remove the diseased part, whereas nursing places the patient in an environment in which nature can assist postoperative patients to reach their optimum health condition. This approach to nursing is as valid today as it was over one hundred years ago, in spite of the fact that both in homes and in hospitals the environment today is more sophisticated in structure. This should be kept in mind as the theory is viewed in more detail. Much of Nightingale's theory is noted in her writing, *Notes on Nursing.*[4]

Table 3–1 demonstrates her major areas of environmental concentration: ventilation, warmth, effluvia, noise, and light. Keep in mind that it is the interrelationship of this concept of a healthy environment with the practice of nursing, as seen by Florence Nightingale, that offers us a basic theory of nursing practice.

Ventilation, especially with increased fresh air, provided without drafts, is of primary importance. *Light* refers to sunlight for the most part, and is secondary. *Warmth, noise,* and *effluvia* (smells) are seen as areas in which attention must be given in order to provide a positive environment.

In utilizing this basic concept—the environment—within the nursing process, it becomes evident that the practitioner must view the patient in a particular context. For example, review the following situation:

Situation I.   Mrs. Anderson, a public health nurse, has just visited Mrs. Rose, an eighty-year-old arthritic patient who lives alone in a small rural community. Since Mrs. Rose has difficulty ambulating, her neighbors visit her often to assist her in any way they can.

Table 3–1

Nightingale's Environmental Concepts

Major Areas of Concentration	Examples
Ventilation	Fresh air, which is of primary importance, can be achieved through open windows. Corrupt, stagnant, and musty air breeds disease. An outlet is needed for impure air. Drafts caused by open windows and doors are to be avoided. Dirty carpets and furniture are a source of impurity in the air.
Warmth	Guarding against the loss of vital heat is essential to the patient's recovery. Chilling is to be avoided. Hot bottles, bricks, and drinks should be used to restore lost heat.
Effluvia (smells)	Sewer air is to be avoided, and care is needed to get rid of noxious body odor caused by disease. Chamber utensils should be odor-free and out of sight. Fumigations and disinfectants should not be used but the offensive substance removed.
Noise	Intermittent sudden noise causes greater excitement than continuous noise, especially during the patient's first sleep. The more the patient sleeps peacefully, the greater his ability to sleep will be. Walking lightly, whispering, or discussing a patient's condition just outside his room is cruel.
Light	Second only to the need for fresh air is the value of light. Beds should be placed in such a position as to allow the patient to see out the window—the sky and sunlight.

One of these neighbors requested that Mrs. Anderson visit to assess the situation.

On entering Mrs. Rose's home, Mrs. Anderson was made aware of the lack of fresh air, the darkness in the environment caused by old dusty drapes covering the windows, and a draft in the bedroom. Mrs. Rose was found sitting in an old chair that provided little or no view of the world around her.

After her visit, Mrs. Anderson contacted Mrs. Rose's neighbors to set up a plan to improve her environment. The drapes were to be removed and replaced by simple curtains that would let the morning sun enter the home. The windows were to be opened in keeping with the weather during specific periods of the day, with care given to reduce drafts. Mrs. Rose's favorite chair was to be placed in such a way that she could look out the window to watch the neighbors coming and going.

This example is not to be viewed as offering a complete assessment of Mrs. Rose, but to point out how Nightingale's basic environmental concept, interrelated with the nursing process, can give us specific directions.

To Nightingale the environment of the patient was quite encompassing. Although she did not specifically distinguish among the physical, social, or psychological environments as such, she speaks of all three in the practice of nursing.

Admittedly, emphasis is placed on the physical environment of the patient. In the context of her time this was essential if lives were to be saved and nursing was to take its proper place as a profession. It is when an optimum physical environment exists that greater attention can be given to the emotional needs of the patient as well as to the prevention of disease.

Figure 3–1 offers a view of the theory created by Nightingale. The key point is diagrammed in the center of the triangle—patient

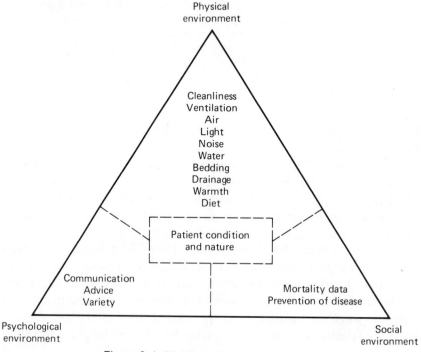

Figure 3-1. Nightingale's theory of nursing.

condition and nature. Here the thrust of environment is on the patient and nature functioning together to allow the reparative process to occur. The three components—physical, social, and psychological—need to be viewed as interrelating rather than as separate distinct parts. The cleanliness of the physical environment has a direct bearing on the prevention of disease and mortality rates within the social environment of the community. (Also, all patients' psychological environments are strongly affected by physical surroundings.)

Physical Environment

As noted in Table 3-1, the basic environmental components are physical in nature and relate to such things as ventilation and warmth. These basic factors affect one's approach to all other aspects of the environment. Cleanliness is an encompassing notion related to all aspects of the physical environment in which the patient is found. The walls and entire room should not be dusty, smoky, or have a close odor.

A patient's bed must be clean, aired, warm, dry, and free from odor. One should provide an environment in which the patient can be easily cared for by others or self. The width, height, and placement of the bed should facilitate the activities of the patient. The bed should be placed in the best lighted spot, away from sudden noises and the odor of drainage. The position of the patient on the bed should be viewed in the context of supporting ventilation.

Psychological Environment

The effect of the mind on the body was fairly well accepted in Nightingale's time. However, there was a lack of understanding of exactly how the condition of the body as affected by the environment could affect the mind. Nightingale did recognize that a negative environment could cause physical stress, thereby affecting the patient's emotional climate. Therefore emphasis is placed on offering the patient a variety of activities to keep his mind stimulated. The view of the sunlight, the attractiveness of the food, and the offering of manual activities that stimulate the need to labor are all factors that assist the patient to survive emotionally. Boredom is viewed as painful.

Communication with the patient is viewed in the context of

the total environment. Communication should not be hurried or allow for interruptions. When speaking with patients, it is important to sit down in front of them, unless other activities such as eating are occurring. The place one communicates with the physician and family about the patient is in the context of the environment of the patient. Outside the patients' rooms or within their hearing distance is viewed as inappropriate.

One should not encourage the sick by false hopes and advice about their illness. Rather, the emphasis here is on communicating about the world around them that they miss, or about good news that visitors can share. Again, patients are viewed in the context of the total environment.

Socal Environment

Observation of the social environment, especially as related to specific data collections relating to illness, is essential to preventing disease. Thus, each nurse must use observational powers in dealing with specific cases rather than be comfortable with data addressing the "average" patient.

Closely related to the community-social environment are those notions already discussed in relation to the individual patient—that is, physical environment such as clean air and water and proper drainage or sewage. The patient's *total* environment not only includes the patient's home or hospital room but the total community influencing that specific environment.

NIGHTINGALE'S THEORY
AND THE FOUR MAJOR CONCEPTS

In reviewing how Nightingale relates her theory to the four major concepts, it becomes evident once again that the environment is the main focus of her theory. Figure 3–2 identifies the four major concepts as they are related in Nightingale's Theory. The *environment* affects the *human* condition, with *nursing* having the role of affecting that environment, so that *health/disease* becomes a reparative process.

Each of the major concepts impacts on the others. *Nursing* functions to influence the human environment to affect health. The *in-*

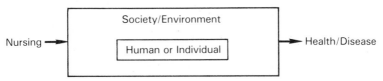

Figure 3-2. Nightingale's theory and the four major concepts.

dividual is affected by the environment and by the nurse who influences his/her health. *Society/environment* has an impact on the nurse and on the health of the individual. *Health* is a process affected by nursing and by environmental and human conditions. These relationships give meaning to the theory by providing a view of the world in which we nurse.

The following list reflects Nightingale's view of the major concepts:

> *Human or Individual*—Has vital reparative powers to deal with disease.
>
> *Nursing*—The goal is to place the individual in the best condition for nature to act by basically affecting the environment.
>
> *Health/Disease*—The focus is on the reparative process of getting well.
>
> *Society/Environment*—Involves those external conditions that affect life and the development of the individual. The focus is on ventilation, warmth, odors, noises, and light.

Basically, these concepts are implicit rather than explicit, and thus they may be misunderstood and misinterpreted by those attempting to use the theory. The concept that is most clearly defined is the *society/environment*. Yet it is unclear how extensively or globally Nightingale viewed the environment. Other theories that will be discussed later within this book view the environment from a broad universal standpoint. Nightingale probably focused on the immediate environment in which humans find themselves. During her time, society was viewed from a rather narrow perspective. Today's view of clean air and water with our concern over environmental pollution is quite different than that held during the nineteenth century. Thus, although Nightingale's main focus is on the environment, she defines that concept in the context of her time only.

It is difficult to understand what the concept of *human/individual* really means to Nightingale. She is descriptive of humans only in terms of their healing process. However, one can draw certain assumptions that are basic to her theory such as humans need clean air, clean water, and proper nutrition. Thus, it is safe to describe individuals as responsive to the environment and having a healing power within themselves.

The concept of *health* is probably the most poorly defined. A view of health as the lack of disease offers us little understanding of what health really encompasses for Nightingale. One might assume that a healthy person is merely an individual who lacks a disease.

Nursing is described in relation to the other three concepts. Nightingale was the first to give clarity to the purpose of nursing. Thus, any description or explanation of this concept needs to be reviewed as an initial attempt to explain a professional role. By today's standards she gives a limited but rather clear picture of the meaning of nursing as a noncurative practice in which the patient is put in the best position for nature to act.

NIGHTINGALE'S THEORY AND THE NURSING PROCESS

In general, although Nightingale's theory has only rather vaguely defined concepts, it offers a lot in terms of guiding practice and research in its generalizability and simplicity. An example of application to practice follows.

Situation II.   Mrs. Kerr is a seventy year-old resident who lives in an old local nursing home. She is rarely visited by her only living relative, a brother who is several years older. Several years ago she became partially immobile on her right side and continues to have difficulty walking around the home. When reminded, she is able to go to the dining room for meals but eats very little. Her environment consists of a two-bed room, which she shares with an eighty-year-old woman who is unaware of her surroundings. On admission, Mrs. Kerr was not able to bring any of her own belongings except for a few clothes. When communicating with her, she remembers the "old" days when she taught at the local elementary school. She seldom initiates a conversation and spends most of her time sitting in a chair in the lounge, apparently watching television.

The above situation is quite typical of a resident within today's nursing homes. In utilizing the nursing process with a focus on Nightingale's theory, it is essential to focus on Mrs. Kerr's environment and her reaction to it, rather than specifically on her as a resident. Table 3–2 reflects the use of the Nightingale theory.

The major emphasis in this situation is to restructure the immediate environment around Mrs. Kerr so that nature can act to main-

Table 3–2
Nightingale's Theory Applied to the Nursing Process

Nursing Process Phases	Case Example of Mrs. Kerr
Assessment— Data collection	Seventy-year-old woman who has partial paralysis of her right side. Can move about the environment. The home offers some alternatives to the resident's surroundings—a dining room, bedroom, and television lounge. Visitors from the outside are allowed. Residents are not encouraged to bring meaningful things with them to the home. The only sensory stimulation is one television set. During periods of eating, food intake is poor.
Analysis of data	Basically, there is a lack of specific data, especially relating to the total environment of the nursing home. Thus, an analysis at this time must be viewed as tentative in nature until a reassessment can be done.
Data gaps	Inadequate information on the following: adequacy of ventilation, presence of drafts, sudden noises, cleanliness of surroundings, variety of dietary offerings, opportunities to communicate with others, variety of stimulus provided, specific physical limitations, previous nursing observation, odors present throughout the home, method of disposal of human wastes, amount of sunlight and artificial light.
Nursing diagnosis	Nonstimulating environment.
Implementation	Increase communication. Provide for an optimum environment that will facilitate health.
	Increase stimulus through a greater exposure to sunlight and fresh air. Place Mrs. Kerr in a room that will increase the amount of interaction she has with others.
Evaluation	Observe effect of a changing environment on her health state.

tain her optimum condition. With additional reassessment and evaluation, much can be done to prolong a healthy life and promote total comfort. It is possible, after such assessment, that the environment of the nursing home may be destructive to Mrs. Kerr's health. Alternatives may need to be sought. By the application of adaptation, need, and stress theories to this situation, in terms of the environment, the base for the practice of nursing becomes more theoretically sound.

Some of the questions that might be used to guide the practitioner in implementing Nightingale's theory in situations like Mrs. Kerr's are:

1. Is the environment the most crucial factor in the effective care of Mrs. Kerr?
2. What adaptations can be made within such environments that will facilitate optimum nursing care?
3. Do adjustments within the environment lead patients to a more optimum state of health and prolong their life?
4. Does the amount of stress within such environments affect both the residents and the nurse?
5. What hierarchy of needs is met in such an environment?

As an approach to the practice of nursing, Nightingale's theory is as valid today as it was over one hundred years ago. Within the hospital environment, much can be done to reduce stress, improve adaptation, and meet patient needs through minor adjustments that can be made by the professional nurse. Some examples are the following: the placement of a patient's bed within the room to provide a view of the outside world or sunlight; the encouraging and educating of visitors to provide a greater amount of variety or stimulation within the environment; the less frequent, sudden awakening of patients; and the provision for a quiet, unhurried atmosphere. Although today's hospitals have clean air through the air conditioning system, and clean water through more sophisticated plumbing systems, they still have drafty, odorous environments created by the lack of attention to such details.

Much of Nightingale's theory might be viewed as involving basic common sense, such as giving attention to the cleanliness of a patient's surroundings, keeping chills away, and providing adequate lighting to read. Yet such things are frequently taken for granted and are often forgotten.

NIGHTINGALE'S WORK AND THE
CHARACTERISTICS OF A THEORY

Nightingale's theory of nursing has its strengths and weaknesses in relation to the characteristics of a sound theory presented in Chapter 1, as noted below.

1. Theories can interrelate concepts in such a way as to create a different way of looking at a particular phenomenon. As mentioned earlier, the four major concepts are not explicit in Nightingale's theory, and yet they do offer nursing a specific way of looking at a particular phenomenon. This is evident in the two examples described in this chapter. Viewed very simply, the theory does offer a prediction in relation to the outcomes of nursing care. Creating a positive environment will allow humans to become healthy. Yet we know today that although the human environment is critical in relation to health, other variables such as genetics are also very significant.

2. Theories must be logical in nature. The relationship between each of the concepts is logical and consistent with similar assumptions. The assumption that the environment affects humans is consistent within Nightingale's explanation of the purpose and goal of nursing and the meaning of health.

3. Theories should be relatively simple yet generalizable. Nightingale's theory, although limited, has a lot of generalizability. It can be utilized in any environment such as hospitals, nursing homes, schools, the individual's home, or wherever human beings may be found. The ideas are also basically simple to apply and easy to measure in terms of outcomes.

4. Theories can be the bases for hypotheses that can be tested.

5. Theories contribute to and assist in increasing the general body of knowledge within the discipline through the research implemented to validate them.

6. Theories can be utilized by the practitioners to guide and improve their practice.

7. Theories must be consistent with other validated theories, laws, and principles but will leave open unanswered questions that need to be investigated.

Due to their similarity, these last four characteristics will be discussed together as they relate to Nightingale's theory. In spite of the simplicity and generalizability of her theory, nursing has not yet adequately incorporated much of it into practice or research. For example, in a way, her theory has been researched by scientists such as environmentalists. That is, we are increasingly becoming aware of how environmental pollution affects our health in a negative way. From a broad perspective this should give Nightingale's theory validity. However, we have not yet adequately validated the theory within the context of the health care and nursing environment. Research questions that can lead to hypotheses need to be tested within clinical nursing. For instance, What effect does the hospital environment have on the pace of the healing process? Does the nurse have the authority to impact on the patient's environment adequately? Do sudden, frequent environmental changes affect patients' perceptions of their reparative process? These are only a few of the many possible questions that can be used to guide research. The answers to these questions could well be used to develop guidelines for nursing education and practice.

NIGHTINGALE'S THEORY OF NURSING AS RELATED TO SCIENTIFIC THEORIES

Nightingale's theory of nursing is closely related to scientific theories frequently used in nursing practice today. Most significant are the theories of adaptation, need, and stress.

Adaptation Theory

Adaptation reflects man's adjustments to forces that confront him. Such forces are viewed in the context of the total environment in which man finds himself. The success or nonsuccess of the adaptive responses of man can be seen by reviewing the environmental forces described by Nightingale. Man's ability to allow nature to act on his behalf as influenced by his environment may lead to either adaptive or maladaptive response. For example, a patient who finds himself in a cold, dusty, poorly ventilated environment will have to use much of his available energy for adapting to his environment rather than for recovering from his illness.

To put this in the context of the present, one should note that during the Vietnam War, injured soldiers were quickly airlifted to casualty stations in which they were treated before being sent to nearby hospitals for more complete care. In comparison to previous treatment of the injured, this led to a much lower death rate. Admittedly, this closely relates to improved medical care, but it should also be noted that removing the injured from a poor environment as soon as possible allowed nature to act on the patient's behalf—the Nightingale theory.

Need Theory

Need theories, especially Maslow's,[5] basically recognize theories given emphasis by Nightingale: for example, the need for oxygenation viewed in the context of fresh air, ventilation, and the need for a safe environment as related to proper drainage and clean water. Need theories stress the ability of humans to survive in the context of how well these needs are met. An environment that strongly supports basic human physiological needs is essential. Maslow's emphasis on a hierarchical order of needs places physiological needs as primary, whereas emotional and social needs have less significance for survivial.[6] Again, Nightingale's emphasis on the physical environment that affects the physiological functioning of humans supports Maslow's theory.

Need theories frequently emphasize providing novelty and activities and encouraging exploration of the environment. Nightingale advised against having the patient suffer boredom from staring at four blank walls all day long. Today the literature speaks of sensory deprivation—demonstrated by boredom, daydreaming, and a lack of concentration.

Stress Theory

Stress involves a threat or a change in the environment in which an individual must cope. Stress can be positive or negative depending on its end result. Stress can encourage a person to take positive action toward a desired goal or need, or it can cause exhaustion if the stress is so intense that the individual is unable to cope. Nightingale emphasized placing the patient in an optimum environment so that there would be a minimum of outside stressors. For example, slow quiet movements, whispering, or sudden noises were viewed as causing stress, whereas purposeful quick actions were seen as more appropriate. However, suddenly waking the patient causes great excitement and can be viewed as a negative stressor.

The number and duration of stressors also have a strong influence on the individual's ability to cope. In reviewing the major components of Nightingale's theory, the greater the degree of poor air, poor water, poor light, and other negative environmental factors, and the longer the duration, the lesser the potential for the patient to cope with his illness. As a matter of fact, given a healthy individual within a poor environment with multiple stressors of long duration, illness would soon occur.

SUMMARY

Nightingale's major focus was on the environment of the patient. Nursing was viewed as distinct from medicine and focused on providing an environment that allowed nature to act on behalf of the patient. Environmental factors involved clean air and water, control of noise, proper drainage, reduction of chills, and a variety of activities. Nightingale emphasized fresh air as primary and good lighting as secondary to the effective care of the patient. Other theories most closely related to her writings are adaptation, need, and stress. In utilizing her theory within the nursing process, the focus is on how the environment affects the patient. Implementation involves adjustments to inadequate environments. Nightingale's theory is as appropriate today as a theoretical base for practice as it was during her time of practice in the mid-1800s. It is the foundation on which all other theories in nursing should be viewed.

NOTES

1. Florence Nightingale, *Notes on Nursing* (New York: Dover Publications, Inc., 1969).
2. Ruth Murray and Judith Zentner, *Nursing Concepts for Health Promotion* (Englewood Cliffs, N.J.: Prentice-Hall, Inc., 1975), p. 149.
3. Nightingale, *Notes on Nursing.*
4. Ibid.
5. Abraham Maslow, *Motivation and Personality* (New York: Harper & Row, Publishers, Inc., 1954).
6. Ibid.

ADDITIONAL REFERENCES

AULD, MARGARET E., and LINDA HULTHEN BIRUM, *The Challenge of Nursing: A Book of Readings.* St. Louis, Mo.: The C. V. Mosby Company, 1973.

BYRNE, MARJORIE L., and LIDA F. THOMPSON, *Key Concepts for the Study and Practice of Nursing.* St. Louis, Mo.: The C. V. Mosby Company, 1972.

4

HILDEGARD E. PEPLAU

Janice Ryan Belcher and Lois J. Brittain Fish

Hildegard Peplau was born in Reading, Pennsylvania, on September 1, 1909. Dr. Peplau graduated from a diploma program in nursing in Pottstown, Pennsylvania, in 1931. She graduated from Bennington College with a B.A. in Interpersonal Psychology in 1943, and from Columbia University in New York with a M.A. in Psychiatric Nursing in 1947, and an Ed.D. in Curriculum Development in 1953. Dr. Peplau's nursing experience includes private and general duty hospital experience, two years in the U.S. Army, nursing research, and part-time private practice in psychiatric nursing. She has taught graduate psychiatric nursing for many years and is a retired Professor Emeritus from Rutgers University. The first postbaccalaureate nursing program in central Europe was facilitated by Dr. Peplau in Belgium.

Hildegard Peplau published the book Interpersonal Relations in Nursing *in 1952.[1] She has also published numerous articles in professional magazines on topics ranging from interpersonal concepts to current issues in nursing. Her pamphlet "Basic Principles of Patient Counseling" was derived from her research and workshops.[2]*

Dr. Peplau has served with many organizations, including the World Health Organization, the National Institute of Mental

Health, and the Nurse Corps. She is past Executive Director and past President of the American Nurses' Association. She has served as a nursing consultant to various foreign countries and to the Surgeon General of the Air Force. Her many contributions to nursing are the result of her pioneer qualities in communicating her perceptions concerning nursing.

Hildegard Peplau published *Interpersonal Relations in Nursing,* referring to her book as a "partial theory for the practice of nursing."[3] In this source, Peplau discussed the phases of the interpersonal process, roles in nursing situations, and methods for studying nursing as an interpersonal process. This chapter defines the crux of her nursing theory to be the phases of the interpersonal process and relates the other ideas to this central core.

According to Peplau, nursing is therapeutic in that it is a healing art, assisting an individual who is sick or in need of health care. Nursing can be viewed as an interpersonal process because it involves interaction between two or more individuals with a common goal. In nursing, this common goal provides the incentive for the therapeutic process in which the nurse and patient* respect each other as individuals, both of them learning and growing as a result of the interaction. Learning takes place when an individual selects stimuli in an environment and develps more fully as a result of reactions to these stimuli.[4]

The attainment of this goal, or any goal, is achieved through the use of a series of steps following a certain pattern. As the relationship of the nurse to patient develops in this therapeutic pattern, there is flexibility in the way in which the nurse functions in practice—by making judgments, by utilizing skills founded in scientific knowledge, by utilizing technical abilities, and by assuming roles.

When the nurse and patient first identify a problem and begin to focus on a course of action, they approach this path from diverse backgrounds and individual uniqueness. Each individual may be viewed as a unique biological-psychological-spiritual-sociological structure, one that will not react the same as any other. Each individual has learned differently from the distinct environment, mores, customs, and beliefs of that individual's given culture. Each person comes with

---

Patient will be used throughout this chapter since it is Peplau's definition of the individual who is in need of health care.

preconceived ideas that influence perceptions, and it is these differences in perception that are so important in the interpersonal process. In addition, the nurse, from an educational background, contributes an understanding of developmental theories, of concepts of
life's adaptations, and of conflict responses, as well as a greater insight of nursing's professional role in the interpersonal process. As
nurse and patient continue the relationship, an understanding of one
another's roles and the factors surrounding the problem increases
until both nurse and patient are mutually sharing in a collaborative
manner toward resolution of the problem.

The nurse and the patient work together, and as a result both
become more knowledgeable and mature in the process. Peplau views
nursing as a "maturing force" and an "educative instrument."[5] She
feels nursing is a learning experience of oneself as well as of the other
individual involved in the interpersonal action. This concept is supported by Genevieve Burton, another nursing author from the 1950s,
who states, "Behavior of others must be understood in light of self
understanding."[6] Thus, persons who are more in touch with themselves will be more aware of the various types of reactions induced
in another individual.

As the nurse guides the patient toward the solutions of the everyday encounters, the methods and principles utilized in the professional practice become increasingly more effective. Each encounter
influences the nurse's personal and professional development. Thus,
the kind of person the nurse becomes has a direct influence on the
therapeutic, interpersonal relationship.

Peplau identifies four sequential phases in interpersonal relationships: (1) *orientation,* (2) *identification,* (3) *exploitation,* and (4)
resolution. Each of these phases overlaps and interrelates as the process evolves toward a solution. Different nursing roles are assumed
during the various phases.

These roles can be broadly described in the following manner:

Teacher: One who imparts knowledge in reference to a need
or interest.

Resource: One who provides specific, needed information
that aids in the understanding of a problem or new
situation.

Counselor: One who, through the use of certain skills and attitudes, aids another in recognizing, facing, accept-

ing, and resolving problems that are interfering with the other person's ability to live happily and effectively.

Leader: One who carries out the process of initiation and maintenance of group goals through interaction.

Technical expert: One who provides physical care by displaying clinical skills and has the ability to operate equipment in this care.

Surrogate: One who takes the place of another.

PEPLAU'S PHASES IN NURSING

Orientation

In the initial phase of *orientation*, the nurse and patient meet as two strangers. The patient and/or the family has a "felt need";[7] therefore professional assistance is sought. However, this need may not be readily identified or understood by the individuals who are involved. For example, a sixteen-year-old girl may call the community mental health center just because she feels "very down." It is in this phase that the nurse needs to assist the patient and family in realizing what is happening to the patient.

It is of the utmost importance that the nurse work collaboratively with the patient and family in analyzing the situation, so that they together can recognize, clarify, and define the existing problem. Take the previous example: The nurse, in the counselor role, helps the teen-age girl who feels "very down" to realize that these feelings are the result of an argument with her mother over last evening's date. As the nurse continues to listen, there is a pattern established of the girl arguing with her mother and feeling depressed. As these feelings are discussed, the girl recognizes the arguing as the precipitating factor that causes the depression. Thus the nurse and the patient have defined the problem. Then, the daughter and the parents agree to discuss the concern with the nurse. Thus, by mutually clarifying and defining the problem in the orientation phase, the patient can direct the accumulated energy from the anxiety of unmet needs to more constructively dealing with the presenting problem.

Rapport is established and continues to be strengthened while concerns are being identified.

While the patient and family are talking to the nurse, a mutual decision needs to be made regarding what type of professional assistance should be pursued. The nurse, as a resource person, may work with the patient and family. As an alternative the nurse might, upon mutual agreement of all parties involved, refer the family to another source such as a psychologist, psychiatrist, or social worker. In the orientation phase, the nurse, patient, and family plan what type of services are needed.

The orientation phase is directly affected by the patient's and nurse's attitudes about giving or receiving aid from a reciprocal person. Therefore, in this beginning phase, the nurse needs to be aware of her personal reactions to the patient. For example, the nurse may react differently to the forty-year-old man with abdominal pain who enters the emergency room quietly than to the forty-year-old man with a history of regular alcohol abuse who enters the emergency room boisterously after a few drinks. The nurse's, as well as the patient's, culture, religion, race, educational background, past experiences, and preconceived ideas and expectations all play a part in the nurse's reaction to the patient. The same influencing factors play a part in the patient's reaction to the nurse. See Figure 4–1. For example, the patient may have stereotyped the nurse into performing

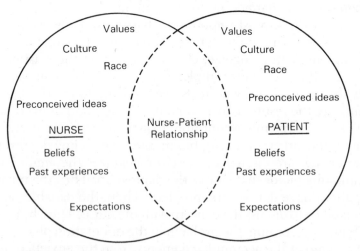

Figure 4-1. Factors influencing the blending of the nurse-patient relationship.

only technical skills such as giving medications or taking blood pressures and therefore may not perceive the nurse as a resource person who can help define the problem. Nursing is an interpersonal process, and both the patient and nurse have an equally important part in the therapeutic interaction.

The nurse, the patient, and the family work together to recognize, clarify, and define the existing problem. This in turn decreases the tension and anxiety associated with the "felt need"[8] and the fear of the unknown. Decreasing tension and anxiety prevents future problems that might arise as a result of repressing an event. Stressful situations are identified through therapeutic interaction. It is imperative that the patient recognize and begin to work through feelings connected with the events leading up to an illness.

Thus, in the beginning of the orientation phase, the nurse and the patient meet as strangers. At the end of the orientation phase, they are concurrently striving to identify the problem and are becoming more comfortable with one another. The patient is settling into the helping environment. The nurse and the patient are now ready to logically progress to the next phase.

Identification

The next phase, referred to as *identification,* is one in which the patient responds selectively to people who can meet his needs. Each patient responds differently in this phase. The patient might actively seek the nurse out or stoically wait until the nurse seeks him out. The response to the nurse is threefold: (1) participate with and be interdependent with the nurse, (2) be autonomous and independent from the nurse; or (3) be passive and dependent on the nurse.[9] An example would be that of a seventy-year-old man who wants to plan his new 1600 calorie diabetic diet. If the relationship is interdependent, the nurse and patient collaborate on the meal planning. Should the relationship be independent, the patient would plan the diet himself with minimal input from the nurse. In a dependent relationship, the nurse does the meal planning for the patient.

Throughout the identification phase, both the patient and nurse must clarify each other's perceptions and expectations.[10] Past experiences of both the patient and the nurse will have a bearing on what their expectations will be during this interpersonal process. As mentioned in the orientation phase, the initial attitudes of the patient and the nurse are important in building a working relationship for identifying the problem and deciding on appropriate assistance.

The perception and expectations of the patient and nurse in the identification phase are even more complex than in the preceding phase. The patient is now responding to the helper selectively. This requires a more intense therapeutic relationship.

To illustrate, a patient who has had a mastectomy may mention to the nurse her inability to understand the arm exercises that have been previously explained to her as an important regimen following surgery. The nurse observes the affected arm to be edematous (swollen). While the nurse is exploring possible reasons for the edema, the patient admits to not doing her arm exercises. The patient's reasoning is the result of being told by a friend that exercising after surgery delays healing. In order to facilitate the patient's understanding and subsequent resumption of the exercises, the nurse can identify professional people, such as the physical therapist, the nurse, and the physician, who will clarify the patient's misconceptions. Generally it is best if the nurse objectively discusses each person's role and the advantages and disadvantages of consulting with each of them. However, in this case, the patient may state that she does not care to discuss the exercises with the nurse or physical therapist because she perceives only the physician as having the necessary information. Thus, previous perceptions of nursing and physical therapy can influence the patient's current decision on the selection of a professional person. In this situation, the nurse needs to be supportive of the patient's decision.

While working through this identification phase, the patient begins to have a feeling of belonging and a capability of dealing with the problem, which decreases her feelings of helplessness and hopelessness. This in turn creates an optimistic attitude from which inner strength ensues.

Exploitation

Following identification, the patient moves into the *exploitation* phase, in which advantage of all available services is taken. The degree to which these services are utilized is based on the interests and needs of the patient. The individual begins to feel an integral part of the helping environment. She/he feels as though some control over the situation is gained by extracting help from the services offered. Take the example of the woman with the edematous arm. During this phase the patient begins to absorb the information given to her for the arm exercises. She reads pamphlets and watches a film describing the exercises; she discusses questions with the nurse; and she may inquire about joining an exercise group through the physical therapy department.

During this phase some patients may make more demands than they did when they were seriously ill. They may make many minor requests or may apply other "attention-getting" techniques depending on their individual needs. These actions may often be difficult, if not impossible, for the health care provider to completely understand. The nurse must deal with the unconscious forces causing the patient's actions. The principles of interviewing techniques must be used in order to explore, understand, and adequately deal with the underlying problems. It is important that the nurse explore the possible causes for the patient's behavior. A therapeutic relationship must be maintained by conveying an attitude of acceptance, concern, and trust. The nurse must encourage the patient to recognize and explore feelings, thoughts, emotions, and behaviors by providing a nonjudgmental atmosphere and a therapeutic emotional climate.

Some patients may take an active interest in, and become involved in, self-care. Such a patient will become more self-sufficient and will demonstrate initiative by establishing appropriate behavior for goal attainment. Through self-determination, the patient progressively develops responsibility for self, belief in potentialities, and adjustment toward self-reliance and independence. These patients realistically begin to establish their own goals toward improved health status. They strive to achieve a pattern or direction to their lives and a feeling of wellness. This is accomplished by becoming productive, by trusting and depending on their own capabilities, and by becoming responsible for their own actions, thus becoming more fully themselves. As a result, as their unique personality continues to form, they develop sources of inner strength with which to face new problems or challenges.

Most patients fluctuate between dependence on others, as in the impaired health role, and the independence of functioning at an optimal health level. Using the previous example, this individual may want to actively exercise on schedule one day but will state she is too tired the next day. The nurse then needs to take the initiative to remind the patient of her scheduled exercises.

This type of intermittent behavior can be compared to the

adjustment reaction of the adolescent in a dependency-independency conflict. The patient may temporarily be in a dependent role while the simultaneous need for independence exists. Various causes may trigger the onset of this psychological disequilibrium. The patient will vacillate unpredictably between the two states and will appear confused and anxious, protesting dependence while fearing independence. In caring for patients who fluctuate between dependence and independence, the nurse must deal with the particular behavior presented rather than attempting to handle the composite problem of inconsistency. The nurse should provide an atmosphere that carries no threat, one in which a person can face himself, recognize his weaknesses, use his strengths without imposing them on others, and accept help from others.

The nurse must also be fully aware of the various facets of communication including clarifying, listening, accepting, and interpreting. Correct use of all these factors will assist the patient to meet his challenges and will pave the way toward maximum wholesome adjustment. Thus, the nurse aids the patient in exploiting all avenues of help, and progress is made toward the final step—the resolution phase.

Resolution

The last phase of Peplau's interpersonal process is *resolution*. The patient's needs have already been met by the collaborative efforts of the nurse and patient. Now, the patient and nurse must terminate their therapeutic relationship and must dissolve the links between them.

Sometimes dissolving these links is very difficult for both the patient and the nurse. Dependency needs in a therapeutic relationship often continue on psychologically after the physiological needs are met. The patient may feel that it "is just not time yet" to end the relationship. For example, a new mother has a desire to learn to take her baby's temperature. During the first home visit, the community health nurse and the new mother set their goal of having the mother take the baby's temperature correctly. After instruction and demonstration by the community health nurse on the first visit, the mother takes the temperature correctly on the second visit. Their goal is met. The relationship is ended because the mother's problem was solved. However, one week after the resolution, the mother

Table 4-1
Phases of the Nurse-Patient Relationship

Phase	Focus
Orientation	Problem-defining phase
Identification	Selection of appropriate professional assistance
Exploitation	Utilization of professional assistance for problem-solving alternatives
Resolution	Termination of the professional relationship

telephones the community health nurse three times concerning minor questions on infant care. The mother at this point has not dissolved the dependency link with the community health nurse.

The final resolution may also be difficult for the nurse. In the above example, the mother may be willing to terminate the relationship, but the community health nurse may continue to visit the home to see how the baby is progressing. The nurse may be unable to become free of this bond in their relationship. In resolution, as in the other phases, anxiety and tension will increase in the patient and in the nurse if there is unsuccessful completion of the phase.

During successful resolution, the patient drifts away from identifying with the helping person, the nurse. This phase is a direct outgrowth of the successful completion of the other phases. The patient then breaks the bond with the nurse. A healthier emotional balance is demonstrated. The nurse also must establish independence from the patient. When the dissolving of the therapeutic interpersonal process is sequential to the previous phases, the patient and the nurse both become stronger maturing individuals. The patient's needs are met, and movement can be made toward new goals. Table 4-1 indicates the focus of each phase.

PEPLAU'S THEORY AND THE FOUR
MAJOR CONCEPTS

Theories of nursing usually evolve around the four concepts of individual, health, society, and nursing. Peplau defines *man** as an orga-

*Peplau uses *man* and *he* in the generic sense.

nism who "strives in its own way to reduce tension generated by needs."[11] *Health* is defined as "a word symbol that implies forward movement of personality and other ongoing human processes in the direction of creative, constructive, productive, personal, and community living."[12] *Society* is not mentioned as such, but Peplau does encourage nursing to consider culture and mores when the person changes environments, for example, when the person is adjusting to the hospital routine.[13] Peplau's lack of a clear definition of society comes from her focus on the specific nurse/patient relationship.

Hildegard Peplau considers *nursing* a "significant therapeutic, interpersonal process."[14] She defines it as a "human relationship between an individual who is sick, or in need of health services, and a nurse especially educated to recognize and to respond to the need for help."[15]

RELATIONSHIP BETWEEN PEPLAU'S PHASES AND THE NURSING PROCESS

Peplau's continuum of the four phases of *orientation, identification, exploitation,* and *resolution* can be compared to the nursing process as discussed in Chapter 2. See Table 4-2. The nursing process in Chapter 2 is defined as "a deliberate, intellectual activity whereby the practice of nursing is approached in an orderly, systematic manner."*

There are basic similarities between the nursing process and Peplau's interpersonal phases. Both Peplau's phases and the nursing process are sequential and focus on therapeutic interactions. Both utilize problem-solving techniques for the nurse and patient to collaborate on, with the end purpose of meeting the patient's needs. Both go from general to specific, for example, the patient's vague feelings to specific facts concerning the vague feelings. And both include observation, communication, and recording as basic tools utilized by nursing.

There are differences, too, between Peplau's phases and the nursing process. When considering differences, it must be taken into account that Peplau's book *Interpersonal Relations in Nursing* was published in 1952. Professional nursing today is functioning with more

*See p. 15.

Table 4-2

Comparison of Nursing Process and Peplau's Phases

Nursing Process	Peplau's Phases
Assessment Data collection and analysis. Need not necessarily a "felt need"; may be nurse-initiated.	*Orientation* Nurse and patient come together as strangers; meeting initiated by patient who expresses a "felt need"; work together to recognize, clarify, and define facts related to need. (*Note:* Data collection is continuous.)
Nursing Diagnosis Summary statement based on analysis.	Patient clarifies "felt need."
Planning Mutually set goals.	*Identification* Interdependent goal setting. Patient has feeling of belonging and selectively responds to those who can meet needs. Patient-initiated.
Implementation Plans initiated toward achievement of mutually set goals. May be accomplished by patient, health care professional, and/or patient's family.	*Exploitation* Patient actively seeking and drawing on knowledge and expertise of those who can help. Patient-initiated.
Evaluation Based on mutually established expected end behaviors. May lead to termination or initiation of new plans.	*Resolution* Occurs after other phases are successfully completed and have been met. Leads to termination.

defined goals. Movement is away from the nurse as the physician's helper and toward the nurse as a consumer advocate. For instance, today part of the nursing process is nursing diagnosis. The American Nurses' Association, in the *Standards of Nursing Practice,* states: "Nursing diagnoses are derived from health status data."[16] Peplau, however, stated (in 1952) that the physician's primary function was "recognizing the full impact of the patient's nuclear problem and the kind of professional assistance that is needed," which results, for the physician, in "the task of evaluating and diagnosing emergent problems."[17] This is in opposition to the present recognition of the independent nursing function.

Nursing functions, according to Peplau, include clarification of the information the physician gives the patient as well as collection of data about the patient that may point out other problem areas.[18] Today, however, with nursing's expanded roles, we have independent nurse practitioners who may or may not refer the patient to the physician, depending on the patient's need. Through expanded roles such as this, nursing is becoming more accountable and responsible, giving professional nursing greater legal independence. The nursing process provides a mode for evaluating the quality of nursing care rendered, which is the core of legal accountability.

Peplau gives the variables in nursing situations as needs, frustration, conflict, and anxiety. She further relates that these variables must be dealt with for growth to occur, as the nurse facilitates healthy development of each personality. It is readily seen that Peplau was influenced by some of the theories of the time, especially Harry S. Sullivan's interpersonal theory[19] and Sigmund Freud's theory of psychodynamics.[20]

In nursing today, variables such as intrafamily dynamics, socioeconomic forces (e.g., financial resources), personal space considerations, and community social service resources should be taken into account for each patient. These variables provide a broader perspective for viewing nursing situations than Peplau's personal factors of needs, frustration, conflict, and anxiety. Currently, even a family, a group, or a community may be collectively defined as the patient.

Nursing has also broadened its perspective in helping the patient reach a fuller health potential through a greater emphasis on health maintenance and promotion. Martha Rogers states, "Maintenance and promotion of health, prevention of disease, nursing diagnosis, intervention, and rehabilitation encompass the scope of nursing's goals."[21] Nurses are actively seeking to identify health problems in a variety of community and institutional settings today.

The specific components of the nursing process and Peplau's phases will now be discussed. Refer again to Table 4–2. Peplau's orientation phase parallels the beginning of the *assessment phase* in that both the nurse and patient come together as strangers. This meeting is initiated by the patient who expresses a need, although the need is not always understood. Conjointly, the nurse and patient begin to work through recognizing, clarifying, and defining facts related to this need. This step is presently referred to as the data collection in the assessment phase of the nursing process.

In the nursing process the need is not necessarily a "felt need."[22] For example, the nurse may be currently functioning in the community by doing health assessments of people who perceive themselves to be healthy. A school nurse may do hearing screening for school children. If a hearing deficit is discovered, a referral is initiated by the nurse. The children do not usually seek out the nurse for this deficit. In this situation, the need must be identified for the child and for his parents in order to persuade them to seek assistance regarding the hearing deficit. Supplying the data on a note sent home to the parents might precipitate the parents' and child's perception of the need. This is congruent with the first part of Edgar H. Schein's model of change, the unfreezing of the established equilibrium so change can take place. Schein states, "If change is to occur, therefore, it must be preceded by an alteration of the present stable equilibrium which supports the present behavior and attitudes.[23] Supplying the data would be one stimulus for change. The nurse may also have to follow up the child's note with a telephone call or a home visit and additional data such as poor grades in order to facilitate the family's entry into the unfreezing stage or into Peplau's "felt need" phase of orientation.[24]

Orientation and assessment are not synonymous and must not be confused. Collecting data is continuous throughout Peplau's phases. In the nursing process, the initial collection of data is the nursing assessment, and further collection of data becomes an integral part of reassessment (see Chapter 2, Figure 2-1).

The *nursing diagnosis* evolves once the health problems or deficits are identified. The nursing diagnosis is a summary statement of the data collected. It delineates the patient's problem or potential problem. Peplau states that "during the period of orientation the patient clarifies his first whole impression of his problem";[25] whereas in the nursing process, the nurse's judgment forms the diagnosis from the data collected.

Mutually set goals evolve from the nursing diagnosis. These goals give direction to the plan and indicate the appropriate helping resources. When helping resources are discussed, the patient then can selectively identify with the resource persons. According to Peplau, the patient is viewed as being in the identification phase.

When the nurse and patient collaborate on goals, there may be a clash based on the preconceptions and expectations of each person, as described earlier in Peplau's identification phase. These discrepancies must be resolved before mutually stated goals can be agreed on. Goal setting should be an interdependent action between nurse and patient.

In the *planning* phase of the nursing process, the nurse must specifically formulate how the patient is going to achieve the mutually set goals. Patient input is actively sought by the nurse so that the patient feels an integral part of the plan and compliance is more likely to take place. In this step the nurse considers the patient's own skills for handling his personal problems. Peplau stresses that the nurse wants to develop a therapeutic relationship so that the patient's anxiety will be channeled constructively to seek resources, thus decreasing feelings of hopelessness. This step in planning can still be considered within Peplau's identification phase.

The patient also begins to have a feeling of belonging because of mutual respect, communication, and interest. The feeling of belonging must be analyzed and should be a thrust toward a healthier personality and not imitative behavior.[26] Peplau states, "Some patients identify too readily with nurses, expecting that all of their wants will be taken care of and that nothing will be expected of them."[27] In Peplau's identification phase, the patient selectively responds to people who can meet his personal needs. Therefore, the identification phase is patient-initiated.

The planning stage of the nursing process gives direction and meaning to the nursing action toward resolving the patient's problems. The nurse utilizes the knowledge from her/his educational background to scientifically base the plan of nursing action.

In the *implementation phase,* as in exploitation, the patient is finally reaping benefits from the therapeutic relationship by drawing on the nurse's knowledge and expertise. In both phases (implementation and exploitation) the individualized plans have already been formed, based on the patient's interest and needs. Therefore, in both phases the plans are initiated toward completion of desired goals. There is a difference, however, between exploitation, where the patient is the one who actively seeks varying types of services in obtaining the maximal benefits available, and implementation, where there is a prescribed plan or procedure, holistic in nature, to achieve mutually predetermined goals or objectives based on the nurse's intellectual knowledge and technical skills. Exploitation is patient-oriented, whereas implementation can be accomplished by the patient or by other persons including health professionals and the patient's family.

In Peplau's resolution phase, the other phases have been successfully worked through, the needs have been met, and resolution and termination are the end result. Although Peplau does not discuss *evaluation* per se, evaluation is an inherent factor in determining the status of readiness for the patient to proceed through the resolution phase.

In the nursing process the evaluation is a separate step, and mutually established expected end behaviors are utilized as tools for evaluation. Time limits on attainment of these behaviors are set for the purposes of evaluation, although these limits need not be strictly adhered to. Circumstances may arise that require an adjustment on the time constraints.

In evaluation, if the situation is clear-cut, the problem moves toward termination. However, if the problem is unresolved, goals and objectives are not met; and if care is ineffective, a reassessment must be done. New goals, planning, and implementation are then established.

PEPLAU'S WORK AND THE CHARACTERISTICS OF A THEORY

Peplau's interpersonal approach to nursing has the characteristics of a theory described in Chapter 1 of this text.* For the first characteristic, concepts are interrelated in such a way as to create a different way of looking at a particular phenomenon. The phases of orientation, identification, exploitation, and resolution interrelate the different components of each phase. This interrelation creates a different perspective of viewing the nurse-patient interaction and the transaction of health care. Peplau broadly relates these four phases to the interpersonal concepts of individual, health, society, and nursing. For example, in the phase of orientation there are components of nurse, patient, strangers, problems, and anxiety.

For the second characteristic, the phases progress in a logical way from initial contact through termination. The names given to the phases are also logically derived and are meaningful.

*See pages 5–8, for a list of these characteristics.

The third and sixth characteristics speak to simplicity, generalizability, and utilization by practitioners to guide and improve practice. Peplau's phases provide simplicity in the view of the natural progression of the nurse-patient relationship. This simplicity leads to an ease of adaptability in any nurse-patient interaction, and thus provides generalizability. Today, nursing is still defined as an interpersonal process. Also, communication and interviewing skills are basic tools of nursing, and thus the phases and the techniques used in them can be and are utilized by practitioners.

The fourth and fifth characteristics speak to the generation of hypotheses and the contribution to general knowledge through research. Peplau's work has contributed greatly to the body of knowledge not only in psychiatric-mental health nursing but in nursing in general. With regard to Peplau's contribution to research in psychiatric-mental health nursing, Professor Grayce Sills states that in the 1950s, two-thirds of research concentrated on relationships.[28] Dr. Sills says, "At Teachers College, Columbia University, Peplau's (1952) work influenced the interpersonal nature and direction of clinical work and studies."[29] Presently, as in the past, researchers are attempting to test Peplau's theory. However, the difficulty of obtaining unbiased observations of relationships in a natural environment can create limitations in testing hypotheses based on an interpersonal process. This problem in testing Peplau's theory is shared by all of the social sciences that deal with human behavior.

In considering the seventh and final characteristic, Peplau's phases are consistent with other theories such as Maslow's need theory[30] and Selye's stress theory.[31] General system theory could be broadly related to the four phases.[32] For instance, the nurse and patient could each be defined as a system with the interaction of the four phases being energy exchanges of input, throughput, and output of each nurse and patient system.

SUMMARY

Peplau's text *Interpersonal Relations in Nursing*, published in 1952, is still applicable in theory and practice. The core of Peplau's theory of nursing is the interpersonal process, which is an integral part of present-day nursing. This process consists of the sequential phases of orientation, identification, exploitation, and resolution. These phases overlap, interrelate, and vary in time duration. The nurse and patient first clarify the patient's problem, and mutual expectations and goals are explored while deciding on appropriate plans for improved health status. This process is influenced by both the nurse's and patient's perceptions and preconceived ideas emerging from their individual uniqueness.

Both Peplau's phases and the nursing process are sequential and focus on therapeutic interactions. Through mutual exploration of the patient's difficulty and the nurse-patient relationship, a broader understanding of the patient's problem and new alternative approaches toward reaching the solution are uncovered.

When two persons meet in a creative relationship, there is a continuing sense of mutuality and togetherness throughout the experience. Both individuals are involved in a process of self-fulfillment, which becomes a growth experience.

Peplau focuses on a specific nurse and patient relationship. Today's nursing process, however, may view the patient collectively as a group, family, or community. Thus, today's nursing process takes the total environment more into account.

Peplau's nursing theory, the interpersonal process, has as its foundation, theories of interaction. It has contributed to nursing in the areas of clinical practice, theory, and research, adding to today's nursing knowledge base. Thus, Peplau's theory has facilitated increased understanding of the patterns of interactions and the nurse/patient value systems, giving fuller resources from which nurses can draw for future encounters with patients who have similar needs.

NOTES

1. Hildegard E. Peplau, *Interpersonal Relations in Nursing* (New York: G. P. Putnam's Sons, 1952).
2. Hildegard E. Peplau, "Basic Principles of Patient Counseling," n.d.; and "Profile: Hildegard E. Peplau, R.N., Ed.D.," *Nursing '74*, 4, no. 2 (February 1974), 13.
3. Peplau, *Interpersonal Relations*, p. 261.
4. Ibid., p. 35.
5. Ibid., p. 8.
6. Genevieve Burton, *Personal, Impersonal, and Interpersonal: A Guide for Nurses* (New York: Springer New York, Inc., 1958), p. 7.
7. Peplau, *Interpersonal Relations*, p. 18.
8. Ibid.
9. Ibid, p. 33.

10. Ibid., p. 36.
11. Ibid., p. 82.
12. Ibid., p. 12.
13. Ibid., p. 28.
14. Ibid., p. 16.
15. Ibid., pp. 5–6.
16. Congress for Nursing Practice, *Standards of Nursing Practice* (Kansas City, Mo.: American Nurses' Association, 1973), p. 2.
17. Peplau, *Interpersonal Relations*, p. 23.
18. Ibid.
19. Harry S. Sullivan, *Conceptions of Modern Psychiatry* (Washington, D.C.: William Alanson White Psychiatric Foundation, 1947).
20. Sigmund Freud, *The Problem of Anxiety* (New York: W. W. Norton & Co., Inc., 1936).
21. Martha E. Rogers, *An Introduction to the Theoretical Basis of Nursing* (Philadelphia: F. A. Davis Company, 1970), p. 86.
22. Peplau, *Interpersonal Relations*, p. 18.
23. Edgar H. Schein, "The Mechanisms of Change," in *The Planning of Change*, 2nd ed., Warren G. Bennis et al., eds. (New York: Holt, Rinehart and Winston, 1969), p. 99.
24. Peplau, *Interpersonal Relations*, p. 18.
25. Ibid., p. 30.
26. Ibid., p. 35.
27. Ibid., p. 32.
28. Grayce M. Sills, "Research in the Field of Psychiatric Nursing, 1952–1977," *Nursing Research*, 26, no. 3 (May-June 1977), 203.
29. Ibid.
30. Abraham Maslow, *Motivation and Personality* (New York: Harper & Row, Publishers, Inc., 1954).
31. Hans Selye, *The Stress of Life* (New York: McGraw-Hill Book Company, 1956).
32. Ludwig von Bertalanffy, *Main Currents in Modern Thought*, cited by Mary Elizabeth Hazzard, in "An Overview of Systems Theory," *Nursing Clinics of North America*, 6, no. 3 (September 1971), 385.

5

VIRGINIA HENDERSON

Chiyoko Yamamoto Furukawa and Joan K. Howe

Virginia Henderson was born in Kansas City, Missouri, in 1897, the fifth child of a family of eight children. Most of her formative years were spent in Virginia, where the family resided during the period her father practiced law in Washington, D.C.

Henderson's interest in nursing evolved during World War I from her desire to help the sick and wounded military personnel. She enrolled in the Army School of Nursing in Washington, D.C., and graduated in 1921. In 1926, Henderson embarked upon the continuation of her education at Columbia University Teachers College, where she completed her B.S. and M.A. degrees in nursing education. She remained at Teachers College from 1930 to 1948 to teach clinical nursing practice with a strong emphasis on the use of the analytical process.

Henderson is a recipient of numerous recognitions for her outstanding contributions to nursing. She is a Professor Emeritus at Yale University School of Nursing and has received honorary doctoral degrees from Rush University, Chicago, Illinois; the University of Rochester, Rochester, New York; the University of Western Ontario, London, Ontario; the Catholic University of America, Washington, D.C.; and Yale University, New Haven, Connecticut.

Her writings are far-reaching and have made an impact on nursing throughout the world. The publications The Nature of Nursing *and* Basic Principles of Nursing Care *are widely known, and the latter has been translated into several languages for the benefit of non-English-speaking nurses.*[1] *Henderson's more recent articles in the* Nursing Times *and* Journal of Advanced Nursing *exemplify her beliefs about nursing and contribute to clarifying nursing practice in view of current technological and societal advances.*[2]

Questions about the exclusive functions of nurses stimulated and prompted Virginia Henderson to devote her career to defining nursing practice. Some of these questions were: What is the practice of nursing? What specific functions do nurses perform? What are nursing's unique activities? Henderson developed her definition of nursing to communicate her thoughts on these questions. She believed an occupation that affects human life must outline its functions, particularly if it is to be regarded as a profession.[3] Her ideas about the definition of nursing were influenced by her nursing education and practice, by her students and colleagues at Columbia University School of Nursing, and distinguished by other nursing leaders. Although all of these experiences contributed to her ideas and beliefs, her personal educational experiences and nursing practice were the dominating forces that gave her insight into what nursing should be and how it should be focused. A review of Henderson's educational preparation and nursing practice furnishes the basis on which to examine her definition of nursing.

EDUCATIONAL AND PRACTICE BACKGROUND

Henderson's interpretation of the nurse's function is the synthesis of many positive and negative influences.[4] A major influence was her basic nursing education in a general hospital, primarily at the Army School of Nursing. Her education involved learning by doing, speed of performance, technical competence, and ability determined by successful mastery of procedures such as catheterizations. As a result, an impersonal approach to care giving emerged and was interpreted as professional behavior. On the other hand, students were also taught the importance of ethics in nursing and a compassion for humanity.

Classroom learning for the nursing students consisted of physician lectures that were simplified versions of instructions given to medical students. The emphasis on disease, diagnosis, and treatment regimens took a cut-and-dried approach to learning. With support from Annie W. Goodrich, dean of the school, Henderson recognized her discontent with the regimentalized mode of care. She concluded this kind of care was simply an extension of medical practice.[5]

At this educational stage, there was a yearning to see her teachers practice because the student's experiences did not include observing a graduate nurse giving care. This was an era when the students were used to staff the hospital in return for their educational experiences. Henderson suggests that the lack of a role model was a serious void in her education. In her case, clinical practice was viewed as a self-learned process while students cared for the sick and wounded soldiers. She perceived this atmosphere as one of indebtedness to the patient for having served the country on the battlefields. Henderson described the nurse-patient relationship as warm and generous with the nurse wanting to do all she could while the soldiers asked for little. This experience was believed to be unique and special because the opportunity for the nurse to express indebtedness to patients was almost nonexistent in a civilian hospital.

In her next experience, Henderson was disappointed with the psychiatric affiliation segment of her preparation for nursing. The human relations skills that could have been learned in this setting failed to materialize. As in her previous experiences, the approach to psychiatric patient care continued to focus on disease entities and treatment. She was dismayed by the lack of understanding regarding the nurse's role in the prevention of mental illness or in the curative aspects of care for the psychiatric patient. This experience left her with a sense of failure as a nurse. Henderson claims the only value of the psychiatric affiliation was the opportunity to gain some appreciation of mental illness.

Her pediatric nursing experience at the Boston Floating Hospital was more positive and introduced the concepts of patient-centered care, continuity of care, and tender-loving care. The task-oriented and regimented approach to care was discarded in this setting. However, she identified other shortcomings such as the failure to use family-centered care. Parents were not allowed to visit their sick child, thus isolating the child from parental support when such support was most needed. Henderson also did not see any effort to assess the home environment to identify the needs of the child and family.

The final student experience at the Henry Street Visiting Nurse Agency in New York allowed her to view the community approach to nursing care. The formal approach to patient care that she had learned earlier was replaced with care that considered the life style of the sick. Henderson had concerns about people being discharged to the same environment that originally led them to hospitalization. She believed that the formal approach to care only served as a stop-gap measure without getting to the cause of the problem. She recognized that this type of care failed to consider the person living outside the behavioral controls existing within the institution.

As a graduate nurse, Henderson worked for several years at the Instructive Visiting Nursing Agency in Washington, D.C., because she was unable to accept the hospital system of nursing. This agency experience was rewarding and included the opportunity to try out her ideas about nursing.

The next position she held was teaching nursing students in a diploma program at the Norfolk Protestant Hospital in Virginia. This five-year responsibility was accepted without further education because she was needed by the institution. Such a situation was not unusual because many diploma schools at that time did not require high academic standards for teaching. During this period, she recognized her need for more knowledge and for clarification of the functions of nursing. Subsequently, she enrolled at Columbia University Teachers College to learn about the sciences and humanities relevant to nursing. These courses enabled Henderson to develop an inquiring and analytical approach to nursing.

After graduation, she accepted the position of teaching supervisor in the clinics of Strong Memorial Hospital in Rochester, New York, for a brief time. Then she returned to Columbia where her distinguished teaching career continued until 1948. While at Columbia, she implemented several ideas on nursing in her courses on medical-surgical nursing. The concepts included patient-centered approach, use of the nursing problem method replacing the medial model, emphasis on field experience for students, family follow-up care, and chronic illness care. She also established nursing clinics and encouraged coordination of care with other health professionals.

THE NEED FOR A DEFINITION OF NURSING

Two factors provide the basis for Henderson's development of a definition of nursing. First, she participated in the revision of a nursing textbook. Second, she was concerned that many states had no provision for the licensure of nurses to ensure the public of safe and competent care.

In preparing the 1939 revision of the *Textbook of the Principles and Practice of Nursing*, which she co-authored with the Canadian nurse Bertha Harmer, Henderson recognized the need to be clear about the functions of the nurse.[6] She believed a textbook that serves as a main learning source for the practice of nursing should present a sound and definitive description of nursing. Furthermore, she asserted that the principles and practice of nursing must be built upon and derived from the definition of the profession.

Her interest in defining nursing coincided with the problems associated with licensure of the practitioner. The process of regulating nursing practice through licensure in each state requires a definition of nursing explicitly stated within the Nurse Practice Acts. These acts provide the legal parameters for the nurse's functions in caring for consumers. The primary purpose of this legislative process is the protection of the public from practitioners who are unprepared or otherwise incompetent.

Although official statements on the nursing function were available from the American Nurses' Association (ANA) in 1932 and 1937, Henderson viewed these statements as nonspecific and unsatisfactory definitions of nursing practice.[7] Then, in 1955, the earlier ANA definition was modified to read:

> The practice of professional nursing means the performance for compensation of any act in the observation, care, and counsel of the ill, injured, or infirm, or in the maintenance of health or prevention of illness of others, or in the supervision and teaching of other personnel, or the administration of medications and treatments as prescribed by a licensed physician or dentist; requiring substantial specialized judgment and skill and based on knowledge and application of the principles of biological, physical, and social science. The foregoing shall not be deemed to include arts of diagnosis or prescription of therapeutic or corrective measures.[8]

This statement was an improvement because it incorporated the concept of function,* but Henderson still maintained that the definition was very general and too vague. The new statement suggested the nurse could observe, care for, and counsel the patient and could supervise other health personnel without herself being supervised by the physician. However, it limited the nurse to giving medications and doing treatment prescribed by the physician, and prohibited the nurse from diagnosing, prescribing, or correcting nursing care problems. Thus Henderson viewed the statement as another unsatisfactory definition of nursing.

THE DEVELOPMENT OF HENDERSON'S DEFINITION OF NURSING

Henderson's definition of nursing was a culmination of her extensive experience as a student, teacher, practitioner, and author. Another important influence was her participation in conferences that investigated and debated the nurse's function. However, she was disappointed that the publications of these gatherings were only circulated to the participants and to a few nursing leaders of the time.

Henderson's first definition of nursing was published in the 1955 revision of Bertha Harmer's nursing textbook. It read:

Henderson's First (1955) Definition

Nursing is primarily assisting the individual (sick or well) in the performance of those activities contributing to health, or its recovery (or a peaceful death) that he would perform unaided if he had the necessary strength, will or knowledge. It is likewise the unique contribution of nursing to help the individual to be independent of such assistance as soon as possible.[9]

This statement on nursing conveys the essence of her definition of nursing as it is known today. Since there was collaboration, it is noteworthy to compare Henderson's definition with Harmer's 1922 definition, which read as follows:

Harmer's 1922 Definition

Nursing is rooted in the needs of humanity and is founded on the ideal of service. Its object is not only to cure the sick and

*Independent functions are those actions that are self-directed.

heal the wounded but to bring health and ease, rest, and comfort to mind and body, to shelter, nourish and practice and to
minister to all those who are helpless or handicapped, young,
aged or immature. Its object is to prevent disease and to preserve health. Nursing is, therefore, linked with every other social
agency which strives for the prevention of disease and the preservation of health. The nurse finds herself not only concerned with
the care of the individual but the health of people.[10]

Some relationship can be seen between the two definitions of
nursing. Henderson's definition abbreviated and consolidated
Harmer's beliefs about nursing. Harmer's definition focused on
disease prevention, health preservation, and the need for linkage with
other social agencies to strive for preventive care. Henderson placed
more emphasis on the care of the sick and well individual but did
not mention nursing's concern for the collective health and welfare
of the people.

Henderson's focus on individual care is evident in the stress she
placed on assisting individuals with essential activities to maintain
health, to recover, or to achieve peaceful death. She delineated
specific nursing activities into fourteen components of basic nursing care to augment her definition. These components provide a list
to help the individual with the activities or provide conditions under
which he or she can perform them without aid.[11] The components
are as follows:

1. Breathe normally.
2. Eat and drink adequately.
3. Eliminate body wastes.
4. Move and maintain desirable postures.
5. Sleep and rest.
6. Select suitable clothing—dress and undress.
7. Maintain body temperature within normal range by adjusting clothing and modifying the environment.
8. Keep the body clean and well-groomed and protect the in-
   tegument.
9. Avoid dangers in the environment and avoid injuring others.
10. Communicate with others in expressing emotions, needs,
    fears, or opinions.
11. Worship according to one's faith.
12. Work in such a way that there is a sense of accomplishment.

13. Play or participate in various forms of recreation.
14. Learn, discover, or satisfy the curiosity that leads to normal development and health and use of the available health facilities.

In 1966, Henderson outlined her ultimate statement on the definition of nursing in *The Nature of Nursing*. She viewed this statement as "the crystallization of my ideas."[12]

> The unique function of the nurse is to assist the individual, sick or well, in the performance of those activities contributing to health or its recovery (or to peaceful death) that he could perform unaided if he had the necessary strength, will or knowledge. And to do this in such a way as to help him gain independence as rapidly as possible.[13]

It can be seen that except for some wording changes, the 1955 and 1966 definitions are quite similar. However, by itself, Henderson's definition of nursing fails to fully communicate the main ideas and views she proposes. To comprehend the breadth of her thoughts about nursing functions as described in the definitions and the fourteen components of basic nursing care, it is necessary to study *Basic Principles of Nursing Care*, a 1972 publication of the International Council of Nurses (Geneva). This publication eloquently describes each of the basic nursing care components so that they can be used as a guide to delineate the unique nursing functions. Henderson believed her two statements, the definition of nursing and the fourteen components, together outline the functions the nurse can initiate and control.

Henderson contended that the nurse is expected to carry out the therapeutic plan of the physician because the nurse is a member of the medical team and prime helper to the ill person in assuring that the medical prescriptions are instituted. This nursing function is believed to foster the therapeutic nurse-patient relationship. The nurse functions as a member of an interdisciplinary health team chiefly for the benefit of the individual to aid recovery from illness or to provide support in dying. The ideal situation for a nurse is full participation as a team member with no interference with the nurse's unique functions. Henderson thinks the nurse should identify and serve as a substitute for what the person lacks in order to make him "complete," "whole," or "independent," taking into account his available physical strength, will, or knowledge to reach good health.[14]

She cautions the nurse about undertaking tasks that detract from the professional role and stresses that priority must be given to the nurse's unique functions. On the other hand, Henderson foresees situations where the nurse may need to assume the role of other health workers or function as a cook or plumber in order to meet the person's obvious needs.[15] This is especially applicable on a worldwide basis, since nursing functions could differ from country to country or even within countries. For example, a nurse working in any area that is underserved in relation to health care would function quite differently from a nurse in a large city hospital. The ratio of nurses to physicians as well as to other health care providers affects what nurses do and continues to create confusion for the public regarding the nurse's role.[16]

Figure 5–1 illustrates the main concepts of Henderson's definition of nursing. It demonstrates nursing as assisting the sick and well individual to perform those activities contributing to health, recovery of health, or peaceful death. Figure 5–1 also identifies nursing as assisting individuals in becoming independent as soon as possible in

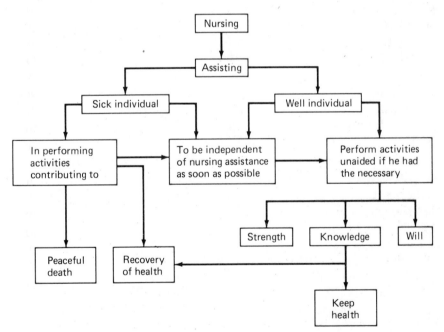

Figure 5–1. Conceptualization of Henderson's definition of nursing. [Modified from Nursing Development Conference Group, *Concept Formalization in Nursing Process and Product* (Boston: Little, Brown & Company, 1973), p. 56. Used with permission.]

the performance of the activities of daily living. Furthermore, to help an individual perform activities unaided, the nurse needs to consider that person's strength, knowledge, and will.

HENDERSON'S THEORY AND THE FOUR MAJOR CONCEPTS

In viewing the concept of the human or individual, Henderson considers the biological, psychological, sociological, and spiritual components. Her first nine components of basic nursing care reflect the physiological aspect, the tenth and fourteenth components speak to the psychological aspect of communicating and learning, the eleventh component reflects the spiritual aspect of religion and morals, and the twelfth and thirteenth components relate to the sociological aspect of occupation and recreation. She refers to humans as having basic needs that are reflected in the fourteen components. However, she goes on to state, "It is equally important to realize that these needs are satisfied by infinitely varied patterns of living, no two of which are alike.[17] Henderson also believes that mind and body are inseparable.[18] The mind and body are interrelated, and the effects of one part are reflected in the other part.

Henderson does not emphasize the concept of society/environment. In her writing she discusses primarily individuals. She looks at them in relation to their families but does not discuss much about the community or the impact the community has on the individual and the family. Her student pediatric affiliation and her experience with the Visiting Nurses agency increased her concern for people. In the textbook she wrote with Harmer, she discusses the tasks of private and public agencies in keeping people healthy.[19] She believes that society wants and expects the nurse's service of acting for the individual who is unable to function independently.[20] She also believes that

> the nurse needs the kind of education that, in our society, is only available in colleges and universities. Training programs operated on funds pinched from the budgets of service agencies cannot provide the preparation the nurse needs.[21]

This generalized education gives the nurse a better understanding of the people receiving nursing care and the various factors that influence people.

Henderson's beliefs about health are related to human functioning. Her definition of health is based on the individual's ability to function independently in relation to the fourteen components. Because good health is a challenging goal for individuals, she believes it is difficult for the nurse to help the individual reach it.[22] She also refers to the fact the nurses tend to stress promotion of health and prevention and cure of disease.[23] Henderson explains how the factors of "age, cultural background, physical and intellectual capacities, and emotional balance affect one's health."[24] These conditions are always present and affect basic needs.

Henderson's view of the concept of nursing is interesting from the time perspective of her writings. She believes nurses need a liberalized education to gain knowledge about the sciences, social sciences, and humanities. The nurse's practice is based on Henderson's definition of nursing, her fourteen components of basic nursing care, and carrying out the physician's therapeutic plan. The creative implementation of nursing care makes the care individualized. It is the nurse's responsibility to improve patient care through nursing research.

> The nurse who operates under a definition that specifies an area of independent practice, or an area of expertness, must assume responsibility for identifying problems, for continually validating her function, for improving the methods she uses, and for measuring the effect of nursing care. In this era research is the name we attach to the most reliable type of analysis.[25]

For Henderson, the nurse must be knowledgeable, have a theoretical base for practicing individualized and humane care, and be a scientific problem solver.

HENDERSON AND THE NURSING PROCESS

Henderson viewed the nursing process as "really the application of the logical approach to the solution to a problem. The steps are those of the scientific method."[26] With this approach, each person can receive individualized care. Likewise, with the nursing process, individualized care is the outcome.

Even though Henderson's definition and explanation of nursing do not directly fit with the steps of the nursing process, a relationship between the two can be demonstrated. Although Henderson does not refer directly to assessment, she implies it in her description of the fourteen components of basic nursing care. The nurse uses the fourteen components to assess the needs of the individual. For example, in assessing the first component, "breathe normally," the nurse would gather all pertinent data about the person's respiratory status. After the first component was assessed, the nurse would move to the next component and gather data in relation to that component. The gathering of data about the person continues until all components are assessed.

To complete the assessment phase of the nursing process, the nurse needs to analyze the data. According to Henderson, the nurse must have knowledge about what is normal in health and disease. Using this knowledge base, then, the nurse would compare the assessment data with what was known about that area. For example, if respirations were observed to be 40/minute in an adult aged forty, the nurse would conclude that this person's respiration rate is faster than normal. Or if a laboratory report showed that the urine was highly concentrated, the nurse would know, "This means that the patient's fluid intake is inadequate, unless he is losing body fluids by other routes."[27] With a scientific knowledge base, the nurse can make some sense from the assessment date. Henderson states,

> The nursing needed by the individual is affected by age, cultural background, emotional balance and his physical and intellectual capacities. All of these should be considered in the nurse's evaluation of the patient's needs for her help.[28]

Following the analysis of the data according to these factors, the nurse then determines the nursing diagnosis. Henderson does not specifically discuss nursing diagnoses. She believes the physician makes the diagnosis, and the nurse acts upon that diagnosis. However, if one looks at Henderson's definition, it can be seen that the nursing diagnosis would deal with identifying the individual's ability to meet human needs with or without assistance, taking into consideration that person's strength, will, and knowledge. Based on the assessment data and the analysis of that data, the nurse can identify actual problems such as abnormal respirations. In addition, potential problems may be identified. For example, in looking at component 11, which deals with one's faith, a potential problem could develop because of hospitalization and a change in the person's normal activities of daily living. If, based on the nurse's assessment and analysis of the data, a person was unable to meet this need, then a nursing diagnosis regarding an actual problem would be made.

Once the nursing diagnosis is made, the nurse proceeds to the planning phase of the nursing process. When discussing the planning phase of nursing care, Henderson states:

> All effective nursing care is planned to some extent. A written plan forces those who make it to give some thought to the individual's needs—unless the person's regimen is made to fit into the routines of the institution in which he may be.[29]

She also contends that the making of a plan for a person going home, known as *discharge planning,* is influenced by the other members of the family.[30] Furthermore, she stresses that plans need to have continuing modification, based on the individual's need. Henderson believes the nursing care plan should be written so others giving nursing care can follow the planned sequence.[31] She also emphasizes that "nursing care is always arranged around, or fitted into, the physician's therapeutic plan."[32] According to Henderson, the planning phase involves making the plan fit the individual's needs, up-dating the plan as necessary based on those needs, making the plan specific so others can implement it, and making sure it fits with the physician's prescribed plan. When writing the plan so others can implement it, the nurse is, in effect, identifying the nursing care needs of the person. Thus, even though Henderson does not apply the terminology used today regarding nursing plans, she uses the same ideas.

Once the nursing care is planned, it can then be implemented. Henderson directly refers to the concept of nursing implementation. She states:

> The modification of care is the creative element which makes nursing an art. The basic technique, or elements of an art, can be described but an artistic achievement demands that the artist manipulate these elements in a unique arrangement. Just so each patient's plan of care should be different from any other.[33]

In giving this creative care, the nurse is assisting the individual to perform activities of daily living as independently as possible. The nursing care is based on physiological principles, age, cultural background, emotional balance, and physical and intellectual capacities. Henderson also states, "This primary function of the practicing nurse, of course, must be performed in such a way that it promotes the physician's therapeutic plan."[34] In other words, the nurse needs to carry out the physician's orders of treatment.

Another important aspect of implementation that Henderson discusses is the relationship between nurse and patient. The nurse "gets inside his skin" to better understand the patient's needs and carry out measures to meet those needs.[35] Henderson also speaks about the quality of nusing care:

> The quality of care is drastically affected by the preparation and native ability of the nursing personnel whether they are giving one, two, three, four, or five hours of care. Standards for "basic nursing" must therefore attempt to include at least some guiding statements on the conditions that demand more and those that demand less attention from highly qualified nurses, also to identify the aspects of care that require more or less nursing competence. The danger of turning over the physical care of the patient to relatively unqualified nurses is twofold. They may fail to assess the patient's needs adequately but, perhaps more important, the qualified nurse, being deprived the opportunity while giving physical care to assess needs, may not find any other chance to do so. In this connection it should also be pointed out that it is easier for any person to develop an emotional supportive role with another if he can perform a tangible service.[36]

This statement clearly supports that the competent nurse utilizes both the interpersonal process and assessment while giving care.

The nursing implementation is based on helping the patient meet the fourteen components. For example, in helping the individual with the sleep and rest component, the nurse tries the known methods of inducing rest and sleep before giving sleeping medication. In *The Nature of Nursing*, Henderson summarizes, "I see nursing as primarily complementing the patient by supplying what he needs in knowledge, will or strength to perform his daily activities and to carry out the treatment prescribed for him by the physician."[37]

Henderson bases the evaluation of each person "according to the speed with which, or the degree to which, he performs independently the activities that make, for him, a normal day."[38] This goes back to the definition that outlines the unique function of the nurse. For evaluation purposes, changes in a person's level of functioning need to be observed and recorded. Therefore, during the initial interaction, the nurse would determine how independently a person was performing the activities listed in the fourteen components of basic nursing care. Then the nurse would compare that data to how independently the person was functioning after the nursing care plan was implemented. All changes would be utilized for the evaluation.

To summarize the stages of the nursing process as applied to Henderson's definition of nursing and to the fourteen components of basic nursing care, refer to Table 5-1.

To further illustrate the use of Henderson's fourteen components, a case study (Mr. L.) is presented in Table 5-2. Using the components as a guide, a sample nursing process is displayed. The nursing process presented demonstrates a limited example and is not intended to be an ultimate or finished process.

HENDERSON'S WORK AND THE CHARACTERISTICS OF A THEORY

Henderson wrote her definition of nursing prior to the development of concepts and theories about nursing. Her intent was to identify the specific functions the nurse performs rather than to describe the theoretical basis for nursing practice. However, in looking at the characteristics of a theory discussed in Chapter 1, some of Henderson's work can be applied.

The first characteristic of a theory is that it interrelates concepts in such a way as to create a different way of looking at a particular phenomenon. Henderson incorporates the concepts of fundamental human needs, biophysiology, culture, and interaction-communication. Maslow's hierarchy of human needs fits well with the fourteen basic components.[39] The first nine components are physiological and safety needs. The remaining five components deal with the love and belonging, social esteem and self-actualization needs. Henderson uses the biophysiology concept when she stresses the importance of physiology and physiological balances in making decisions about nursing care. The concept of culture as it affects human needs is learned from the family and other social groups. Because of this, Henderson suggests that a nurse is unable to fully interpret or supply all the requirements for the individual's well-being. At best the nurse can merely assist the individual in meeting human needs.

Table 5-1

A Summary of the Nursing Process
and of Henderson's Fourteen Components
and Definition of Nursing

Nursing Process	Henderson's Fourteen Components and Definition of Nursing
Nursing assessment	Assess needs of human being based on the fourteen components of basic nursing care:

1. Breathing normally	8. Keep body clean and well-groomed
2. Eat and drink adequately	9. Avoid dangers in environment
3. Elimination of body wastes	10. Communication
4. Move and maintain posture	11. Worship according to one's faith
5. Sleep and rest	12. Work accomplishment
6. Suitable clothing dress/undress	13. Recreation
7. Maintain body temperature	14. Learn, discover, or satisfy curiosity

Nursing Process	Henderson's Fourteen Components and Definition of Nursing
	Analysis: Compare data to knowledge base of health and disease.
Nursing diagnosis	Identify individual's ability to meet own needs with or without assistance, taking into consideration strength, will, or knowledge.
Nursing plan	Document how the nurse can assist the individual, sick or well.
Nursing implementation	Assist the sick or well individual in the performance of activities in meeting human needs to maintain health, recover from illness, or to aid in peaceful death. Intervention based on physiological principles, age, cultural background, emotional balance, and physical and intellectual capacities. Carry out treatment prescribed by the physician.
Nursing evaluation	Utilize the acceptable definition of nursing and appropriate laws related to the practice of nursing. The quality of care is drastically affected by the preparation and native ability of the nursing personnel rather than the amount of hours of care. Successful outcomes of nursing care are based on the speed with which or degree to which the patient performs independently the activities of daily living.

Table 5-2

The Nursing Process for Mr. L.
Using Henderson's Fourteen Components

Case study: Mr. L. is 25 years old, married, and the father of two preschool-age children. His wife is 6 months pregnant. Mr. L. quit school in the 10th grade. He works 16 hours a day as a skilled laborer in a factory and holds a second job washing dishes at a restaurant to meet the family expenses.

Nursing Process	*Data and Relevant Information*
Assessment	**Assessment**
(Assess needs of Mr. L. based on the 14 components of basic nursing care)	
1. Breathing normally.	1. Respiration rate—18, regular; smokes 2 packs of cigarettes/day; dry cough in A.M.; no shortness of breath. (Data about work environment needed.)
2. Eat and drink adequately.	2. Takes sandwich, fruit, potato chips for lunch; skips breakfast; buys soft drink; eats evening meals at the restaurant. (Results of 72-hour diet recall needed.)
3. Elimination of body wastes.	3. Reports no problems related to elimination.
4. Move and maintain posture.	4. Reports pain in both legs after 8 hours of washing dishes. No problems with mobility.
5. Sleep and rest.	5. Reports 5–6 hours sleep/night. "Feels tired most of the time."
6. Suitable clothing dress/undress.	6. Wears jeans and shirt to work—both jobs. Owns ski jacket and boots for cold weather wear. (Work environment data needed.)
7. Maintain body temperature.	7. Temperature 98.6 F. Reports no problem with being hot or cold.
8. Keep body clean and well-groomed.	8. Showers and shampoos hair daily.
9. Avoid environment hazards.	9. Wears clothes to match weather conditions. (Home environment safety—need more data.)
10. Communication.	10. Able to speak to be understood. (Communication with family—need further data.)
11. Worship according to faith.	11. Attends church (Baptist) with family every other Sunday.
12. Work accomplishment.	12. Reports happy with jobs.
13. Recreation	13. "Need more time to spend with family."
14. Learn, discover, or satisfy curiosity.	14. Reports interested in finishing high school. Plans to pursue college education.

Table 5–2 *(continued)*

Nursing Process	Data and Relevant Information
Analysis	According to Erikson's developmental stage theory,[a] Mr. L. is in the intimacy stage. He is able to support his family and take care of most of their needs, except for recreational needs. Physiologically, Mr. L. is functioning within the normal range. Three concerns are: the amount of cigarettes he smokes, pains in his legs, and the inadequate sleep and rest pattern. Mr. L. plans for the future to upgrade his education and to seek better employment.
Nursing diagnosis	1. Inadequate sleep and rest pattern resulting in feeling tired and no time to spend with family. 2. Lack of knowledge regarding cigarette smoking resulting in potential health hazard. 3. Discomfort in legs resulting from standing 8 hours on the job.
Nursing plan	1. Explore with Mr. L. and wife: a. Alternatives to working two jobs. b. Adjust schedule to include recreation with family. 2. Determine information Mr. L. has re smoking and its hazards. 3. Formulate isometric exercises for leg pains.
Nursing implementation	Assist Mr. L. in the performance of activities in meeting his human needs to maintain health. Intervention based on physiological principles, age, cultural background, emotional balance, and physical and intellectual capacities.
Nursing evaluation	Success of the nurse based on speed with which or degree to which Mr. L. is able to carry out the activities selected.

[a]Erik H. Erikson, *Childhood and Society*, 2nd ed. (New York: W. W. Norton & Co., Inc., 1963), pp.247–74.

Finally, the concept of interaction-communication can be seen. Henderson states the nurse must be sensitive to nonverbal communication and must encourage the expression of feelings.[40] The natural development of a constructive nurse-patient relationship is important in the validation of patient needs. Henderson uses several concepts in her definition of nursing and all fourteen components to describe the particular phenomenon called *nursing*. Each of the concepts shows an interrelationship that describes and explains nursing as it is viewed by Henderson. Thus she created a new way of understanding the relationships of several concepts in her definition of nursing.

Just as theories must be logical in nature (characteristic 2), so are Henderson's definition and components. According to Henderson, the nurse assists the individual to perform those activities contributing to health, its recovery, or peaceful death and encourages independence as quickly as possible. The fourteen components provide a list for the individual and nurse to use in reaching that goal. The components start with physiological functioning and move to the psychosocial functioning.

Henderson's work is relatively simple yet generalizable (characteristic 3). Her work can be applied to the health of all individuals regardless of age. Nurses functioning at different levels can utilize Henderson's definition and components in their practice.

If Henderson's definition of nursing and the fourteen components can be viewed as a theory, it is possible to generate hypotheses that can be tested (characteristic 4). Some examples may be:

1. Do nurses in their practice follow the sequence of the fourteen components as outlined?
2. Are basic human functions taken for granted except in emergency situations where life support is a priority?
3. Do nurses give care to presenting problems initially and then move on to other unique functions?
4. What clinical specialty areas of nursing practice include or exclude components ten through fourteen?

Henderson supports hypothesis testing and states that she hopes hypotheses selected by researchers are worth being tested and that the findings can be used to improve practice rather than simply for academic respectability.[41]

Another characteristic of a theory is whether it serves to increase the general body of knowledge within the discipline (characteristic 5). Since Henderson's ideas of nursing practice are well accepted throughout the world as a basis for nursing care, the extent and impact of the definition and the components may be elicited through research. Well-designed research could assist in determining Henderson's contribution to the knowledge of what nurses worldwide believe about nursing practice. Such research would help validate Henderson's beliefs about the unique function of nursing. Such a project may be an appropriate undertaking for the International Council of Nurses.

Consistent with a theory, nurses can use the definition and fourteen components of basic nursing care to guide and improve their practice (characteristic 6). Ideally, the nurse would improve nursing practice by using Henderson's definition and the fourteen components to improve the health of individuals and, thus, reduce illness. The final outcome would be increased health promotion and maintenance or peaceful death.

Finally, there is potential for the comparison of Henderson's definition and components with validated theories, laws, and principles (characteristic 7). The concepts of fundamental human needs, biophysiology, culture, and interaction-communication as they apply to nursing practice are being investigated by many nurse researchers as well as by those in other professional health and social science disciplines. Although the research topics may not be specifically related to Henderson's interpretation of the concepts, they are validating the basis of her work as well as seeking answers to human problems that affect nursing practice. Henderson is an avid supporter of nursing research and would welcome the validation of her ideas of the unique function of nursing. She believes nursing must accept the responsibility to conduct research to investigate problems specifically related to the practice of nursing.

LIMITATIONS

Although Henderson based her ideas about nursing care on the fundamental human needs and the physical and emotional aspects of the individual, the concept of the holistic nature of human beings does not clearly emerge in her publications. For example, the fact that a person's oxygenation needs will have an effect on the other remaining components of basic nursing care is unclear. Also, if the assumption is made that the fourteen components are prioritized, it is of significance to note there is an interrelationship among the components since each component does affect the next one on the list. If priority according to individual needs is implied in the listing of the components, does the presenting emotional problem take a back seat to physical care, and is this area of care deferred until such time the physiological need areas are given proper attention? Henderson specifies that the nurse must consider such factors as age, temperament, social or cultural status, and physical and intellectual capacity in the use of the components, thus emphasizing differences in the individual but not necessarily the interrelationship of these factors. However, the reader must keep in mind Henderson wrote her ideas about nursing before the emergence of the concept of holism. She has since stated her belief in a holistic approach to the client.[42]

The fact that the majority of the fourteen components are focused on the physiological needs gives the impression that nursing care considerations are more on the physical than the psychosocial needs. This is not to say that there must be a balance, but a misunderstanding that nursing care emphasis is more on the physical aspects than on the psychosocial aspects may be a possible conclusion.

In assisting the individual in the dying process, Henderson acknowledges that the nurse helps, but there is little explanation as to what is done in this area. In her statement of the definition of nursing, the placing of a parenthesis around the words *peaceful death* brings questions as to why this was done.

CONCLUSIONS

The concept of nursing presented by Henderson in her definition of nursing and the fourteen components is self-explanatory. Therefore, it could be used as a guide by most without difficulty. Many of Henderson's thoughts and ideas continue to be useful today. This can be validated by the demand of her ICN publication, which in 1972 was in its seventh printing.

If a suggestion to improve Henderson's concept of nursing can be made, the incorporation of holism and system theory might provide a more complete explanation of the relationship of the components. Also confirmation of the priority listing of the components is needed to clarify what the nurse is to do if the presenting problem is other than a physical one.

When one considers the time in which Henderson wrote about her ideas and beliefs about nursing, she deserves much credit as one of the pioneers giving direction to the development of nursing theories.

SUMMARY

Henderson states,

> I believe that the function the nurse performs is primarily an independent one—that of acting for the patient when he lacks knowledge, physical strength, or the will to act for himself as he would ordinarily act in health, or in carrying our prescribed therapy. The function is seen as complex and creative, as offering unlimited opportunity for the application of the physical, biological, and social sciences, and the development of skills based on them.[43]

The fourteen components of basic nursing are viewed by Henderson as the unique function of the nurse. This together with her definition of nursing provides the basis for nursing practice.

NOTES

1. Virginia Henderson, *The Nature of Nursing* (New York: Macmillan Publishing Co., Inc., 1966); idem, *Basic Principles of Nursing Care* (Geneva: International Council of Nurses, 1972).
2. Virginia Henderson, "Preserving the Essence of Nursing in a Technological Age, Part I," *Nursing Times*, 75 (November 22, 1979), 2012–13; idem, "Preserving the Essence of Nursing in a Technological Age, Part II," *Nursing Times*, 75 (November 29, 1979), 2056–58; and idem, "The Concept of Nursing," *Journal of Advanced Nursing*, 3 (1978), 16–17.
3. Henderson, *The Nature of Nursing*, p. 1.
4. Ibid., p. 6
5. Ibid., p. 7.
6. Bertha Harmer and Virginia Henderson, *Textbook of the Principles and Practice of Nursing*, 4th ed. (New York: Macmillan Publishing Co.,

Inc., 1939); Gwendolyn Safier, *Contemporary American Leaders in Nursing* (New York: McGraw-Hill Book Company, 1977), p. 119.

7. Henderson, *The Nature of Nursing*, p. 3.

8. "ANA Statement on Auxiliary Personnel in Nursing Service," *The American Journal of Nursing*, 62, no. 7 (1962).

9. Bertha Harmer and Virginia Henderson, *Textbook of the Principles and Practice of Nursing*, 5th ed. (New York: Macmillan Publishing Co., Inc., 1955), p. 4; and Nursing Development Conference Group, *Concept Formalization in Nursing: Process and Product* (Boston: Little, Brown & Co., 1973), pp. 41–42.

10. Bertha Harmer, *Textbook of the Principles and Practice of Nursing* (New York: Macmillan Publishing Co., Inc., 1922), p. 3; Nursing Development Conference Group, *Concept Formalization in Nursing: Process and Product* (Boston: Little, Brown & Company, 1973), p. 40.

11. Henderson, *The Nature of Nursing*, pp. 16–17.

12. Ibid., p. 15.

13. Ibid.

14. Ibid., p. 16.

15. Henderson, *Basic Principles*, p. 3.

16. Henderson, "The Concept of Nursing," pp. 16–17.

17. Henderson, *Basic Principles*, p. 7.

18. Henderson, *The Nature of Nursing*, p. 11.

19. Harmer and Henderson, *Textbook of the Principles*, 5th ed., p. 33.

20. Henderson, *The Nature of Nursing*, p. 68.

21. Ibid. p. 69.

22. Henderson, *Basic Principles*, p. 5.

23. Henderson, *The Nature of Nursing*, pp. 21–22.

24. Henderson, *Basic Principles*, p. 10.

25. Ibid., p. 38.

26. Virginia Henderson, "Nursing—Yesterday and Tomorrow," *Nursing Times*, 76 (May 22, 1980), 905–7.

27. Henderson, *Basic Principles*, p. 25.

28. Ibid., p. 10.

29. Ibid., p. 14.

30. Ibid.

31. Ibid.

32. Ibid., p. 15.

33. Ibid., p. 14.

34. Henderson, *The Nature of Nursing*, p. 27.

35. Ibid., p. 24.

36. Henderson, *Basic Principles*, p.13.

37. Henderson, *The Nature of Nursing*, p. 21.

38. Ibid., p. 30.

39. Abraham Maslow, *Motivation and Personality* (New York: Harper & Row, Publishers, Inc., 1954).
40. Henderson, *The Nature of Nursing*, p. 14.
41. Virginia Henderson, "We've Come a Long Way But What of the Direction?" *Nursing Research*, 26 (May-June 1977), 163–64.
42. Virginia Henderson, speech at History of Nursing Museum, Philadelphia, May 1982.
43. Henderson, *The Nature of Nursing*, p. 68.

ADDITIONAL REFERENCE

HENDERSON, VIRGINIA, and others, *Reference Resource for Research and Continuing Education in Nursing.* Kansas City, Mo.: American Nurses' Association Publication No. 6125, 1977.

6

ERNESTINE WIEDENBACH

Agnes M. Bennett and Peggy Coldwell Foster

Ernestine Wiedenbach, a 1922 graduate of Wellesley College, Wellesley, Massachusetts, received her nursing diploma from the Johns Hopkins School of Nursing, Baltimore, Maryland in 1925. Her Master's degree is from Teachers College, Columbia University, New York, in 1934. She also obtained a certificate in nurse midwifery from the Maternity Center Association in New York in 1946. She has practiced as a nurse midwife and a public health nurse and has taught in a number of schools of nursing. She is an Associate Professor Emeritus from Yale University School of Nursing.

According to Ernestine Wiedenbach, nursing is nurturing and caring for someone in a motherly fashion. That care is given in the immediate present and can be given by any caring person.[1] Nursing is a helping service that is rendered with compassion, skill, and understanding to those in need of care, counsel, and confidence in the area of health.[2]

Nursing wisdom is acquired through meaningful experience. Sensitivity alerts the nurse to an awareness of inconsistencies in a situation that might signify a problem. It is a key factor in assisting the nurse to identify the patient's* need for help.[3]

The nurse's beliefs and values regarding the significance of life, the worth of the individual, and the aspirations of each human being determine the quality of nursing care. The nurse's purpose in nursing represents a professional commitment.[4]

Wiedenbach states that the characteristics of a professional person that are essential for the professional nurse include: (1) *clarity* of purpose, (2) *mastery* of skills and knowledge essential for fulfilling her purpose, (3) *ability* to establish and sustain purposeful working relationships with others in the health care field, (4) *interest* in advancing knowledge in her area of interest and in researching new knowledge, and (5) *dedication* to furthering the good of man.[5]

The practice of nursing comprises a wide variety of services, each directed toward the attainment of one of its three components: (1) *identification* of the patient's need for help, (2) *ministration* of the help needed, and (3) *validation* that the help provided was indeed helpful to the patient.[6]

WIEDENBACH'S PRESCRIPTIVE THEORY

After her work with J. Dickoff and P. James in the late 1960s in which they jointly presented a symposium on "Theory in a Practice Discipline,"[7] Wiedenbach began to develop her own theory of nursing.

Theory may be described as a system of conceptualizations invented to some purpose. Prescriptive theory (a situation-producing theory) may be described as one that conceptualizes both a desired situation and the prescription by which it is to be brought about. Thus, a prescriptive theory directs action toward an explicit goal.[8] Wiedenbach's prescriptive theory is made up of three factors:[9]

1. The *central purpose*, which the practitioner recognizes as essential to the particular discipline.
2. The *prescription* for the fulfillment of the central purpose.
3. The *realities in the immediate situation* that influence the fulfillment of the central purpose. See Figure 6–1.

*Wiedenbach consistently uses the term *patient* and refers to the nurse as *her* in all her writings. This approach will be used in this chapter.

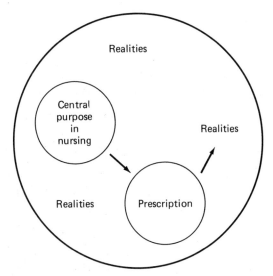

Figure 6-1. Wiedenbach's prescriptive theory. [Adapted from Ernestine Wiedenbach, *Meeting the Realities in Clinical Teaching* (New York: Springer Publishing Co., Inc., 1969), p. x.]

The Central Purpose

"The nurse's central purpose defines the quality of health she desires to effect or sustain in her patient and specifies what she recognizes to be her special responsibility in caring for him."[10] This central purpose (or commitment) is based on the individual nurse's philosophy. Wiedenbach states:

> Purpose and philosophy are, respectively, goal and guide of clinical nursing. Purpose—that which the nurse wants to accomplish through what she does—is the overall goal toward which she is striving, and so is constant. It is the nurse's reason for being and doing. . . . Philosophy, an attitude toward life and reality that evolves from each nurse's beliefs and code of conduct, motivates the nurse to act, guides her thinking about what she is to do, and influences her decisions. It stems from both her culture and subculture and is an integral part of her. It is personal in character, unique to each nurse, and expressed in her way of nursing. Philosophy underlies purpose, and purpose reflects philosophy.[11]

Wiedenbach identifies three essential components for a nursing philosophy: (1) a reverence for the gift of life, (2) a respect for the dignity, worth, autonomy, and individuality of each human being, and (3) a resolution to act dynamically in relation to one's beliefs.[12] Any of these concepts might be further developed. However, Wiedenbach emphasizes the second in her work.

Wiedenbach formulated the following beliefs about the individual:[13]

1. Each human being is endowed with unique potential to develop within himself the resources that enable him to maintain and sustain himself.
2. The human being basically strives toward self-direction and relative independence, and desires not only to make the best use of his capabilities and potentialities but to fulfill his responsibilities as well.
3. The human being needs stimulation in order to make the best use of his capabilities and realize his self-worth.
4. Whatever the individual does represents his best judgment at the moment of doing it.

Thus, the central purpose is a concept the nurse has thought through—one she has put into words, believes in, and accepts as a standard against which to measure the value of her action to the patient. It is based on her philosophy and suggests the nurse's reason for being, the mission she believes is hers to accomplish.[14]

The Prescription

Once the nurse has identified her own philosophy and recognizes that the patient has autonomy and individuality, she can work *with* the individual to develop a *prescription* or plan for his care.

A *prescription* is a directive to activity.[15] It specifies both the *nature of the action* that will most likely lead to fulfillment of the nurse's central purpose and the *thinking process* that determines it.[16] A prescription may indicate the broad general action appropriate to implementation of the basic concepts as well as suggest the kind of behavior needed to carry out these actions in accordance with the central purpose. These actions may be voluntary or involuntary. Voluntary action is an intended response, whereas involuntary action is an unintended response.[17]

A prescription is a directive to at least three kinds of voluntary action: (1) *mutually understood and agreed upon* action (the practitioner has evidence that the recipient understands the implications of the intended action and is psychologically and/or physiologically receptive to it); (2) *recipient-directed* action (the recipient of the action essentially directs the way it is to be carried out); and (3) *practitioner-directed* action (the practitioner carries out the action).[18] Once the nurse has formulated a central purpose and has accepted it as a personal commitment, she not only has established the prescription for her nursing but is ready to implement it.[19]

The Realities

When the nurse has determined her central purpose and has developed the prescription, she must then consider the *realities* of the situation in which she is to provide nursing care. Realities consist of all factors—physical, physiological, psychological, emotional, and spiritual—that are at play in a situation in which nursing actions occur at any given moment.[20] Wiedenbach defines the five realities as: (1) the agent, (2) the recipient, (3) the goal, (4) the means, and (5) the framework.

The *agent* who is the practicing nurse or her delegate is characterized by personal attributes, capacities, capabilities, and most importantly, commitment and competence in nursing. As the agent, the nurse is the propelling force that moves her practice toward its goal. In the course of this goal-directed movement, she may engage in innumerable acts called forth by her encounter with actual or discrepant factors and/or situations within the realities of which she herself is a part.[21]

The agent or nurse has four basic responsibilities:[22]

1. To reconcile her assumptions about the realities with her central purpose.
2. To specify objectives of practice in terms of behavioral outcomes that are realistically attainable.
3. To practice nursing in accordance with her objectives.
4. To engage in related activities which contribute to her self-realization and to the improvement of nursing practice.

The *recipient* is the patient who is characterized by personal attributes, problems, capacities, aspirations, and most importantly, the ability to cope with the concerns or problems being experienced. He is the recipient of the nurse's actions or the one on whose behalf the action is taken. The patient is vulnerable. He is dependent on others for help and risks losing his individuality, dignity, worth, and autonomy.[23]

The *goal* is the desired outcome the nurse wishes to achieve. The goal is the end result to be attained by nursing action. The stipulation of an activity's goal gives focus to the nurse's action and implies her reason for taking it.[24]

The *means* comprise the activities and devices through which the practitioner is enabled to attain her goal. The means include skills, techniques, procedures, and devices that may be used to facilitate nursing practice. The nurse's way of giving treatments, of expressing concern, of using the means available is individual and is determined by her central purpose and the prescription.[25]

The *framework* consists of the human, environmental, professional, and organizational facilities that not only make up the context within which nursing is practiced but also constitute its currently existing limits. The framework is composed of all the extraneous factors and facilities in the situation that affect the nurse's ability to obtain the desired results. It is a conglomerate of objects existing or missing, policies, setting, atmosphere, time of day, humans, and happenings that may be current, past, or anticipated.[26]

The realities offer uniqueness to every situation. The success of professional nursing practice is dependent on them. Unless the realities are recognized and are dealt with, they may prevent the achievement of the goal.

Central purpose, prescription, and realities (components of prescriptive theory) are interdependent on one another as depicted in Figure 6–1. The prescription is derived by the nurse from her central purpose and is affected by the realities of the situation. The nurse develops a prescription based on her central purpose, which is implemented in the realities of the situation. Together these components constitute the substance of Wiedenbach's prescriptive theory. This theory when articulated serves as the guiding light of professional practice.[27]

WIEDENBACH'S
CONCEPTUALIZATION OF NURSING
PRACTICE AND PROCESS

According to Wiedenbach, nursing practice is an art in which the nursing action is based on the principle of helping. Nursing action may be thought of as consisting of four distinct kinds of actions:[28]

1. Reflex   (spontaneous)
2. Conditioned (automatic)
3. Impulsive   (impulsive)
4. Deliberate   (responsible)

Nursing as a practice discipline is goal-directed. The nature of the nursing act is based on thought. The nurse thinks through the kind of results she wants, gears her actions to obtain those results, then accepts responsibility for the acts and the outcome of those acts.[29] Since nursing requires thought, it can be considered a deliberate responsible action.

Nursing practice has three components: (1) identification of the patient's need for help; (2) ministration of the help needed, and (3) validation that the action taken was helpful to the patient.[30] Within the identification component, there are four distinct steps. First, the nurse observes the patient. She looks for an inconsistency between the expected behavior of the patient and the apparent behavior. Second, she attempts to clarify what the inconsistency means. Third, she determines the cause of the discomfort that she has ascertained the patient is experiencing. Finally, she validates with the patient that her help is needed.

The second component is the ministration of the help needed. In ministering to her patient, the nurse may give advice or information, make a referral, apply a comfort measure, or carry out a therapeutic procedure. Should the patient become uncomfortable with what is being done, the nurse will need to identify the cause and, if necessary, make an adjustment in the plan of action.

The third component is validation. After help has been ministered, the nurse validates that the actions were, indeed, helpful. Evidence must come from the patient that the purpose of the nursing actions has been fulfilled.[31]

Wiedenbach views the nursing process essentially as an internal personalized mechanism. As such, it is influenced by the nurse's culture, purpose in nursing, knowledge, wisdom, sensitivity, and concern.[32]

In Wiedenbach's nursing process (see Figure 6-2), she identifies seven levels of awareness: sensation, perception, assumption, realization, insight, design, and decision.[33] Her nursing process begins with an activating situation. This situation exists among the realities and serves as a stimulus to arouse the nurse's consciousness. This consciousness leads to a subjective interpretation of the first three levels, which are defined as: *sensation* (experienced sensory impression), *perception* (the interpretation of a sensory impression), and *assumption* (the meaning the nurse attaches to the perception). These three levels of awareness are obtained through the focus of the nurse's attention on the stimulus; they are intuitive rather than cognitive and may initiate an involuntary response.

For example, a nurse enters a patient's room and states, "My, it's hot in here!" She immediately goes to the window and opens it. The *sensation* is: the room temperature. The *perception* is: "It feels hot." The *assumption* is: "If I am hot, then the patient must be hot." The involuntary response is to open the window.

Progressing from intuition to cognition, the nurse's actions become voluntary rather than involuntary. The next four levels of awareness occur in the voluntary phase. These are: *realization* (in which the nurse begins to validate the assumption previously made about the patient's behavior); *insight* (which includes joint planning and additional knowledge about the cause of the problem); *design* (the plan of action decided upon by the nurse and confirmed by the patient); and *decision* (the nurse's performance of a responsible action.[34]

To continue with the previous example: The nurse asks, "Are you too warm?" and the patient replies, "No, I'm not. I have felt cold since I washed my hair." The nurse responds, "I will close the window and get you a blanket." The patient agrees, "That would be fine." The nurse shuts the window and gets a blanket for the patient.

The *realization* is: the validation of the patient's perception of warmth. The *insight* is: the additional information that the patient had washed his hair. The *design* is: the plan to close the window and get a blanket as confirmed by the patient. The *decision* is: the nurse shuts the window and gets a blanket for the patient.

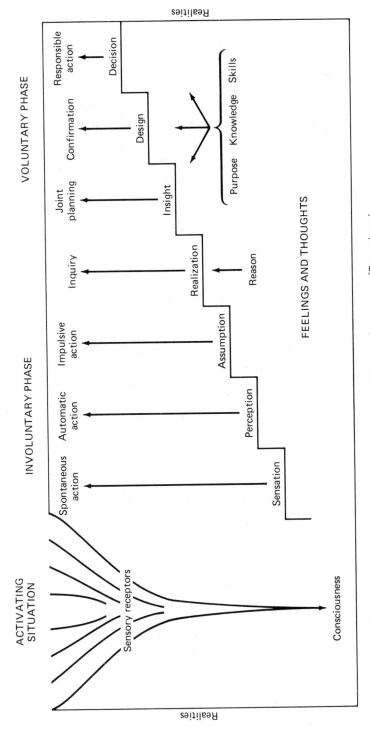

Figure 6-2. Conceptualization of the nursing process. [Reproduced from Joy P. Clausen and others, *Maternity Nursing Today* (New York: McGraw-Hill Book Company, 1977), p. 43.]

WEIDENBACH'S THEORY AND THE
FOUR MAJOR CONCEPTS

Weidenbach emphasizes that the human or *individual* possesses unique potential, strives toward self-direction, and needs stimulation. Whatever the individual does represents his best judgment at that moment. She believes these characteristics require respect from the nurse.[35]

Wiedenbach does not define the concept of *health*. However, she supports the World Health Organization's definition of health as a state of complete physical, mental, and social well-being and not merely the absence of disease and infirmity.[36]

The third concept concerns the *environment*. In Wiedenbach's work she refers to the nurse giving care to an individual patient wherever that contact between the health professional and patient may occur. She also identifies the environment as a component of the realities in which that care is given.

The fourth concept, *nursing*, is the application of knowledge and skill toward meeting a need for help expressed by a patient. Nursing is a helping process with action directed toward providing something the patient requires or desires, a process that will restore or extend the patient's ability to cope with demands implicit in his healthy situation.[37]

COMPARISON OF THE NURSING
PROCESS WITH WIEDENBACH'S
NURSING PROCESS AND NURSING
PRACTICE

The comparison of the nursing process described in Chapter 2 and Wiedenbach's conceptualization of the nursing process and nursing practice yields some similarities and several significant differences (see Table 6–1). In Wiedenbach's nursing process, the steps of (1) observation, (2) ministration of help, and (3) validation are comparable with the nursing process's phases of *assessment, implementation,* and *evaluation.*

Assessment, the first phase of the nursing process, considers the person holistically and requires extensive data collection. In Wiedenbach's model (see Figure 6–3), the nurse is stimulated, then reacts to the stimulus at the levels of sensation or perception. These levels

Table 6-1

Comparison of the Nursing Process with
Wiedenbach's Nursing Process and Nursing
Practice

Nursing Process	Wiedenbach's Nursing Process		Wiedenbach's Nursing Practice
1. Nursing assessment	Stimulus		1. Observation
	Involuntary 1. Sensation 2. Perception 3. Assumption	Voluntary	
1. (a) Analysis and synthesis 2. Nursing Diagnosis		4. Realization with reason —Inquiry	
3. (a) Goals and objectives 3. (b) Plans		5. Insight— Joint planning 6. Design— Confirmation	
4. Implementation with scientific rationale	1. (a) Spontaneous Action 2. (a) Automatic action 3. (a) Impulsive action	7. Decision with responsible action	2. Ministration of help
5. Nursing evaluation			3. Validation

are involuntary and intuitive. The nurse then makes an assumption about the situation and may act involuntarily. Such acts are spontaneous, automatic, or impulsive. They occur on the spur of the moment and are precipitated by unchecked, rampant thoughts and feelings. Occasionally in an emergency they may be lifesaving. However, these involuntary acts can frequently do more harm than good.[38]

If the nurse makes an assumption, she might act impulsively. However, Wiedenbach points out that the nurse needs to willfully apply a strategy brake (see Figure 6-3). This provides time for her

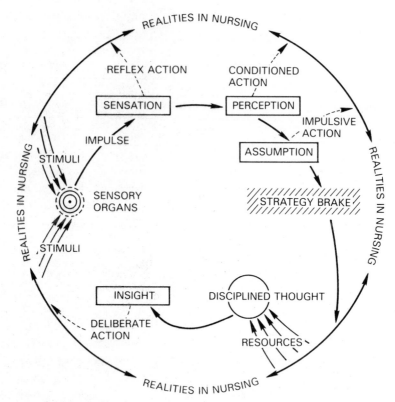

Figure 6-3. Genesis of Nursing Action. Diagrammatic presentation of how an impulse to act originates and how it is converted into action. Broken lines represent overt processes; solid lines represent covert processes. [Reprinted by permission of G.P. Putnam's Sons from *Family-Centered Maternity Nursing*, 2nd edition by Ernestine Wiedenbach. Copyright © 1967 by G.P. Putnam's Sons.]

to assemble the resources necessary for disciplined thought to control her action.[39] This strategy brake then is applied just prior to Wiedenbach's realization level. At the realization level the process becomes voluntary as the nurse uses reason and inquiry.

In the nursing process the assessment phase components of analysis and synthesis require much conscious thought and deliberation about the data before the nurse can make a *nursing diagnosis*. Once the nursing diagnosis has been determined, the nurse sets goals and objectives and *plans* the nursing care. This planning phase can be compared to Wiedenbach's levels of insight and design, which are part of her voluntary phase. The insight level of her model includes joint planning. This joint planning is between the nurse and the patient and does not involve other health care professionals.

Wiedenbach does not directly incorporate the concept of goal as part of the nursing process. However, the nurse's central purpose could be considered a goal.[40] On the design level the nurse plans a course of action. After the plan is decided on, the nurse confirms it with the patient. Once the plan has been decided on and confirmed, the nurse performs the responsible, deliberate nursing action. This level is comparable to the *implementation* phase of the nursing process.

In Wiedenbach's model of the nursing process, she does not identify *evaluation*. However, she does refer to evaluation in her discussion of nursing practice, emphasizing that the nurse needs "validation that the help provided was indeed helpful to the patient."[41]

WIEDENBACH'S WORK AND THE CHARACTERISTICS OF A THEORY

As required by the characteristics of a theory, Wiedenbach's work does interrelate concepts in such a way as to create a different way of looking at a particular phenomenon. She defines and interrelates the concepts of realities and central purpose to devise a prescription for nursing care.

A theory should also be logical in nature. When using Wiedenbach's theory, it is difficult, if not impossible, to follow a logical thought process and predict the outcome of nursing care because the prescription and desired outcome will vary from one nurse to another depending on each nurse's central purpose. However, Wiedenbach identified she was presenting a prescriptive rather than a predictive theory.

Wiedenbach's theory does meet the characteristic of being relatively simple yet generalizable to all of nursing. Although the theory is situation-producing, it is not situation-specific. The situation is produced by the nurse's central purpose and prescription within the existing realities. The situation is not site-oriented and thus could be a hospital, a community setting, a school, or a newborn nursery.

Theories should be able to be used as the bases for testable hypotheses. Theories also should contribute to and assist in increasing the general body of knowledge within the discipline through research implemented to validate them. Although Wiedenbach's theory presents a philosophical approach that has not been tested, hypotheses can be formed. For example: What is the influence of various sets of realities on the outcome with a given central purpose and prescription?

Theories should be able to be utilized by practitioners to guide and improve their practice. Wiedenbach's theory can be used to support, guide, and assist the nurse to fulfill her commitment to nursing. The nurse's commitment to nursing is her central purpose that will influence prescriptions within the situational realities. Thus the nurse whose central purpose is holistic support of the optimal development of the individual will develop prescriptions that deal with a multitude of aspects of the individual rather than focusing solely on the problem that led to initial contact.

Theories should be consistent with other validated theories, laws, and principles but should leave open unanswered questions that need to be investigated. Wiedenbach does not utilize theories or support her theory from other disciplines.

SUMMARY

As a pioneer in nursing, Ernestine Wiedenbach began her nursing career as a staff nurse in the 1920s. Her first nursing textbook was published in 1958.

Wiedenbach's theory for nursing, a prescriptive theory, contains three concepts: *central purpose, prescription,* and *realities.* The interrelationship of these three concepts would be as follows: Within the realities, the nurse develops a prescription for nursing care based on her central purpose. The central purpose is the nurse's philosophy for care; the prescription is the directive to activity; the realities are the matrix in which the action occurs. These concepts are all interdependent.

Wiedenbach's theory is a philosophical, altruistic approach to nursing. The nurse is viewed as a loving, caring individual. The nurse's philosophy about the value and worth of the individual directs her care. Wiedenbach states: "Nursing [is] a service which ideally exemplifies man's humanity to man."[42]

The reader perceives that the nurse acts with a self-sacrificing commitment to nursing. If a nurse values the life and dignity of human beings, then she will provide quality nursing care.

Wiedenbach does not identify what is unique about nursing. She recognizes that nursing is a goal-directed practice discipline. She states that "Although recognized as a humanitarian service, nursing in its entirety is hard to describe, and the nurse's responsibilities are hard to delineate."[43]

Nursing practice, defined by Wiedenbach as observation, ministration of help, and validation, closely correlates with the nursing process. However, Wiedenbach's conceptualization of the nursing process varies greatly from the nursing process presented in Chapter 2 of this text.

Wiedenbach identifies the nursing process as being activated by a stimulus. This stimulus may cause an involuntary response unless the reflexive action is stopped by a strategy brake. This brake allows the nurse to think and reason before performing a voluntary or deliberate nursing action.

Although Wiedenbach's work does not fulfill all the characteristics of a theory, it is innovative within the nursing profession. Her classic writings, as well as those written with Dickoff and James,[44] serve as a basis for the development of nursing theory. Wiedenbach is a "mother" of nursing theory development.

NOTES

1. Ernestine Wiedenbach, *Clinical Nursing, A Helping Art* (New York: Springer Publishing Co., Inc., 1964), p. 1.
2. Joy P. Clausen and others, *Maternity Nursing Today* (New York: McGraw-Hill Book Company, 1977), p. 39.
3. Wiedenbach, *Clinical Nursing*, p. 53.
4. Ernestine Weidenbach, "Nurses' Wisdom in Nursing Theory," *American Journal of Nursing*, 70, no. 5 (1970), 1058.
5. Wiedenbach, *Clinical Nursing*, p. 2.
6. Clausen and others, *Maternity Nursing Today*, p. 39.
7. James Dickoff, Patricia A. James, and Ernestine Wiedenbach, "Theory in a Practice Discipline II: Practice-Orientated Research," *Nursing Research*, 17 (November-December 1968), 545–54.
8. Ernestine Wiedenbach, *Meeting the Realities in Clinical Teaching* (New York: Springer Publishing Co., Inc., 1969), p. 2.
9. Ibid.
10. Wiedenbach, *Clinical Nursing*, p. 16.
11. Ibid., p. 13.
12. Wiedenbach, *Clinical Nursing*, p. 16.
13. Ibid., p. 17.

14. Wiedenbach, "Nurses' Wisdom in Nursing Theory," pp. 1059–62.
15. Wiedenbach, *Meeting the Realities*, p. 3.
16. Wiedenbach, "Nurses' Wisdom in Nursing Theory," p. 1059.
17. Wiedenbach, *Meeting the Realities*, p. 3.
18. Ibid.
19. Wiedenbach, "Nurses' Wisdom in Nursing Theory," p. 1060.
20. Ibid.
21. Ernestine Wiedenbach, *Family-Centered Maternity Nursing*, 2nd ed. (New York: G. P. Putnam's Sons, 1967), p. 6.
22. Wiedenbach, "Nurses' Wisdom in Nursing Theory," p. 1060.
23. Ibid.
24. Ibid., p. 1061.
25. Ibid., p. 1062.
26. Ibid., p. 1061.
27. Wiedenbach, *Meeting the Realities*, p. 5.
28. Clausen and others, *Maternity Nursing Today*, p. 43; and Wiedenbach, *Family-Centered Maternity Nursing*, p. 8.
29. Wiedenbach, "Nurses' Wisdom in Nursing Theory," p. 1059.
30. Clausen and others, *Maternity Nursing Today*, p. 39.
31. Wiedenbach, *Clinical Nursing*, pp. 52–58.
32. Clausen and others, *Maternity Nursing Today*, p. 44.
33. Ibid., pp. 41–44.
34. Ibid.
35. Wiedenbach, *Family-Centered Maternity Nursing*, p. 8.
36. Wiedenbach, *Meeting the Realities*, p. 95.
37. Clausen and others, *Maternity Nursing Today*, p. 39.
38. Wiedenbach, *Clinical Nursing*, p. 17.
39. Clausen and others, *Maternity Nursing Today*, p. 39.
40. Wiedenbach, *Clinical Nursing*, p. 17.
41. Wiedenbach, *Meeting the Realities*, p. 42.
42. Wiedenbach, *Family-Centered Maternity Nursing*, p. 5.
43. Wiedenbach, *Clinical Nursing*, p. 1.
44. James J. Dickoff and Ernestine Wiedenbach, "Theory in a Practice Discipline I: Practice-Orientated Discipline," *Nursing Research*, 17 (September-October 1968), 415–35; and James J. Dickoff, Patricia A. James, and Ernestine Wiedenbach, "Theory in a Practice Discipline II: Practice-Orientated Research," *Nursing Research*, 17 (November-December 1968), 545–54.

ADDITIONAL REFERENCES

Books

GRIFFITH, JANET W., and PAULA J. CHRISTENSEN, eds., *Nursing Process—Application of Theories, Frameworks and Models.* St. Louis, Mo.: The C. V. Mosby Company, 1982.
Nursing Development Conference Group, *Concept Formalization in Nursing.* Boston: Little, Brown & Company, 1973.

Articles

DICKOFF, JAMES J., "Symposium in Theory Development in Nursing, Researching Research's Role in Theory Development," *Nursing Research,* 17 (May–June 1968), 204–6.
DICKOFF, JAMES J., and PATRICIA A. JAMES, "Symposium of Theory Development in Nursing: A Theory of Theories: A Position Paper," *Nursing Research,* 17 (May–June 1968), 197–203.
WIEDENBACH, E., "Childbirth as Mothers Say They Like It," *Public Health Nursing,* 51 (August 1949), 417–21.
_____, "Nurse-Midwifery, Purpose, Practice and Opportunity," *Nursing Outlook,* 8 (May 1960), 256.
_____, "The Helping Art of Nursing," *American Journal of Nursing,* 63 (November 1963), 54–57.
_____, "Family Nurse Practitioner for Maternal and Child Care," *Nursing Outlook,* 13 (December 1965), 50 ff.
_____, "Genetics and the Nurse," *Bulletin of the American College of Nurse Midwifery,* 13 (May 1968), 8–13.
_____, "The Nurse's Role in Family Planning—A Conceptual Base for Practice," *Nursing Clinics of North America,* 3 (June 1968), 355 ff.
_____, "Comment on Beliefs and Values: Basis for Curriculum Design," *Nursing Research,* 19 (September-October 1970), 427.

7

LYDIA E. HALL

Julia B. George

Lydia E. Hall received her basic nursing education at York Hospital School of Nursing in York, Pennsylvania. Both her B.S. in Public Health Nursing and M.A. in teaching Natural Sciences are from Teachers College, Columbia University, New York.

Lydia Hall was the first director of the Loeb Center for Nursing and Rehabilitation and continued in that position until her death in 1969. Her experience in nursing spans the clinical, educational, research, and supervisory components. Her publications include several articles on the definition of nursing and quality of care. Lydia Hall put forth what she considered a basic philosophy of nursing upon which the nurse may base patient care. This philosophy is still used as a working reality at the Loeb Center for Nursing.

LOEB CENTER FOR NURSING AND REHABILITATION

Lydia Hall originated the philosophy of care of Loeb Center at Montefiore Hospital, Bronx, New York. Loeb Center opened in January 1963 to provide professional nursing care to persons who are past

Gratitude is expressed to Kathleen Hale for her contributions to this chapter in the first edition.

the acute stage of illness. The center's functioning concept is that the need for professional nursing care increases as the need for medical care decreases.

Those in need of continued professional care who are sixteen years of age or older and are no longer experiencing an acute biological disturbance are transferred from the acute care hospital to Loeb Center. Good candidates for care at Loeb are those who have a desire to come to Loeb, are recommended by their physicians, and possess a favorable potential for recovery and return to the community.

Physically, Loeb Center has a capacity of eighty beds and is attached to Montefiore Hospital. The rooms are arranged with patient comfort and maneuverability as first priority. The patients also have access to a large communal dining room. The primary care givers are registered professional nurses. Nonpatient care activities are supplied by messenger-attendants and ward secretaries.

> Loeb's primary purpose was and is to demonstrate that high quality nursing care given by registered nurses, in a non-directive setting, offers a supportive service to people in the post-acute phase of their illness that enables them to recover sooner, and to leave the center able to cope with themselves and what they must face in the future.[1]

To create a nondirective setting, there are very few rules or routines, no schedules, and no dictated mealtimes or specified visiting hours.[2] The nurses at Loeb strive to help the patient determine and clarify goals and, with the patient, work out ways to achieve the goals at the individual's pace, consistent with the medical treatment plan and congruent with the patient's sense of self.[3]

LYDIA HALL'S THEORY OF NURSING

Lydia Hall presents her theory of nursing visually by drawing three interlocking circles, each circle presenting a particular aspect of nursing. The circles represent *care*, *core*, and *cure*.

The Care Circle

The care circle (Figure 7-1) represents the nurturing component of nursing and is exclusive to nursing. Involved in nurturing is the utilization of the factors that make up the concept of mother-

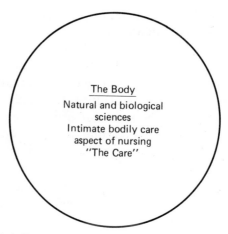

Figure 7-1. The care circle of patient care. [From Lydia Hall, *Nursing—What Is It?* p. 1. Publication of the Virginia State Nurses' Association, Winter 1959. Used with permission.]

ing (care and comfort of the person) and provide for teaching-learning activities.

The professional nurse provides bodily care for the patient and helps complete such basic daily biological functions as eating, bathing, and dressing. When providing this care, the nurse has as a main goal the comfort of the patient.

Providing care for a patient at the basic needs level presents the nurse and patient with an opportunity for closeness. When this opportunity is developed to the fullest, the patient is given an opportunity to share and explore feelings with the nurse. This opportunity to explore feelings represents the teaching-learning aspect of nurturing.

When functioning in the care circle, the nurse applies knowledge of the natural and biological sciences to provide a strong theoretical base for nursing implementations. In interactions with the patient the nurse's role must be clearly defined. A strong theory base allows the nurse to maintain a professional status rather than a mothering status, while at the same time incorporating closeness and nurturance in giving care. The patient views the nurse as a potential comforter, one who provides care and comfort through the laying on of hands.

The Core Circle

The core circle (Figure 7–2) of patient care involves the therapeutic use of self and is shared with other members of the health team. The professional nurse, by developing an interpersonal relationship with the patient, is able to help the patient verbally express feelings regarding the disease process. Through such expression the patient is able to gain self-identity and further develop toward maturity.

The professional nurse, by use of the reflective technique (acting as a mirror for the patient), helps the patient look at and explore feelings regarding his or her current health status and related potential changes in life style. The nurse uses a freely offered closeness to help the patient bring into awareness the verbal and nonverbal messages being sent to others. Motivations are discovered through the process of bringing into awareness the feelings being experienced. The patient is now able to make conscious decisions based on understood and accepted feelings and motivations. The motivation and energy necessary for healing exist within the patient rather than in the health care team.

> To look at and listen to self is often too difficult without the help of a significant figure (nurturer) who has learned how to hold up a mirror and sounding board to invite the behaver to

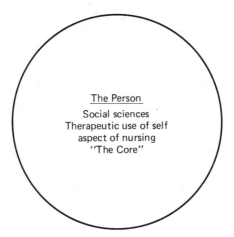

Figure 7-2. The core circle of patient care. [From Lydia Hall, *Nursing—What Is It?* p. 1. Used with permission.]

look and listen to himself. If he accepts the invitation, he will explore the concerns in his acts and as he listens to his exploration through the reflections of the nurse, he may uncover in sequence his difficulties, the problem area, his problem and eventually the threat which is dictating his out-of-control behavior.[4]

The Cure Circle

The cure circle of patient care (Figure 7–3) is shared with other members of the health team. The professional nurse helps the patient and family through the medical, surgical, and/or rehabilitative prescriptions made by the physician. During this aspect of nursing care the nurse is an active advocate of the patient.

The nurse's role during the cure aspect is different from the care circle since many of the nurse's actions take on a negative quality of avoidance of pain rather than a positive quality of comforting. This is negative in the sense that the patient views the nurse as a potential cause of pain, involved in such actions as administering injections, versus the potential comforter who provided care and comfort.

Interaction of the Three Aspects of Nursing

Since Hall emphasizes the importance of a total person approach, it is important that the three aspects of nursing (see Figure 7–4) are not viewed as functioning independently but rather as inter-

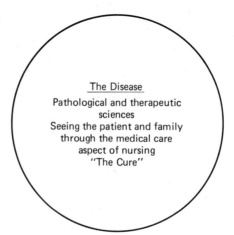

The Disease

Pathological and therapeutic
sciences
Seeing the patient and family
through the medical care
aspect of nursing
"The Cure"

Figure 7-3. The cure circle of patient care. [From Lydia Hall, *Nursing—What Is It?* p. 1. Used with permission.]

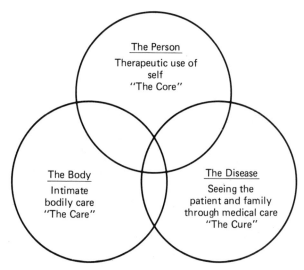

Figure 7-4. Hall's three aspects of nursing.

related. The three aspects interact and the circles representing them change size depending on the patient's total course of progress.

In the philosophy of Loeb Center, the professional nurse functions most therapeutically when patients have entered the second stage of their hospital stay (i.e., they are recuperating and are past the acute stage of illness).

During this recuperation stage, the care and core aspects are the most prominent, and the cure aspect is less prominent (see Figure 7-5). The size of the circles represents the degree to which the pa-

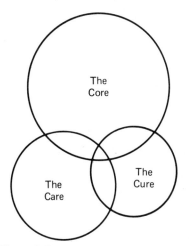

Figure 7-5. Care and core predominate.

tient is progressing in each of the three areas. The professional nurse at this time is able to help the patient reach the core of his problem through the closeness provided by the care aspect of nursing.

HALL'S THEORY AND THE FOUR MAJOR CONCEPTS

Although the concept of nursing is identified by Hall, she does not speak directly to the other three concepts of human, health, or society/environment. However, inferences can be made from her work, as noted below.

The *individual* human who is sixteen years of age or older and past the acute stage of a long-term illness is the focus of nursing care in Hall's work. The source of energy and motivation for healing is the individual care recipient, not the health care provider. Hall emphasizes the importance of the individual as unique, capable of growth and learning, and requiring a total person approach.

Health can be inferred to be a state of self-awareness with conscious selection of behaviors that are optimal for that individual. Hall stresses the need to help the person explore the meaning of his or her behavior to identify and overcome problems through developing self-identity and maturity.

The concept of *society/environment* is dealt with in relation to the individual. Hall is credited with developing the concept of Loeb Center because she assumed the hospital environment during treatment of acute illness creates a difficult psychological experience for the ill individual.[5] Loeb Center focuses on providing an environment that is conducive to self-development. The focus of the action of nurses is the individual, so that any actions taken in relation to society or environment would be for the purpose of assisting the individual in attaining a personal goal.

Nursing is identified as consisting of participation in the care, core, and cure aspects of patient care. Care is the sole function of nurses, whereas core and cure are shared with other members of the health care team. However, the major purpose of care is to achieve an interpersonal relationship with the individual that will facilitate the development of core, i.e., the development of self-identity and self-direction by the patient.

HALL'S THEORY AND THE NURSING PROCESS

Hall places the motivation and energy needed for healing within the patient. This aspect of her theory influences the nurse's total approach to the five phases of the nursing process: assessment, diagnosis, planning, implementation, and evaluation.

The *assessment* phase involves collection of data about the health status of the individual. According to Hall, the process of data collection is directed for the benefit of the patient rather than for the benefit of the nurse. Data collection should be directed toward increasing the patient's self-awareness. Through use of observation and reflection, the nurse is able to assist the patient in becoming aware of both verbal and nonverbal behaviors. In the individual, increased awareness of feelings and needs in relation to health status increases his ability for self-healing.

The assessment phase also pertains to guiding the patient through the cure aspect of nursing. The health team collects biological data (physical and laboratory) to help the patient and family understand and progress through the medical regime.

The second phase is the *nursing diagnosis,* or statement of the patient's need or problem area. How a nurse envisions the nursing role will influence the interpretation of assessment data and conclusions reached. Viewing the patient as the power for self-healing will direct conclusions differently than if the healing power rests in the physician or nurse. The patient will be the one in control.

Planning involves setting priorities and mutually establishing patient-centered goals. The patient will decide what is of highest priority and also what goals are desirable.

The core is involved in planning. The role of the nurse is to use reflection to help the patient become aware of and understand needs, feelings, and motivations. Once motivations are clarified, Hall indicates the patient is the best person to set goals and arrange priorities. The nurse seeks to increase patient awareness and to support decision making based on the patient's new level of awareness. The nurse works with the patient to help keep the goals consistent with the medical prescription. The nurse needs to draw on a knowledge base in the social and scientific areas to present the patient with creative alternatives from which to choose.

Implementation involves the actual institution of the plan of care. This phase is the actual giving of nursing care. In the care circle, intimate bodily care is given to the patient by the nurse. The nurse works *with* the patient, helping with bathing, dressing, eating, and other care and comfort needs.

The nurse also helps the patient and family through the cure aspect of nursing. She works with the patient and family to help them understand and implement the medical plan.

The professional nurse uses a "permissive non-directive teaching-learning approach" to implement nursing care, thus helping the patient reach the established goals.[6] This includes "helping the patient with his feelings, providing requested information and supporting patient-made decisions."[7]

Evaluation is the process of assessing the patient's progress toward the health goals. The evaluation phase of the process is directed toward deciding whether or not the patient is successful in reaching the established goals. The following questions would apply to the use of Hall's theory in the evaluation phase:

1. Is the patient learning "who he is, where he wants to go, and how he wants to get there?"[8]
2. Is the patient learning to understand and explore the feelings that underlie behavior?
3. Is the nurse helping the patient see motivations more clearly?
4. Are the patient's goals congruent with the medical regime? Is the patient successful in meeting the goals?
5. Is the patient physically more comfortable?

Whether or not a person is growing in self-awareness regarding his feelings and motivations can be recognized through changes in his outward behavior.

HALL'S WORK AND THE CHARACTERISTICS OF A THEORY

Hall's work can be compared to the characteristics of a theory as presented in Chapter 1.

1. Theories can interrelate concepts in such a way as to create a different way of looking at a particular phenomenon. The use of the terms *care, core,* and *cure* is unique to Hall. She interrelated these concepts and, in 1963, provided a different way of looking at the phenomenon of care of the individual with a long-term illness, which was an acute social problem of the time. Although other developments in health care have altered the need to some extent, her ideas are still relevant and useful, particularly if some of the limitations she imposed are removed. For example, care, core, and cure needs exist in acute and ambulatory settings and in individuals younger than sixteen.

2. **Theories must be logical in nature.** On first reading, Hall's work appears to be completely and simply logical. However, closer scrutiny reveals that although Hall indicates that care, the bodily laying on of hands, is the only aspect that is solely nursing—implying that it is the major focus for nursing, her major emphasis is on core. The care aspect is a means to achieving core rather than an end in itself.[9] Although this is not illogical, the initial impression is not the true logic of the work.

3. **Theories should be relatively simple yet generalizable.** Hall's work is simple in its presentation. However, the openness and flexibility required for its application may not be so simple for nurses whose personality, educational preparation, and/or experience have not prepared them to function with minimal structure. This and the self-imposed age and illness requirements limit the generalizability. Although the need for structure is a personal characteristic of the nurse, the limitations of age and stage of illness do not necessarily apply outside of Loeb Center.

4. **Theories are the bases for hypotheses that can be tested,** and 5. **Theories contribute to and assist in increasing the general body of knowledge within the discipline through the research implemented to validate them.** These two characteristics are certainly true for Hall's work and have been demonstrated in the research conducted to evaluate the effectiveness of Loeb Center. This research was conducted at Mrs. Hall's insistence, in spite of the enthusiastic acceptance of Hall's philosophy by those in the Montefiore health care community.[10] This research is evidence that hypotheses can be developed and tested. In addition, the sharing of a report about the Loeb Center in a Congressional hearing is evidence of an increase in the general body of knowledge.[11]

6. **Theories can be utilized by practitioners to guide and improve their practice.** If no other characteristic of a theory was met

by Hall's work, Loeb Center is an ideal demonstration of this characteristic. Hall's work was designed for practice and has been implemented by practitioners successfully for two decades.

**7. Theories must be consistent with other validated theories,
laws, and principles but will leave open unanswered questions that
need to be investigated.** Hall recognized the importance of knowledge of validated theories, laws, and principles. She indicated the
theoretical base for each of the aspects of patient care. The care aspect
is based in the natural and biological sciences, core in the social sciences, and cure in the pathological and therapeutic sciences. The
specific applications of these sciences provide a source of unanswered
questions to be investigated.

Hall's work presents interrelated concepts in a way that provides
a new view of a particular phenomenon. It is logical in nature, simpler
in presentation than application but capable of being generalized,
can be the basis of testable hypotheses, has led to research, is utilized by practitioners to guide practice, and is consistent with other
validated theories, laws, and principles. Thus her work may be considered a theory.

APPLICATION AND LIMITATIONS
OF THE THEORY

In reviewing Hall's theory of nursing there are several areas that limit
its application to patient care.

The first of these areas is the stage of illness. Hall applies her
ideas of nursing to a patient who has passed the acute stage of biological stress; i.e., the patient who is experiencing the acute phase
of illness is not included in Hall's approach to nursing care. However, it is possible to apply the care, core, and cure ideas to the care
of those who are acutely ill. The acutely ill individual often needs
care in relation to basic needs; he also needs core awareness of what
is going on and cure understanding of the plan of medical care.

A second limiting factor is age. Hall refers only to adult patients
in the second stage of their illness. This eliminates all younger patients. Based on this theory, Loeb Center admits only patients sixteen years of age and older. However, it would be possible to apply
Hall's theory with younger individuals. Certainly adolescents younger
than sixteen are capable of seeking self-identity.

A third limiting factor is the description of how to help a person toward self-awareness. The only tool of therapeutic communication discussed is reflection. By inference, all other techniques of therapeutic communication are eliminated. This emphasis on reflection arises from the belief that both the problem and the solution lie in the individual, and the nurse's function is to help the individual find them. But reflection is not always the most effective technique to be used. Other techniques such as active listening and non-verbal support may be used.

Fourth, the family is mentioned only in the cure circle. This means the nursing contact with families is used only in regard to the patient's own medical care. It does not allow for helping a family increase awareness of the family's self.

Finally, Hall's theory relates only to those who are ill. This would indicate no nursing contact with healthy individuals, families, or communities, and it negates the concept of health maintenance and health care to prevent illness.

Basically, Hall's theory can be readily applied within the confines of the definition of adults past the acute stage of illness. However, this is too confining for a total view of nursing, which includes working with individuals, families, and communities throughout the life cycle and along a health continuum.

However, it should be noted that the nurse who utilizes Hall's theory will function in a manner similar to the method of assignment known as *primary nursing*. Considering that Hall instituted Loeb Center in the early 1960s, her ideas certainly provided leadership and innovation in nursing practice. She also is deserving of praise for having the courage to create a new environment in which to put her ideas into practice.

SUMMARY

Although Lydia Hall first presented her theory of nursing during the late 1950s and early 1960s, Loeb Center for Nursing and Rehabilitation is still using Hall's theory in providing patient care today.

Hall's theory of nursing involves three interlocking circles, each representing one aspect of nursing. The care aspect represents intimate bodily care of the patient. The core aspect deals with the innermost feelings and motivations of the patient. The cure aspect tells how the nurse helps the patient and family through the medical aspect of care. The main tool the nurse uses to help the patient realize his motivations and to grow in self-awareness is that of reflection.

Of the major concepts, only nursing is defined as the function necessary to carry out care, core, and cure. Hall presents a philosophical view of humans as having the energy and motivation for self-awareness and growth. Definitions of health and society/environment must be inferred.

Her work may be considered a theory since it meets each of the characteristics of theories presented in Chapter 1.

Lydia Hall's theory may be used in the nursing process. The core, care, and cure aspects are applicable to each phase of the nursing process. The limitations of Hall's theory—illness orientation, age, family contact restrictions, and use of reflection only—can be overcome by taking a broader view of care, core, and cure and by emphasizing the aspect that is most appropriate for a particular situation.

NOTES

1. Susan Bowar-Ferres, "Loeb Center and Its Philosophy of Nursing," *The American Journal of Nursing*, 75, no. 5 (May 1975), 810.
2. Ibid., p. 814.
3. Ibid., p. 813.
4. Lydia Hall, "Another View of Nursing Care and Quality," address given at Catholic University Workshop, Washington, D.C., 1965.
5. Bowar-Ferres, "Loeb Center and Its Philosophy of Nursing," p. 813.
6. Ibid.
7. Esther L. Brown, *Nursing Reconsidered, A Study of Change, Part I: The Professional Role in Institutional Nursing.* (Philadelphia: J. B. Lippincott Company, 1970), p. 159.
8. Bowar-Ferres, "Loeb Center and its Philosophy of Nursing" p. 813.
9. Barbara J. Stevens, *Nursing Theory* (Boston: Little, Brown & Company, 1979), pp. 19–28.
10. Brown, *Nursing Reconsidered*, pp. 164–65.
11. "Loeb Center for Nursing and Rehabilitation Project Report," *Congressional Record*, May-June 1963, pp. 1515–62.

ADDITIONAL REFERENCES

ALFANO, GENROSE, "Administration Means Working with Nurses," *The Amerian Journal of Nursing*, vol. 64, no. 6 (June 1964).

_____, "Loeb Center," *Nursing Clinics of North America,* vol. 4, no. 3 (September 1969).

BERNARDIN, ESTELLE, "Loeb Center—As the Staff Nurse Sees It," *The American Journal of Nursing,* vol. 64, no. 6 (June 1964).

ENGLERT, BARBARA, "How a Staff Nurse Perceives Her Role at Loeb Center," *Nursing Clinics of North America,* vol. 6 (June 1971).

HALL, LYDIA, "Quality of Nursing Care," *Public Health News,* New Jersey State Department of Health, June 1955.

_____, *Nursing—What Is It?* Publication of the Virginia State Nurses Assn., Winter 1959.

_____, "A Center for Nursing," *Nursing Outlook,* vol. 2, no. 1 (November 1963).

_____, "Can Nursing Care Hasten Recovery?" *The American Journal of Nursing,* vol. 64, no. 6 (June 1964).

_____, "The Loeb Center for Nursing and Rehabilitation at Montefiore Hospital and Medical Center," *International Journal of Nursing Studies,* vol. 6 (1969).

ISLER, CHARLOTTE, "New Concepts in Nursing Therapy, More Care as the Patient Improves," *R.N.,* June 1964.

8

DOROTHEA E. OREM

Peggy Coldwell Foster and Nancy P. Janssens

Dorothea E. Orem, R.N., M.S.N.Ed., is a consultant in nursing and nursing education with Orem and Shields, Inc., Chevy Chase, Maryland. She has held positions as Professor of Nursing at Catholic University of America, Washington, D.C.; and as scholar-in-residence, School of Nursing, Medical College of Virginia, Richmond, Virginia; and also holds an honorary Doctor of Science from Georgetown University, Washington, D.C. Ms. Orem was Chairperson of the Nursing Development Conference Group, 1968–1978.

If you give a man a fish he will have a single meal;
If you teach him how to fish he will eat all his life.
　　　　　　　　　　　　　　　　　　　　—Kuan-Tzer

Since 1959, Orem's self-care model has evolved as a conceptual framework for nursing education curriculum, clinical nursing practice, nursing administration, and nursing research. Dorothea Orem's concept of nursing as the provision of self-care was first published in 1959 and focused on the individual.[1] Since then she has published two editions of *Nursing: Concepts of Practice*, 1971 and 1980,[2]

In the 1980 publication, she expanded the focus to include multi-person units (families, groups, or communities). The concept of self-care as a model for nursing practice has also been examined by the Nursing Conference Development Group of which she is Chairperson.[3]

OREM'S GENERAL THEORY OF NURSING

According to Orem,

> Nursing has as its special concern the individual's need for self-care action and the provision and management of it on a continuous basis in order to sustain life and health, recover from disease or injury, and cope with their effects.[4]

Orem presents three theoretical constructs of her general theory of nursing: (1) the self-care construct, (2) the self-care deficit construct, and (3) the nursing systems construct.[5]

The Self-Care Construct

> Self-care is the practice of activities that individuals initiate and perform on their own behalf in maintaining life, health, and well-being. Normally adults voluntarily care for themselves. Infants, children, the aged, the ill, and the disabled require complete care or assistance with self-care activities.[6]

Those who provide self-care are self-care agents, whereas those who provide care to infants, children, or dependent adults are dependent-care agents.[7]

Self-care is a deliberate action that has pattern and sequence. It is developed in day-to-day living, aided by intellectual curiosity, by instruction, by supervision from others, and by experience in performing self-care measures.[8] The human ability for engaging in self-care is referred to as *self-care agency*. When self-care by individuals or multiperson units is effectively performed, it contributes to human structural integrity, human functioning, and human development.

Orem presents the three categories of self-care requisites as (1) universal, (2) developmental, and (3) health-deviation. Self-care requisites can be defined as the purposes of actions directed toward the provision of self-care. The totality of these self-care actions is termed *therapeutic self-care demand.*[9]

Universal self-care requisites are associated with life processes and the maintenance of the integrity of human structure and functioning. They are common to all human beings during all stages of the life cycle and should be viewed as interrelated factors, each affecting the others.

Orem identifies the categories of universal self-care requisites as (1) *air, water, food*—resources vital to the continuation of life, to growth and development, to repair of body tissue, and to normal integrated functioning; (2) *care associated with elimination processes and excrements*—substances eliminated by the body for physiological reasons including regulation and control of these substances; (3) *activity and rest*—a pattern of energy with a balance between respite and activities; (4) *solitude and social interaction*—a balance between aloneness and being with others; (5) *prevention of hazards to human life, human functioning, and human well being*—conditions that imperil the life and well-being of humans; and (6) *normalcy*—the state of being normal according to scientific theory (e.g., Piaget) and cultural and societal values.

Before 1980, Orem had included the *developmental self-care requisites* within universal self-care. Developmental self-care requisites comprise maintenance of conditions to support life processes and human development, including needs in the various developmental stages and preventive care for adverse conditions affecting the developmental process (e.g., during the loss of significant others, possessions, or job).

Health deviation self-care is required in conditions of illness, injury, or disease or may result from the medical measures required to diagnose and/or correct the condition (e.g., an individual who has a colostomy resulting from the correction of an obstruction must learn new self-care techniques for elimination). The six health deviation self-care requisites are (1) seeking appropriate medical assistance for conditions of human pathology, (2) attending to the effects of human pathology, (3) carrying out medically prescribed measures effectively, (4) caring for or regulating uncomfortable or deleterious effects of prescribed medical measures, (5) accepting self in relation to a state of health in need of health care and modifying the self-concept, and (6) altering one's life style to promote personal development while living with the effect of pathology and medical measures.[10]

In general, in this first construct, Orem has explained *what* self-care is and the various factors that affect its provision. In the second construct, to be discussed below, Orem specifies *when* nursing is needed to assist the client in the provision of self-care.

The Self-Care Deficit Construct

The self-care deficit construct is the core of Orem's general theory of nursing because it delineates when nursing is needed. A self-care deficit that is health-related is the criterion for identifying one who needs nursing care. Thus, nursing is required in the absence or limitation of the ability of the adult, or parent (guardian) in the case of a child, to meet continuous self-care requirements as well as when the need arises to use special techniques and apply scientific knowledge in the design or provision of care.[11]

The domain of nursing practice can be described in terms of activities in which nurses engage when they provide nursing. Orem has identified five areas of activity for nursing practice:[12]

1. Entering into and maintaining nurse-patient relationships with individuals, families, or groups until patients can legitimately be discharged from nursing.
2. Determining if and how patients can be helped through nursing.
3. Responding to patients' requests, desires, and needs for nurse contacts and assistance.
4. Prescribing, providing, and regulating direct help to patients and their significant others in the form of nursing.
5. Coordinating and integrating nursing with the patient's daily living, other health care needed or being received, and social and educational services needed or being received.

Self-care has been defined and the need for nursing delineated in the first and second constructs. In the next (third) construct, Orem outlines *how* the self-care needs of the patient(s) will be met by the nurse and/or by the patient via the nursing systems.

The Nursing Systems Construct

The nursing system is dependent on the self-care needs and abilities of the patient. Orem has developed three nursing systems to meet

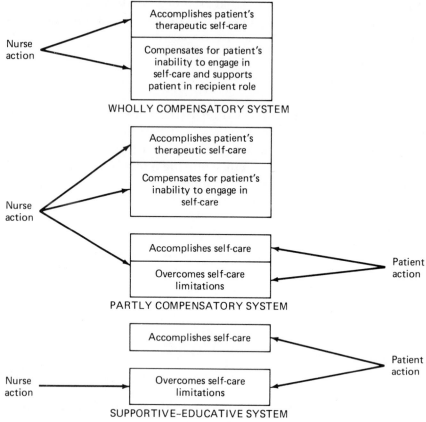

Figure 8–1. Basic nursing systems. [From Dorothy E. Orem, *Nursing: Concepts of Practice* (New York: McGraw-Hill Book Company; 1971), p. 78. Used with permission.]

the self-care requisites of the patient(s) (see Figure 8–1). The design and elements of the nursing system are designated as follows:

A. The specific roles and responsibilities of the patient(s) and of the nurse in the nurse-patient relationship.
B. Specific helping methods to be utilized by the nurse to attain self-care goals. These helping methods are: acting for, guiding, supporting (physically or psychologically), teaching another, or providing an environment to promote development.
C. Classification of patient(s) care.

The three nursing systems are: (1) wholly compensatory, (2) partly compensatory, and (3) supportive-educative.

The *wholly compensatory nursing system* is represented by a situation in which the patient has no active role in the performance of care. The nurse "helps" by acting for or doing for the patient. There are three stages in this system: (1) the patient is totally incapacitated, mentally and physically, (2) the patient is in a state of physical incapacitation but is aware of happenings in the environment, and (3) the patient's psychomotor activity is not directed toward meeting requirements for life, safety, or effective human functioning.[13] An example of a person needing care in the wholly compensatory system would be an individual who is nonresponsive. In this situation, the nurse must ensure that all needs are met, including oxygenation, nutrient intake, elimination, body hygiene, range of motion exercises, and sensory stimulation.

The *partly compensatory nursing system* is represented by a situation in which both the nurse and the patient perform care measures or other actions involving manipulative tasks or ambulation. Either the nurse or the patient may have the major role in the meeting of the needs.[14] An example of a person needing nursing care in the partly compensatory system would be an individual who has had recent surgery. This person might need much assistance with oral hygiene, toilette, or ambulation. Or the individual might be able to meet most self-care needs and actively communicate to the nurse the time, the type, and the degree of assistance that is needed.

The *supportive-educative system* is a system where the person is able, or can and should learn, to perform the required self-care measure but cannot do so without assistance. The methods of helping or assisting in this system would include: support, guidance, the provision of a developmental environment, and teaching.[15] An example of a person needing care in the supportive-educative system would be an adolescent with a metabolic disorder. When the community health nurse visits the home, the nurse would give support to the patient and his family by listening to their concerns. The nurse would then teach all pertinent members of the family the pathophysiology of the impairment, the need for exercise, the technical skills for medication administration, and foot care. The nurse would also guide them in the dietary regime and would encourage them to provide an environment where the adolescent can meet his physical and psychological developmental tasks.

OREM'S THEORY AND THE FOUR
MAJOR CONCEPTS

Orem discusses each of the four major concepts of individual human being, health, society, and nursing in her work. *Human beings* are distinguished from other living things by their capacity to (1) reflect upon themselves and their environment; (2) symbolize what they experience; and (3) use symbolic creation (ideas, words) in thinking, in communicating, and in guiding efforts to do and to make things beneficial for themselves or others.[16] Integrated human functioning includes physical, psychological, interpersonal, and social aspects. Orem believes that individuals have the potential for learning and development. The way an individual meets his self-care needs is not instinctual but is a learned behavior. Factors that affect learning include: age, mental capacity, culture, society, and the emotional state of the individual. If the individual cannot learn self-care measures, others must learn the care and provide it.

Orem supports the World Health Organization's definition of *health* as the state of physical, mental, and social well-being and not merely the absence of disease or infirmity. She states that "the physical, psychological, interpersonal and social aspects of health are inseparable in the individual."[17] Orem also presents health based on the concept of preventive health care. It includes the promotion and maintenance of health (primary prevention), the treatment of disease (secondary prevention), and the prevention of complications (tertiary prevention).

Orem utilizes health as a focus to classify nursing needs as follows: life cycle, recovery, illness of undetermined origin, genetic and developmental problems or biological immaturity, cure or regulation, stabilization of integrated functioning, and terminal illness.[18]

In modern *society*, adults are expected to be self-directed and responsible for themselves and for the well-being of their dependents. Most societies further accept that persons who cannot meet these requirements should be helped in their immediate distress and helped to attain or regain responsibility within their existing capacity. Thus, both self-help and help to others are valued by society as desirable activities. Nursing as a specific type of human service is based on both values. In most communities, people see nursing as a desirable and necessary service.[19]

Orem speaks to several factors related to the concept of *nurs-*

ing. These are the art and prudence of nursing, nursing as a service, role theory related to nursing, and technologies in nursing.

The art of nursing includes a theoretical base in the nursing disciplines and in the sciences, arts, and humanities. This base directs decisions when designing nursing systems within the nursing process.

> Nursing prudence is the quality of nurses that enables them (1) to seek and take counsel in new or difficult nursing situations, (2) to make correct judgments, . . . (3) to decide to act in a particular way, and (4) to take action.[20]

The development of the individual nurse's art and prudence is affected by unique life and nursing experiences.

Orem further defines nursing as:

> a service, a mode of helping human beings and not a tangible commodity. Nursing's form or structure is derived from actions deliberately selected and performed by nurses to help individuals or groups under their care to maintain or change conditions in themselves or their environments.[21]

The specialized abilties that enable nurses to provide nursing care to individuals or multiperson units, when conceptualized as a unit, is termed nursing agency.[22] Nursing agency is analogous to self-care agency in that both are abilities for specialized types of deliberate action. Nursing agency is developed and exercised for the benefit and well-being of others, and self-care agency is developed and exercised for the benefit and well-being of oneself.[23]

The nurse's and patient's roles define the expected behaviors for each in the specific nursing situation. Various factors that influence the expected role behaviors are culture, environment, age, sex, the health setting, and finances. The roles of nurse and patient are complementary. That is, a certain behavior of the patient elicits a certain response in the nurse, and vice versa. Both work together to accomplish the goal of self-care.

In the nurse-patient relationship, the nurse or patient may experience role conflict since each is performing concurrent roles; for example, the patient also has expected behaviors from his roles as a father, a husband, and a construction worker. Thus the conflict in the behaviors required for the various roles may affect the performance of self-care. Knowledge of role theory is useful for the professional nurse to assist in (1) designing a nursing system, (2) defining the role of the nurse and the patient in a specific nursing situation, and (3) implementing the plan to achieve the goal of health care.

Orem states that nursing includes the abilities of a practical and technological nature.[24] It is important to note that although Orem recognizes that specialized technologies are usually developed by members of the health professions, she emphasizes the need for social and interpersonal dimensions in nursing. She states,

> A technology is systematized information about a process or a method of effecting some desired result through deliberate practical endeavor, with or without the use of materials or instruments.[28]

Two categories of technologies used in nursing are (1) social and interpersonal technologies and (2) regulatory technologies.[26]

Social and interpersonal technologies include:

1. Communication adjusted to age and developmental state, to health state, and to sociocultural orientation;
2. Bringing about and maintaining interpersonal, intragroup or intergroup relations for coordination of effort;
3. Bringing about and maintaining therapeutic relations in light of psychosocial modes of functioning in health and disease; and
4. Giving human assistance adapted to human needs and action abilities and limitations.

Regulatory technologies include:

1. Maintaining and promoting life processes,
2. Regulating psychophysiological modes of functioning in health and disease,
3. Promoting human growth and development, and
4. Regulating position and movement in space.

The effective integration of social and interpersonal technologies with the regulatory technologies promotes quality professional nursing.

OREM'S THEORY AND THE NURSING PROCESS

The nursing process according to Orem may be defined as

> determining why a person needs nursing, designing a system of nursing assistance, planning for the delivery of the specified nursing assistance, [and] providing and controlling the delivery of nursing assistance.[27]

Table 8–1 compares the nursing process presented in Chapter 2 and Orem's nursing process.

The steps of Orem's nursing process may be summarized as follows:[28]

> Step 1: The initial and continuing determination of why a person should be under nursing care.
>
> Step 2: The designing of a nursing system and planning for the delivery of nursing according to the designed system.
>
> Step 3: The initiation, conduction, and control of assisting actions.

Step 1 of Orem's nursing process can be considered as the *diagnosis* and prescriptive portion. It is an investigative operation that enables nurses to make judgments about the existing health care situations and decisions about what can and should be done based on collective data.[29] Within Step 1 the nurse would seek answers to the following five questions:[30]

1. What is the patient's therapeutic care demand? Now? At a future time?
2. Does the patient have a deficit for engaging in self-care to meet the therapeutic self-care demand?
3. If so, what is its nature and the reasons for its existence?
4. Should the patient be helped to refrain from engagement in self-care or to protect already developed self-care capabilities for therapeutic purposes?
5. What is the patient's potential for engaging in self-care at a future time period? Increasing or deepening self-care knowl-

Table 8-1

Comparison of Orem's Nursing Process and the
Nursing Process

Nursing Process[a]		*Orem's Nursing Process*	
1.	Assessment	Step 1.	Diagnosis and prescription: Determine why nursing is needed.
2.	Nursing diagnosis		Analyze and interpret—make judgments regarding care.
3.	Plans with scientific rationale	Step 2.	Design of a nursing system and plan for delivery of care.
4.	Implementation	Step 3.	Production and management of nursing systems.
5.	Evaluation		

[a]Five-step process outlined in Chapter 2 of this text.

edge? Learning techniques of care? Fostering willingness to engage in self care? Effectively and consistently incorporating essential self-care measures (including new ones) into the systems of self-care and daily living?

Within *Step 1* the nurse would *assess* the individual's self-care requisites and ability to provide self-care or serve as a self-care agent. After this information is gathered by assessment, it is analyzed by the nurse and interpreted to enable her to design a plan of care.

Step 2 is the designing and *planning* component of the process. The nurse designs a nursing system that is wholly compensatory, partly compensatory, or supportive-educative. The two actions involved in the design of the nursing systems would be: (a) bringing about a good organization of the components of the therapeutic self-care demands, and (b) selecting the ways of helping that will be both effective and efficient in compensating for or overcoming the self-care deficits—that is, planning for the delivery of therapeutic self-care.[31]

Step 3 is the production and management of nursing systems. The nurse *implements* the nursing system design. The role of the nurse in this step is to: (a) assist the patient (or family) in self-care matters to achieve identified and described health-related results, (b) check what was done against what was specified to be done, (c) collect evidence to describe results of care, and (d) use evidence to *evaluate* results achieved against results specified in nursing system design.[32]

Historically, minimal emphasis has been given to Steps 1 and 2 of Orem's nursing process. Orem recommends that a professional nurse be responsible for the total nursing process.[33] This professional nurse may be assisted by other professional, vocational, or technical nurses.

OREM'S WORK AND THE CHARACTERISTICS OF A THEORY

Orem identifies her work as a framework of "concepts of practice." However, when compared with the characteristics of a theory from Chapter 1, it is apparent that this "framework" may be considered a theory.

1. Theories can interrelate concepts in such a way as to create a different way of looking at a particular phenomenon. The premise of self-care is incorporated with nursing in the three broad systems of wholly compensatory, partly compensatory, and supportive-educative to provide a new way of looking at nursing care.

2. Theories must be logical in nature. Orem's theory follows a logical thought process. She states her general theory, presents the concepts of her theory, supports the concepts with suppositions, and then supports the suppositions with presuppositions.

3. Theories should be relatively simple yet generalizable. Orem's theory is used by several schools of nursing as a theory base for a student's basic preparation for practice. The self-care deficits and nursing systems constructs can be comprehended and applied to all individual clients and, with further adaptation, to multiperson units.

4. Theories are the bases for hypotheses that can be tested. Orem's theory of self-care can be used to generate testable hypotheses. For example, hypotheses could be developed about the relationship between selected self-care deficits and the nursing system needed to meet those deficits.

5. Theories contribute to and assist in increasing the general body of knowledge within the discipline through the research implemented to validate them. Orem focuses on nursing as a helping art, assisting the individual to meet self-care needs, as the foundation for nursing practice. Research on self-care needs, and the assistance to meet them, adds to nursing's body of knowledge.

6. Theories can be utilized by the practitioners to guide and improve their practice. Orem's theory is used by an independent practitioner and by practitioners in clinical settings who have published information about their practice.[35]

7. Theories must be consistent with other validated theories, laws, and principles. Orem's theory is consistent with role theory, field theory, and preventive health concepts.

ANALYSIS AND CONCLUSIONS

Dorothea E. Orem's theory of nursing provides a comprehensive base for nursing practice. It has utility for professional nursing in the areas of nursing education curricula, clinical nursing practice, nursing administration, and nursing research.

Orem promotes the concept of professional nursing. She emphasizes that nurses are educated not trained. In the process of that education, nurses must learn to "think nursing" not just perform discrete nursing tasks.[36] Orem utilizes theories from other disciplines to support her general theory of nursing (e.g., Lewin's force-field theory,[37] role theory, and the concepts of preventive health).

Orem has expanded her focus of individual self-care to include multiperson units (families, groups, and communities). Although most of her second edition still focuses on the individual, she recognizes the value of family members and significant others for the individual's provision of self-care.

Her self-care premise is contemporary with the concepts of health promotion and health maintenance. Self-care in Orem's theory is comparable to holistic health in that both promote the individual's responsibility for health care.

In the second edition of *Nursing: Concepts of Practice,* Orem has presented her concepts with expanded explanations that allow for direct application in nursing practice, such as a specific set of nursing actions to meet the universal self-care requirements.[38]

Orem emphasizes the importance of developmental self-care needs by presenting these as a separate category in the self-care requisites. Orem has also expanded her discussion of the nursing process. She has developed assessment questions and sets of nursing actions to meet self-care needs and has elaborated on the application of the methods of helping and on the concept of evaluation. It should be pointed out here that some of Orem's terminology could be confusing to the reader and needs clarification, such as her use of the terms *diagnosis, prescription, therapeutic self-care demand, nursing agency,* and *technologies.*

A major strength of Orem's theory is that she specifies when nursing is needed. She also stresses that nurses should be responsible for continuing education to provide quality professional nursing care.

Orem's concept of self-care has pragmatic application in nursing practice. Some nursing curricula are based on premises of self-care, and Lucille Kinlein in independent practice uses the concept of self-care as the core of her professional nursing practice.[39] Documented use of Orem's theory in clinical practice includes self-care of clients with enterostomal therapy,[40] diabetes,[41] and carcinoma.[42]

Orem's theory offers a unique way of looking at the phenomenon of nursing. Her work contributes significantly to the development of nursing theories.

NOTES

1. Dorothea E. Orem, *Guides for Developing Curricula for the Education of Practical Nurses* (Washington, D.C.: Government Printing Office, 1959).
2. Dorothea E. Orem, *Nursing: Concepts of Practice* (New York: McGraw-Hill Book Company, 1971; and idem, *Nursing: Concepts of Practice,* 2nd ed. (New York: McGraw-Hill Book Company, 1980).
3. Nursing Development Conference Group, *Concept Formalization in Nursing: Process and Product,* 2nd ed. (Boston: Little, Brown & Company, 1979).
4. Orem, *Nursing,* 2nd ed., p. 6.
5. Ibid., p. 26.
6. Ibid., p. 35.
7. Ibid.
8. Ibid., p. 83.
9. Ibid., p. 39.
10. Ibid., pp. 50–51.
11. Ibid., p. 7.
12. Ibid., p. 25.
13. Orem, *Nursing,* 1st ed., pp. 78–79.
14. Ibid., pp. 79–80.
15. Ibid., p. 79.

16. Orem, *Nursing,* 2nd ed., p. 118.
17. Ibid., p. 119.
18. Ibid., p. 137–49.
19. Ibid., p. 6.
20. Ibid., p. 89.
21. Ibid., p. 5.
22. Nursing Development Conference Group, *Concept Formalization,* Chapter 5.
23. Orem, *Nursing,* 2nd ed., p. 88.
24. Ibid., p. 89.
25. Ibid., p. 90.
26. Ibid., pp. 91–92.
27. Ibid., p. 201.
28. Ibid., p. 202.
29. Ibid., p. 203.
30. Ibid.
31. Ibid., p. 210.
32. Ibid., p. 201.
33. Ibid., pp. 202–3.
34. J. E. Backscheider, "Self-Care Requirements, Self-Care Capabilities and Nursing Systems in the Diabetic Nurse Management Clinic," *American Journal of Public Health,* 64 (December 1974), 1138–46; Elizabeth A. McFarlane, "Nursing Theory: The Comparison of Four Theoretical Proposals," *Journal of Advanced Nursing,* 5 (1980), 3–19; Mary Colette Smith, "Proposed Metaparadigm for Nursing Research and Theory Development—An Analysis of Orem's Self-Care Theory," *Image,* 11, no. 3 (October 1979), 75–79.
35. M. Lucille Kinlein, *Independent Nursing Practice with Clients* (Philadelphia: J. B. Lippincott Company, 1977); Barbara Bromley, "Applying Orem's Self-Care Theory in Enterostomal Therapy," *American Journal of Nursing,* 80, no. 2 (February 1980), 245–49.; Sheila Fitzgerald, "Utilizing Orem's Self-Care Model in Designing an Educational Program for the Diabetic," *Topics in Clinical Nursing.* 2, no. 2 (July 1980), 57–65; and P. Murphy, "A Hospice Model and Self-Care Theory," *Oncology Nursing Forum,* 8, no. 2 (Spring 1981), 19–21.
36. Orem, *Nursing,* 2nd ed., p. 14.
37. W. G. Bennis, K. D. Benne, and R. Chin, *The Planning of Change* (New York: Holt, Rinehart and Winston, 1969).
38. Orem, *Nursing,* 2nd ed., p. 43.
39. Kinlein, *Independent Nursing Practice.*
40. Bromley, "Applying Orem's Self-Care Theory."
41. Fitzgerald, "Utilizing Orem's Self-Care Nursing Model."
42. Murphy, "A Hospice Model."

ADDITIONAL REFERENCES

Books

Nursing Development Conference Group, *Concept Formalization in Nursing: Process and Product.* Boston: Little, Brown & Company, 1973.

ROY, CALLISTA, and JOAN P. RIEHL, eds., *Conceptual Models for Nursing Practice,* 2nd ed. East Norwalk, Conn.: Appleton-Century-Crofts, 1980.

9

FAYE G. ABDELLAH

Suzanne M. Falco

*Faye G. Abdellah is the Assistant Surgeon General and Chief
Nurse Officer for the U.S. Public Health Services, Department
of Health and Human Services, Washington, D.C. She holds an
Ed.D. from Teachers College, Columbia University, New York,
and an LL.D. from Columbia University.*

In 1960, influenced by the desire to promote client-centered comprehensive nursing care, Abdellah described nursing as a service to
individuals, to families, and, therefore, to society. According to
Abdellah, nursing is based on an art and science that mold the attitudes, intellectual competencies, and technical skills of the individual
nurse into the desire and ability to help people, sick or well, cope
with their health needs. Nursing may be carried out under general
or specific medical direction. As a comprehensive service, nursing
includes:[1]

1. Recognizing the nursing problems of the client.
2. Deciding the appropriate courses of action to take in terms
   of relevant nursing principles.
3. Providing continuous care of the individual's total health
   needs.

4. Providing continuous care to relieve pain and discomfort and provide immediate security for the individual.
5. Adjusting the total nursing care plan to meet the client's individual needs.
6. Helping the individual to become more self-directing in attaining or maintaining a healthy state of mind and body.
7. Instructing nursing personnel and family to help the individual do for himself that which he can within his limitations.
8. Helping the individual to adjust to his limitations and emotional problems.
9. Working with allied health professions in planning for optimum health on local, state, national, and international levels.
10. Carrying out continuous evaluation and research to improve nursing techniques and to develop new techniques to meet the health needs of people.

These original premises have undergone an evolutionary process. As a result, in 1973, item 3— "providing continuous care of the individual's total health needs"—was eliminated.[2] Although no reason was given, it can be hypothesized that the words *continuous* and *total* render that service virtually impossible to provide. From these premises, Abdellah's theory was derived.

ABDELLAH'S THEORY

Although Abdellah's writings are not specific as to a theoretical statement, such a statement can be derived by using her three major concepts of health, nursing problems, and problem-solving. Abdellah's theory would state that nursing is the use of the problem-solving approach with key nursing problems related to the health needs of people. Such a theoretical statement maintains problem-solving as the vehicle for the nursing problems as the client is moved toward health—the outcome. It is also a relatively simple statement and can be utilized as a basis for nursing practice, education, and research.

Health

Although Abdellah never defined it per se, her concept of health may be defined as the dynamic pattern of functioning whereby there is a continued interaction with internal and external forces that re-

sults in the optimal use of necessary resources that serve to minimize vulnerabilities.[3] By performing nursing services, the nurse
helps the client achieve a state of health. However, in order to effectively perform these services, the nurse must accurately identify
the lacks or deficits regarding health that the client is experiencing.
These lacks or deficits are the client's health needs.

Nursing Problems

The client's health needs can be viewed as problems. These problems may be *overt* as an apparent condition, or *covert* as a hidden
or concealed one. Because covert problems can be emotional, sociological, and interpersonal in nature, they are often missed or perceived
incorrectly. Yet, in many instances, solving the covert problems may
solve the overt problems as well.[4]

Such a view of problems implies a client-centered orientation.
Abdellah, however, seems to imply a different viewpoint. She says
a nursing problem presented by a client is a condition faced by the
client or client's family that the nurse through the performance of
professional functions can assist them to meet.[5] Abdellah's use of
the term *nursing problems* is more consistent with "nursing functions"
or "nursing goals" than with client-centered problems. This viewpoint leads to an orientation that is more nursing-centered than
client-centered.[6]

This nursing-centered orientation to client care seems contrary
to the client-centered approach that Abdellah professes to uphold.
The apparent contradiction can be explained by her desire to move
away from a disease-centered orientation. In her attempt to bring
nursing practice into its proper relationship with restorative and pre-
ventative measures for meeting total client needs,[7] she seems to
swing the pendulum to the opposite pole, from the disease orientation to nursing orientation, while leaving the client somewhere in
the middle (see Figure 9-1).

Problem-Solving

Quality professional nursing care requires that nurses be able
to identify and solve overt and covert nursing problems. This can
be accomplished by the problem-solving approach. The problem-solv-

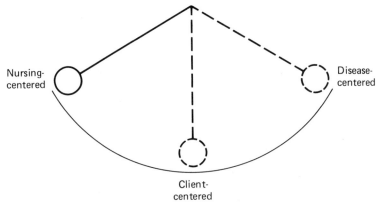

Figure 9-1. The focus of care pendulum.

ing process involves identifying the problem, selecting pertinent data, formulating hypotheses, testing hypotheses through the collection of data, and revising hypotheses where necessary on the basis of conclusions obtained from the data.[8]

Many of these steps parallel the steps in the nursing process of assessment, diagnosis, planning, implementation, and evaluation. The problem-solving approach was selected because of the assumption that the correct identification of nursing problems influences the nurse's judgment in selecting the next steps in solving the client's nursing problems.[9] The problem-solving approach is also consistent with such basic elements of nursing practice espoused by Abdellah as observing, reporting, and interpreting the signs and symptoms that comprise the deviations from health and constitute nursing problems; and with analyzing the nursing problems and selecting the necessary course of action.[10]

THE TWENTY-ONE NURSING PROBLEMS

The crucial element within Abdellah's theory is the identification of correct nursing problems. To assist in this identification, the need was defined for a systematic classification of nursing problems presented by the client. It was felt that such problems could be classified into three major categories:[11]

1. Physical, sociological, and emotional needs of clients.
2. Types of interpersonal relationships between the nurse and client.
3. Common elements of client care.

Over a five-year period, several studies were carried out to establish the classification. As the result of this research, twenty-one groups of common nursing problems were identified (see Table 9–1). It is these twenty-one common nursing problems of Abdellah's that are most widely known, and they will be the focus of the rest of the chapter.

These twenty-one nursing problems focus on the physical, biological, and social-psychological needs of the client and attempt to

Table 9–1
Abdellah's Twenty-One Nursing Problems

---

1. To maintain good hygiene and physical comfort.
2. To promote optimal activity: exercise, rest, and sleep.
3. To promote safety through the prevention of accidents, injury, or other trauma and through the prevention of the spread of infection.
4. To maintain good body mechanics and prevent and correct deformities.
5. To facilitate the maintenance of a supply of oxygen to all body cells.
6. To facilitate the maintenance of nutrition of all body cells.
7. To facilitate the maintenance of elimination.
8. To facilitate the maintenance of fluid and electrolyte balance.
9. To recognize the physiological responses of the body to disease conditions—pathological, physiological, and compensatory.
10. To facilitate the maintenance of regulatory mechanisms and functions.
11. To facilitate the maintenance of sensory function.
12. To identify and accept positive and negative expressions, feelings, and reactions.
13. To identify and accept the interrelatedness of emotions and organic illness.
14. To facilitate the maintenance of effective verbal and nonverbal communication.
15. To promote the development of productive interpersonal relationships.
16. To facilitate progress toward achievement of personal spiritual goals.
17. To create and/or maintain a therapeutic environment.
18. To facilitate awareness of self as an individual with varying physical, emotional, and developmental needs.
19. To accept the optimum possible goals in the light of limitations, physical and emotional.
20. To use community resources as an aid in resolving problems arising from illness.
21. To understand the role of social problems as influencing factors in the case of illness.

Source: From Faye G. Abdellah and others, *Patient-Centered Approaches to Nursing* (New York: Macmillan Publishing Co., Inc., 1960), pp. 16–17. Used with permission.

provide a more meaningful basis for organization than the categories of systems of the body. The most difficult problems were felt to be numbers 12, 14, 15, 17, 18, and 19.[12] Although a rationale is not provided for this, it is interesting to note that all these problems fall into the realm of social-psychological needs and tend to be more covert in nature.

Within the practice of nursing, it was anticipated that these twenty-one problems as broad groupings would encourage the generalization of principles and would thereby guide care and promote the development of the nurse's judgmental ability. Contained in each of the broad nursing problems are numerous specific overt and covert problems. It was also anticipated that the constant relating of the broad basic nursing problems to the specific problems of the individual client and vice versa would encourage the development of increased ability to use theory in clinical practice. Thus, a greater understanding of the relationship between theory and practice would strengthen the usefulness of the nursing problems.[13]

COMPARISON WITH OTHER THEORIES

An examination of these twenty-one problems yields similarities with other theories. Most notable is their similarity to Henderson's fourteen components of basic nursing care.[14] See Table 9-2. As can be seen in this table, Abdellah has consolidated some components, such as number 7—Select suitable clothing, and number 8—Keep body clean and well groomed; and has expanded others, most notably number 14—Learn, discover, and satisfy curiosity. The strong similarity may be the result of both Henderson's and Abdellah's exposure to the same environment—Teachers College, Columbia University, New York. It might be hypothesized that Abdellah moved from the rather simplistic form of Henderson's theory to a more complex structure.

Despite the above similarity, a major difference is evident. Henderson's components are written in terms of client behaviors, whereas Abdellah's problems are formulated in terms of the nursing services that should be incorporated into the determination of the client's needs.[15] This emphasis on nursing services is consistent with Abdellah's apparent nurse-centered orientation mentioned earlier.

Table 9-2

Comparison of Maslow's, Henderson's, and Abdellah's Frameworks

Maslow	Henderson	Abdellah[a]
1. Physiological needs	1. Breathe normally.	5. To facilitate the maintenance of a supply of oxygen to all body cells.
	2. Eat and drink adequately.	6. To facilitate the maintenance of nutrition of all body cells.
		8. To facilitate the maintenance of fluid and electrolyte balance.
	3. Eliminate by all avenues of elimination.	7. To facilitate the maintenance of elimination.
	4. Move & maintain desirable posture.	4. To maintain good body mechanics and prevent and correct deformities.
	5. Sleep & rest.	2. To promote optimal activity: exercise, rest, and sleep.
	6. Select suitable clothing.	10. To facilitate the maintenance of regulatory mechanisms and functions.
	7. Maintain body temperature.	1. To maintain good hygiene and physical comfort.
	8. Keep body clean & well groomed & protect the integument.	
2. Safety needs	9. Avoid environmental dangers & avoid injuring others.	3. To promote safety through the prevention of accident, injury, or other trauma and through the prevention of the spread of infection.
		11. To facilitate the maintenance of sensory function.
3. Belonging and love needs.	10. Communicate with others.	14. To facilitate the maintenance of effective verbal and nonverbal communication.
		15. To promote the development of productive interpersonal relationships.
	11. Worship according to faith.	16. To facilitate progress toward achievement of personal spiritual goals.

Maslow	Henderson	Abdellah[a]
4. Esteem needs	12. Work at something providing a sense of accomplishment.	19. To accept the optimum possible goals in the light of limitations, physical and emotional.
	13. Play or participate in various forms of recreation.	9. To recognize the physiological responses of the body to disease conditions—pathological, physiological, and compensatory.
	14. Learn, discover, or satisfy curiosity.	12. To identify and accept positive and negative expressions. feelings, and reactions.
		13. To identify and accept the interrelatedness of emotions and organic illness.
		17. To create and/or maintain a therapeutic environment.
		18. To facilitate awareness of self as an individual with varying physical, emotional, and developmental needs.
		20. To use community resources as an aid in resolving problems arising from illness.
		21. To understand the role of social problems as influencing factors in the cause of illness.
5. Self-actualization needs		

[a]Numbers in column 3 refer to the twenty-one problems as listed in Table. 9–1.

Henderson seems to have maintained the client orientation, whereas Abdellah seems to have moved beyond it (see Table 9-2).

Abdellah's nursing problems are also comparable to Maslow's hierarchy of needs.[16] In contrast to Henderson's components, which have a strong physiological orientation, Abdellah's expansion in the *esteem needs area* provides a more balanced set of nursing problems between the physical and nonphysical areas (Table 9-2). As with Henderson's components, Abdellah's problems do not meet the self-actualization needs of Maslow. This is not surprising as self-actualization is not a goal to be accomplished but a process that is ongoing—the dynamic process of beginning. To place elements in this area would negate the dynamism of self-actualization. From a different viewpoint, if Henderson's components and Abdellah's problems are fulfilled, then the client will move toward becoming and self-actualization.

ABDELLAH'S THEORY AND THE FOUR MAJOR CONCEPTS

Abdellah does not clearly specify each of the four major concepts—the individual or human, health, environment/society, and nursing. She does describe the recipients of nursing as *individuals* (and families), although she does not delineate her beliefs or assumptions about the nature of human beings. Her twenty-one nursing problems deal with biological, psychological, and social areas of individuals and can be considered to represent areas of importance to them.

Health, or the achieving of it, is the purpose of nursing services. Although Abdellah does not give a definition of health, she speaks to "total health needs" and "a healthy state of mind and body" in her description of nursing as a comprehensive service.[17]

Society is included in "planning for optimum health on local, state, national, and international levels."[18] However, as Abdellah further delineated her ideas, the focus of nursing service is clearly the individual. Society is negated when she discusses implementation.

Nursing is broadly grouped into the twenty-one problem areas to guide care and promote the use of nursing judgment. Abdellah considers nursing to be a comprehensive service that is based on an art and science and aims to help people, sick or well, cope with their health needs.

USE OF THE TWENTY-ONE
PROBLEMS IN THE
NURSING PROCESS

Because of the strong nurse-centered orientation in the twenty-one
nursing problems, their use in the nursing process is primarily to direct
the nurse. Indirectly, the client benefits. If the nurse helps the client
reach all the goals stated in the nursing problems, then the client
will be moved toward health.

Within the *assessment* phase, the nursing problems provide
guidelines for the collection of data. A principle underlying the problem-solving approach is that for each identified problem, pertinent
data are collected. Thus, for each of the identified twenty-one nursing problems, relevant data are collected. The overt or covert nature
of the problems necessitates a direct or indirect approach, respec-
tively. For example, the overt problem of nutritional status can be
assessed by direct measures of weight, food intake, and body size;
whereas the covert problem of maintaining a therapeutic environment requires more indirect approaches to data collection.

The nursing problems can be divided into those that are basic
to all clients and those that reflect sustenal, remedial, or restorative
care needs, as seen in Table 9–3. By facilitating data collection, such
a classification promotes investigating those problems consistent with
the client's stage of illness. However, such a classification promotes
the thinking that the client's stage of illness determines appropriate
or acceptable problems. Such thinking is contrary to the philosophy
of holism. If clients are holistic, then they can have needs in any and
all areas regardless of the stage of illness. A varied multitude of nursing problems could then exist.

The results of the data collection would determine the client's
specific overt and/or covert problems. These specific problems would
be grouped under one or more of the broader nursing problems. This
step is consistent with that involved in *nursing diagnosis*. Within this
framework, the nursing diagnoses are derived from the exhibited nursing problems.

The twenty-one nursing problems can have a great impact on
the *planning* phase of the nursing process. The statements of the
nursing problems most closely resemble goal statements. Therefore,
once the problem has been diagnosed, the goals have been established.
Many of the nursing-problem statements can be considered goals for

Table 9-3

The Relationships among the Classification and Approach of the Twenty-One Nursing Problems and Stages of Illness, Nursing Interventions, and Criterion Measures

Stages of Illness[a]	Nursing Problems	Classification and Approach[b]	Nursing Interventions[c]	Criterion Measures[a]
Basic to all patients	1. To maintain good hygiene and physical comfort. 2. To promote optimal activity: exercise, rest, and sleep. 3. To promote safety through prevention of accident, injury, or other trauma and through the prevention of the spread of infection. 4. To maintain good body mechanics and prevent and correct deformities.	Overt and/or covert problems Direct and/or indirect methods	Measures necessary to maintain hygiene, physical comfort, activity, rest and sleep, safety, and body mechanics.	Related to preventive care needs.
Sustenal care needs	5. To facilitate the maintenance of a supply of oxygen to all body cells. 6. To facilitate the maintenance of nutrition of all body cells. 7. To facilitate the maintenance of elimination. 8. To facilitate the maintenance of fluid and electrolyte balance. 9. To recognize the physiological responses of the body to disease conditions—pathological, physiological, and compensatory. 10. To facilitate the maintenance of regulatory mechanisms and functions. 11. To facilitate the maintenance of sensory function.	Usually overt problems Direct methods	Measures necessary to maintain oxygen supply, nutrition, elimination, fluid and electrolyte balance, regulatory mechanisms, and sensory functions. Interventions imply recognition of body's response to disease.	Related to sustenal and restorative care needs —the normal and disturbed physiological body processes that are vital to sustaining life.

Stages of Illness[a]	Nursing Problems	Classification and Approach[b]	Nursing Interventions[c]	Criterion Measures[a]
Remedial care needs	12. To identify and accept positive and negative expressions, feelings, and reactions.	Usually overt problems Indirect methods	Measures that are helpful to the client and his family during their emotional reactions to client's illness	Related to rehabilitation needs, particularly those involving emotional and interpersonal difficulties.
	13. To identify and accept the interrelatedness of emotions and organic illness.			
	14. To facilitate the maintenance of effective verbal and nonverbal communication.			
	15. To promote the development of productive interpersonal relationships.			
	16. To facilitate progress toward achievement of personal and spiritual goals.			
	17. To create and/or maintain a therapeutic environment.			
	18. To facilitate awareness of self as an individual with varying physical, emotional, and developmental needs.			
Restorative care needs	19. To accept the optimum possible goals in the light of limitations, physical and emotional.	Overt and/or covert problems Direct and/or indirect methods	Measures that will assist the client and his family to cope with the illness and necessary life adjustment.	Related to sociological and community problems affecting client care.
	20. To use community resources as an aid in resolving problems arising from illness.			
	21. To understand the role of social problems as influencing factors in the cause of illness.			

[a]From Faye G. Abdellah and Eugene Levine, *Better Patient Care Through Nursing Research* (New York: Macmillan Publishing Co., Inc., 1965), pp. 78–79, 280–81.
[b]From Faye G. Abdellah and others, *Patient-Centered Approaches to Nursing* (New York: Macmillan Publishing Co., Inc., 1973), pp. 81–82.
[c]From Joan Haselman Carter and others, *Standards of Nursing Care* (New York: Springer Publishing Co., Inc., 1976), pp. 8–9.

either the nurse or the client. Given that these problems are called *nursing problems,* then it becomes reasonable to conclude that these goals are basically nursing goals.

Using the goals as the framework, a plan is developed and appropriate nursing interventions are determined. Table 9–3 summarizes the kinds of interventions that would be appropriate for the categories of nursing problems. Again, holism tends to be negated in *implementation* because of the isolated, particulate nature of the nursing problems.

Following implementation of the plan, *evaluation* takes place. According to the American Nurses' Association *Standards of Nursing Practice,*[19] the plan is evaluated in terms of the client's progress or lack of progress toward the achievement of the stated goals. This would be extremely difficult if not impossible to do for Abdellah's nursing-problem approach since it has been determined that the goals are *nursing* goals, not *client* goals. Thus, the most appropriate evaluation would be the *nurse's* progress or lack of progress toward the achievement of the stated goals.

Abdellah postulates that criterion measures can be determined from the groupings of the nursing problems, as shown in Table 9–3. A criterion is a value-free name of a measurable variable believed or known to be a relevant indicator of the quality of client care.[20] These criteria can be used to measure client care. Although it is not clear in her writings, the measurement of criteria has been substituted for evaluating a client's progress toward goal achievement.

The use of Abdellah's twenty-one nursing problems in an example might be beneficial. Consider the case of Ron who experienced severe crushing chest pain following a board meeting at his place of business. In addition to the pain, he experienced shortness of breath, tachycardia, and profuse diaphoresis. Upon admission to the hospital, assessment indicated that Ron might have sustained some cardiac damage. Investigation into his history revealed that he has been having episodes of chest pain for the past two months. With this as the data base, the specific problems of pain, impaired cardiac functioning, work-related stress, and failure to seek medical assistance can be identified. These specific problems can be related to selected nursing problems defined by Abdellah, and the nursing problems can be related to the stage of Ron's illness. Nursing strategies and criterion measures can then be determined. Table 9–4 illustrates the implemen-

Table 9–4

An Illustration of the Implementation of Abdellah's Framework in Ron's Care

Stages of Illness	Selected Abdellah Nursing Problems	Classification and Approach	Selected Nursing Interventions	Criterion Measures
Basic to care	1. To maintain good hygiene and physical comfort.	Overt problem of pain Direct and indirect methods	1. Administer oxygen 2. Elevate headrest. 3. Reposition client. 4. Administer prescribed analgesic. 5. Remain with client.	Amount of pain
Sustenal care needs	5. To facilitate the maintenance of a supply of oxygen to all body cells.	Overt problem of impaired cardiac functioning Direct methods	1. Promote rest. 2. Place in sitting position. 3. Promote deep breathing and coughing. 4. Implement exercise program as tolerated.	Vital signs
Remedial care needs	13. To identify and accept the interrelatedness of emotional and organic illness.	Covert problem of effects of work-related stress on cardiac functioning Indirect methods	1. Investigate the nature of his job and activities involved. 2. Explore his work-related goals. 3. Explore the kinds of stress associated with his job.	Knowledge of relationship between stress and his illness
Restorative care needs	20. To use community resources as an aid in resolving problems arising from illness.	Overt problem of failure to seek medical assistance when needed Direct methods	1. Teach early warning signs and symptoms of cardiac distress. 2. Teach course of action should specific symptoms occur.	Knowledge of appropriate use of certain community resources

tation of Abdellah's framework. The results of fractionalizing care can be readily seen by the repetition of intervention strategies for the two problems of pain and impaired cardiac functioning. (This table is in no way designed to be inclusive. Rather, it is offered as an attempt to make the theory operational.)

ABDELLAH'S WORK AND THE CHARACTERISTICS OF A THEORY

In comparing Abdellah's work with the characteristics of a theory presented in Chapter 1, it may be seen that Abdellah's theory has interrelated the concepts of health, nursing problems, and problem-solving as she attempts to create a different way of viewing nursing phenomena (characteristic 1). The result was the statement that nursing is the use of the problem-solving approach with key nursing problems related to the health needs of people. Problem-solving is an activity that is inherently logical in nature (characteristic 2).

Because of the failure of the framework to provide a perspective on humans and society in general, the theory cannot be applied to those who do not have health needs or nursing problems. This may well be intentional as the framework seems to focus quite heavily on nursing practice with individuals. This somewhat limits the ability to generalize, although the problem-solving approach is readily generalizable to clients with specific health needs and specific nursing problems (characteristic 3).

One of the most important questions that arises when considering Abdellah's work is the role of the client within the framework. This question could generate hypotheses for testing and thus demonstrates the ability of Abdellah's work to generate hypotheses for testing (characteristic 4). The results of testing such hypotheses would contribute to the general body of nursing knowledge (characteristic 5).

As a logical and simple statement, Abdellah's problem-solving approach can easily be used by practitioners to guide various activities within their nursing practice. This is especially true when considering nursing practice that deals with clients who have specific needs and specific nursing problems (characteristic 6).

Abdellah's theory is consistent with other theories such as those of Maslow and Henderson. Although this consistency exists, many questions remained unanswered (characteristic 7).

LIMITATIONS

The major limitation to Abdellah's theory and the twenty-one nursing problems is their very strong nursing-centered orientation. With this orientation, appropriate uses might be the organization of teaching content for nursing students and/or the evaluation of student's performance in the clinical area. But in terms of client care, there is little emphasis on what the client is to achieve.

Abdellah's framework is inconsistent with the concept of holism. The classification of the twenty-one nursing problems according to stages of illness and the particulate nature of the problems attests to this. As a result, the client may be diagnosed as having numerous problems that would lead to fractionalized care efforts, and potential problems might be overlooked because the client is not deemed to be in a particular stage of illness.

CONCLUSIONS

Abdellah's theory and framework provide a basis for determining and organizing nursing care. If all of the problems are investigated, the client would be likely to be thoroughly assessed. The problems also provide a basis for organizing appropriate nursing strategies. It is anticipated that by solving the nursing problems, the client would be moved toward health. The nurse's philosophical frame of reference would determine whether this theory and the twenty-one nursing problems could be implemented in practice.

SUMMARY

Using Abdellah's concepts of health, nursing problems, and problem-solving, the theoretical statement of nursing that can be derived is the use of the problem-solving approach with key nursing problems related to the health needs of people. From this framework, twenty-one nursing problems were developed. These problems are compared to Henderson's fourteen components of nursing and Maslow's hierarchy of needs. Ways to utilize the nursing problems in the nursing process are explored. The major limitation of Abdellah's theory is its strong nursing-centered orientation. Some modification of the nursing problems to promote a more client-centered orientation would encourage effective utilization of the theory in professional nursing practice.

NOTES

1. Faye G. Abdellah and others, *Patient-Centered Approaches to Nursing* (New York: Macmillan Publishing Co., Inc., 1960), pp. 24–25.
2. Faye G. Abdellah and others, *New Directions in Patient-Centered Nursing* (New York: Macmillan Publishing Co., Inc., 1973), p. 19.
3. Gertrude Torres and Marjorie Stanton, *Curriculum Process in Nursing: A Guide to Curriculum Development* (Englewood Cliffs, N.J.: Prentice-Hall, Inc., 1982), p. 126.
4. Abdellah and others, *Patient-Centered Approaches*, pp. 6–7.
5. Ibid.
6. Marion E. Nicholls and Virginia G. Wessells, eds., *Nursing Standards and Nursing Process* (Wakefield, Mass.: Contemporary Publishing, Inc., 1977), p. 6.
7. Abdellah and others, *Patient-Centered Approaches*, pp. 30–31.
8. Ibid., pp. 6, 26.
9. Faye G. Abdellah and Eugene Levine, *Better Patient Care Through Nursing Research* (New York: Macmillan Publishing Co., Inc., 1965), p. 492.
10. Abdellah and others, *Patient-Centered Approaches*, p. 26.
11. Ibid., p. 11.
12. Abdellah and others, *New Directions*, p. 79.
13. Abdellah and others, *Patient-Centered Approaches*, p. 27.
14. Virginia Henderson and Gladys Nite, *Principles and Practice of Nursing*, 6th ed. (New York: Macmillan Publishing Co., Inc., 1978), p. 94.
15. Lillian DeYoung, *The Foundations of Nursing* (St. Louis, Mo.: The C. V. Mosby Company, 1976), p. 112.
16. Abraham Maslow, *Motivation and Personality* (New York: Harper & Row, Publishers, Inc., 1954).
17. Abdellah and others, *Patient-Centered Approaches*, pp. 24–25.
18. Ibid., p. 25.
19. Congress for Nursing Practice, *Standards of Nursing Practice* (Kansas City, Mo.: American Nurses' Association, 1973).
20. Doris Bloch, "Criteria, Standards, Norms—Crucial Terms in Quality Assurance," *Journal of Nursing Administration*, 7, no. 7 (September 1977), 22.

ADDITIONAL REFERENCES

BYRNE, MARJORIE L., and LIDA F. THOMPSON, *Key Concepts for the Study and Practice of Nursing.* St. Louis, Mo.: The C. V. Mosby Company, 1972.

CARTER, JOAN HASELMAN, and others, *Standards of Nursing Care.* New York: Springer Publishing Co., Inc., 1976.

10

IDA JEAN ORLANDO

Mary Disbrow Crane

*Ida Jean Orlando Pelletier has had a varied career as a practition-
er, educator, researcher, and consultant in nursing. During the early
part of her career she worked as a staff nurse in such areas as ob-
stetrics, medicine and surgery, and the emergency room. She has
also held supervisory positions and the title of Second Assistant
Director of Nurses. In 1954, she received her M.A. in mental health
consultation from Columbia University, New York. She then went
to Yale University where she became a research associate and prin-
cipal investigator on a project studying the integration of mental
health concepts into the basic curriculum. This led to the publication of her first book,* The Dynamic Nurse-Patient Relationship:
Function, Process, and Principles, *in 1961.[1] She has also served
as director of the graduate program in mental health and psychiatric
nursing at Yale.*

*In 1962, Orlando moved to Massachusetts. She became a clinical
nursing consultant to a psychiatric hospital, McLean Hospital, and
at a veterans' hospital. At McLean Hospital, she carried out the
research that led to the publication in 1972 of her second book,*
The Discipline and Teaching of Nursing Process.[2]

*Since 1972, Orlando has been associated intermittently with Boston
University School of Nursing, teaching nursing theory and super-
vising graduate students in the clinical area. The New England*

158

Board of Higher Education has employed her as a project consultant in their Mental Health Project for Associate Degree Faculties. Her most recent position is as a nurse educator at Metropolitan State Hospital in Waltham, Massachusetts.

Throughout her career, Orlando has been active in a variety of organizations including the Massachusetts Nurses' Association and the Harvard Community Health Plan. She has also lectured and offered workshops and consultation to a wide variety of agencies.

Ida Jean Orlando Pelletier is another significant contributor to the developing body of nursing knowledge. She describes a nursing process based on the interaction at a specific time between a patient and a nurse. Two books present her ideas. Her initial work, *The Dynamic Nurse-Patient Relationship: Function, Process and Principles* was published in 1961.[3] *The Discipline and Teaching of Nursing Process,* showing further refinement of her theory, appeared in 1972.[4]

Orlando's educational background and the work that led her to publish provide insight into the content of her theory. Her advanced nursing preparation and area of teaching responsibility and practice were in mental health and psychiatric nursing. Although she applied her ideas to many nursing speciality areas, her interactive focus is dominant. Her position as an educator also influenced her work. Both of her books were the result of studies designed to improve the teaching of nurses.

The Dynamic Nurse-Patient Relationship was written after the completion of a five-year project at Yale University in the mid-1950s. The purpose of this project, supported by a grant from the National Institute of Mental Health, was "to identify the factors which enhanced or impeded the integration of mental health principles in the basic nursing curriculum."[5] The book describes the curriculum content developed from the study. Its stated purpose is "to offer the professional nursing student a theory of effective nursing practice."[6]

After completing her first book, Orlando refined her ideas and put them into practice at a private psychiatric facility, McLean Hospital in Belmont, Massachusetts. Again with a National Institute of Mental Health grant, she studied an objective means to evaluate her process and training in its discipline. This work, done during the 1960s, led to *The Discipline and Teaching of Nursing Process.*[7] In this book, she is concerned with the specific definition of nursing function and with incorporating nursing activities beyond the nurse-patient relationship into a total nursing system. She also developed more readily measured criteria to guide the nurse in her reaction to patient behavior.*

Orlando's work spans a fertile period of nursing thinking. She was probably influenced by, as well as an influence upon, other nursing theorists. For example, Orlando sounds similar to Nightingale when she states, "It is important for the nurse to concern herself with the patient's distress because the treatment and prevention of disease proceeds best when conditions extraneous to the disease itself and its management do not cause the patient additional suffering."[8] Another nursing theorist, Peplau, published her highly interpersonal theory two years before Orlando began her first study.[9] Henderson also was redefining her definition of nursing during Orlando's first study. Henderson's 1955 definition is consistent with Orlando when she states, "Nursing is primarily assisting the individual . . . in the performance of those activities . . . that he would perform unaided if he had the necessary strength, will or knowledge."[10] Thus the majority of the nursing theorists described in this book published during the time that Orlando was actively working on her theory.

ORLANDO'S KEY CONCEPTS

Certain major concepts are evident in Orlando's theory of nursing. She believes that nursing is *unique* and *independent* because it concerns itself with an *individual's need for help*, real or potential, in an *immediate* situation. The process by which nursing resolves this helplessness is *interactive* and is pursued in a *disciplined* manner that requires *training*.

Throughout her career, Orlando has been concerned with identifying that which is *uniquely* nursing. In her first book she presents principles to guide nursing practice.[11] She feels that the use of general principles from other fields is not sufficient to help the nurse in her interaction with patients. In this book, she identifies nursing's role as follows, "It is the nurse's direct responsibility to see to it that the patient's needs for help are met either by her own activity or by calling in the help of others."[12]

---

*In this chapter, the feminine pronoun is used when referring to the nurse and the masculine pronoun when referring to the patient. This is consistent with Orlando's use of these pronouns and terms.

By the time of her second book, Orlando suggests that nursing's failure to establish its uniqueness results from the lack of a clearly identifiable function.[13] This leads to inadequate care and insufficient attention to the patient's reactions to his immediate experiences. Thus, nursing "is concerned with providing direct assistance to individuals in whatever setting they are found for the purpose of avoiding, relieving, diminishing, or curing the individual's sense of helplessness."[14]

It is this unique function that gives nurses the authority to work *independently*. Orlando recommends that "nurses . . . must radically shift their focus from assistance to physicians and institutions to assisting patients with what they cannot do alone."[15] Physicians' orders are directed to patients, not to nurses. Moreover, at times the nurse may even assist the patient *not* to comply with a medical order. She must also resolve conflicts between the patient's need for help and institutional policies. Nursing's unique function allows nurses to work in any setting where persons experience a need for help that they cannot resolve themselves. Thus, nurses may practice with well or ill persons in an independent practice or in an institutional setting.

Orlando's theory focuses on the patient as an *individual*. Each person is different. Thus, appropriate nursing actions for two patients with the same presenting behavior must be individualized. The nurse cannot automatically act based only on principles, past experience, or physicians' orders. She must first ascertain that her action will meet the specific patient's need for help.

Nursing is concerned with "individuals who suffer or anticipate a sense of helplessness."[16] Orlando defines need as "a requirement of the patient which, if supplied, relieves or diminishes his immediate distress or improves his immediate sense of adequacy or well-being.[17]. In many instances, people can meet their own needs and do not require the help of professional nurses. When they cannot do this, or do not clearly understand these needs, a *need for help* is present. The nurse's function is to correctly identify and relieve this need for help.

The *immediacy* of the nursing situation is a vital concept in Orlando's theory. Each patient's behavior must be assessed to determine whether it expresses a need for help. Furthermore, identical behaviors by the same patient may indicate different needs. The nursing action must also be specifically designed for the immediate encounter. Long-term planning has no part in Orlando's theory except as it pertains to providing adequate staff coverage for a job setting.

Thus, Orlando's process is dynamic. In this area, her theory is consistent with Martha Roger's principles of homeodynamics.[18]

Orlando's nursing process is totally *interactive*. It describes, step by step, what goes on between a nurse and a patient in a specific encounter. A patient behavior causes the process to begin. The process involves the nurse's reaction to this behavior and her consequent action. The nurse shares her reaction with the patient to identify the need for help and the appropriate action. Orlando's principles are meant to guide the nurse at various stages of the interaction. She emphasizes the importance of interaction when she writes, "Learning how to understand what is happening between herself and the patient is the central core of the nurse's practice and comprises the basic framework for the help she gives to patients."[19]

The actual *process* of a nurse-patient interaction is the same as that of any interaction between two persons. When the nurse uses this process in caring for patients, Orlando calls it the "nursing process." It is the tool that the nurse uses to fulfill her function to the patient. In an attempt to extend her theory to encompass all nursing activities, Orlando broadens the use of the process beyond the individual nurse-patient relationship in her book *The Discipline and Teaching of Nursing Process*. She applies the process to contacts between a nurse leader and those she supervises or directs. When used in this manner, she refers to the process as the "directive or supervisory job process in nursing."[20]

If the nursing process is the same as the interactive process between any two individuals, how can nursing call itself a profession? The key is *discipline* in utilization of the process. Orlando provides three criteria to evaluate this discipline. These criteria differentiate an "automatic personal response" from a "disciplined professional response."[21] Only the latter leads to effective nursing care, that is, relief of the patient's sense of helplessness. Learning to employ the process discipline requires *training*. This justifies the need for specific education in nursing. Orlando's nursing process and the criteria for its disciplined use provide the content for the following section.

ORLANDO'S NURSING PROCESS

Orlando's nursing process is based on the "process by which any individual acts."[22] The purpose of the process when used between a nurse and a patient is meeting the patient's need for help. Improvement in the patient's behavior that indicates resolution of the need is the result. The process is also used with other persons working in a job setting. The purpose here is to understand how the professional and job responsibilities of each affect the other. This allows each person to effectively fulfill her professional function for the patient within the organizational setting.

Patient Behavior

The nursing process is set in motion by *patient behavior*. All patient behavior, no matter how insignificant, must be considered as expression of need for help until its meaning to a particular patient in an immediate situation is understood. Orlando stresses this in her first principle: "The presenting behavior of the patient, regardless of the form in which it appears, may represent a plea for help."[23]

When the patient experiences a need that he cannot resolve, a sense of helplessness occurs. The patient's behavior reflects this distress. In *The Dynamic Nurse-Patient Relationship*, Orlando describes some categories of patient's distress. These are "physical limitations, adverse reactions to the setting or experiences which prevent the patient from communicating his needs."[24] Feelings of helplessness due to physical limitations may result from incomplete development, temporary or permanent disability, or restrictions of the environment, real or imagined. Adverse reactions to the setting, on the other hand, usually result from incorrect or inadequate understanding of an experience there. Patients may become distressed from a negative reaction to any aspect of the setting despite its helpful or therapeutic intent. Frequently a need for help may also arise from the patient's inability to communicate effectively. This may be due to such factors as ambivalence concerning dependency brought on by illness, embarrassment related to the need, lack of trust in the nurse, and inability to state the need precisely.

Patient behavior may be verbal or nonverbal. Inconsistency between these two types of behavior may be the factor that alerts the nurse that the patient needs help. Verbal behavior encompasses all the patient's use of language. It may take the form of "complaint, requests, questions, refusals, demands, and comments or statements."[25] Nonverbal behavior includes physiological manifestations such as heart rate, perspiration, edema, and urination; and motor activity such as smiling, walking, and avoiding eye contact. Nonverbal patient behavior may also be vocal. This includes such actions as sobbing, laughing, shouting, and sighing.

Although all patient behavior may indicate a need for help, it may not effectively communicate that need. When it does not, problems in the nurse-patient relationship can arise. Ineffective patient behavior "prevents the nurse from carrying out her concerns for the patient's care or from maintaining a satisfactory relationship to the patient."[26] Ineffective patient behavior may also indicate difficulties in the initial establishment of the nurse-patient relationship, inaccurate identification of the patient's need by the nurse, or negative patient reaction to automatic nursing action. Resolution of ineffective patient behavior deserves high priority as the behavior usually becomes worse over time if the need for help that it expresses remains unresolved.

Nurse Reaction.

The patient behavior stimulates a *nurse reaction*, which marks the beginning of the nursing process. This reaction is comprised of three sequential parts. First, the nurse perceives the behavior through any of her senses. Second, the perception leads to thought. Finally, the thought produces an automatic feeling.[27] For example, the nurse sees a patient smile, thinks he is happy, and feels good. This reaction forms the basis for determining the nursing action. However, the nurse must first share her reaction with the patient to ascertain that she has correctly identified the need for help and the nursing action appropriate to resolve it. Orlando offers a principle to guide the nurse in her reaction to patient behavior. The nurse does not assume that any aspect of her reaction to the patient is correct, helpful, or appropriate until she checks the validity of it in exploration with the patient."[28]

Perception, thought and feeling occur automatically and almost simultaneously. Therefore the nurse must learn to identify each part of her reaction. This helps her to analyze the reaction to determine why she reacted as she did. The process becomes logical rather than intuitive. The nurse is able to use her reaction for the purpose of helping the patient.

The discipline in the nursing process prescribes how the nurse shares her reaction with the patient. Orlando offers a principle to explain the usefulness of this sharing:

Any observation shared and explored with the patient is immediately useful in ascertaining and meeting his need for help or finding out that he is not in need at that time.[29]

She provides the following three criteria to ensure that the nurse's exploration of her reaction with the patient is successful:[30]

1. What the nurse says to the individual in the contact must match (be consistent with) any or all of the items contained in the immediate reaction, and what the nurse does non-verbally must be verbally expressed and the expression must match one or all of the items contained in the immediate reaction.
2. The nurse must clearly communicate to the individual that the item being expressed belongs to herself.
3. The nurse must ask the individual about the item expressed in order to obtain correction or verification from the same individual.

Which aspect of her reaction the nurse shares with the patient is not as important as that it be shared in the manner described in the criteria. From a practical standpoint, it may be more expeditious to share a perception than a thought or feeling. "You are grimacing" contains less assumption than "Are you in pain?" In this way the patient can more easily express his need for help without having to correct the nurse's misconception.

Feelings can and should be shared even when they are negative. The nonverbal action of the nurse will usually show her feelings if they are not verbally expressed. Thus, the nurse's verbal and nonverbal behavior will be inconsistent. Proper sharing of feelings can effectively help the patient to express his need for help. For example, a nurse may react to a patient's refusal of a medication with anger. If she says, "I am angry with your refusal of your medication. Could you explain to me why you have refused?" she invites the patient to explain the need for help that his refusal expressed. Her expression meets the three criteria, and the patient's need for help can be identified and resolved.

This example shows the importance of the nurse sharing her reaction as a fact about herself. She states, "I am angry," rather than, "You make me angry." This clear identification of the reaction as her own reduces the chance of patient misinterpretation. It also encourages the patient to share his reaction in a similar manner.

Adequate identification of the three aspects of the nurse's reaction helps to resolve extraneous feelings that may interfere with the patient's care. The nurse may find that her feelings come from her personal belief of how people should act or from stresses in the organizational setting. These feelings or stresses are unrelated to meeting the patient's need. If they are not resolved, the nurse's verbal and nonverbal behavior will again be inconsistent. This same process should be employed with nurses or other professionals in the job setting to resolve any conflicts that interfere with the nurse fulfilling her professional function for the patient.

Orlando used her three criteria in the study described in *The Discipline and Teaching of Nursing Process* and found that use of the process discipline is positively related to improvement in patient behavior.[31] The study also showed a positive relationship between the nurse's use of the process and its use by the patient.[32] Thus, use of the process alone can help the patient communicate his need more effectively.

Orlando offers a diagram depicting open sharing of the nurse's reaction versus keeping the reaction secret (see Figures 10–1 and 10–2). The nurse action that results from the reaction becomes a behavior stimulating a reaction to the patient. Only openness in sharing of the reaction assures that the patient's need will be effectively resolved. This sharing, in the manner prescribed, differentiates professional nursing practice from automatic personal response.

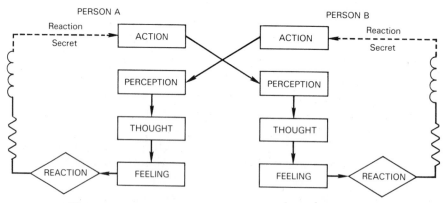

Figure 10-1. The action process in a person-to-person contact functioning in secret. The perceptions, thoughts, and feelings of each individual are not directly available to the perception of the other individual through the observable action. [From Ida Jean Orlando, *The Discipline and Teaching of Nursing Process* (New York: G. P. Putnam's Sons, 1972), p. 26. Used with permission.]

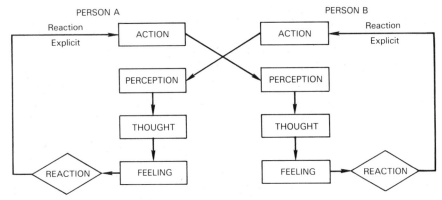

Figure 10-2. The action process in a person-to-person contact functioning by open disclosure. The perceptions, thoughts, and feelings of each individual are directly available to the perception of the other individual through the observable action. [From Ida Jean Orlando, *The Discipline and Teaching of Nursing Process* (New York: G. P. Putnam's Sons, 1972), p. 26. Used with permission.]

Nurse's Action

Once the nurse has validated or corrected her reaction to the patient's behavior through exploration with him, she can complete the nursing process with the *nurse's action*. Orlando includes "only what she [the nurse] says or does with or for the benefit of the patient" as professional nursing action.[33] The nurse must be certain that her action is appropriate to meet the patient's need for help. Orlando's principle guiding nursing action states, "The nurse initiates a process of exploration to ascertain how the patient is affected by what she says or does."[34]

The nurse can act in two ways: automatic or deliberative. Only the second manner fulfills her professional function. Automatic actions are "those decided upon for reasons other than the patient's immediate need," whereas deliberative actions ascertain and meet this need.[35] There is a distinction between the purpose an action actually serves and its intention to help the patient. For example, a nurse administers a sleeping pill because the physician orders it. Carrying out the physician's order is the purpose of the action. However, the nurse has not determined that the patient is having trouble sleeping or that a pill is the most appropriate way to help him sleep. Thus the action is automatic, not deliberative, and the patient's need for help is unlikely to be met.

The following list identifies the criteria for deliberative actions:

1. Deliberative actions result from the correct identification of patient needs by validation of the nurse's reaction to patient behavior.
2. The nurse explores the meaning of the action to the patient and its relevance to meeting his need.
3. The nurse validates the action's effectiveness immediately after completing it.
4. The nurse is free of stimuli unrelated to the patient's need when she acts.

Automatic actions fail to meet one or more of these criteria. Automatic actions are most likely to be done by nurses primarily concerned with carrying out physicians' orders, routines of patient care, or general principles for protecting health or by nurses who do not validate their reactions to patient behaviors.

Professional Function

Nurses often work within organizations with other professionals, and are subject to the authority of the organization that employs them. It is inevitable, therefore, that at times conflicts will arise between the actions appropriate to the nurse's profession and those required by the job. Nonprofessional actions can prevent the nurse from carrying out her professional function, and this can lead to inadequate patient care. A well-defined function of the profession can help to prevent and resolve this conflict.

Nurses should not accept positions that do not allow them to meet their patient's need for help. If a conflict does arise, the nurse must present data to show that nursing is unable to fulfill its professional function. Orlando believes that an employer is unlikely to continue to require job activities that interfere with a well-defined function of a profession. For an agency to do so "would be to completely abandon the whole point of having enlisted the service of that profession in the agency or institution."[36]

Nurses must be constantly aware that their "activity is professional only when it deliberately achieves the purpose of helping the patient."[37] Some automatic activities may be necessary to the running of an institution. These should, however, be kept to a minimum and should be carried out, as much as possible, by support personnel. The nurse must attend to helping the patients resolve any conflict between these routines and their needs for help.

Thus, the nursing process is set in motion by a patient behavior that may indicate a need for help. The nurse reacts to this behavior with perceptions, thoughts, and feelings. She shares an aspect of her reaction with the patient, making sure that her verbal and nonverbal actions are consistent with her reaction, that she identifies the reaction as her own, and that she invites the patient to comment on the validity of her reaction. A properly shared reaction by the nurse helps the patient to use the same process to more effectively communicate his need. Next, an appropriate action to resolve the need is mutually decided upon by the patient and nurse. After the nurse acts, she immediately asks the patient if the action has been effective. Throughout the interaction, the nurse makes sure that she is free of any extraneous stimuli that interfere with her reaction to the patient.

ORLANDO'S THEORY AND THE FOUR MAJOR CONCEPTS

Orlando includes material specific to three of the four major concepts: the human or individual, health, and nursing. The fourth concept, society, is not included in her theory.

She uses the concept of *human* as she emphasizes individuality and the dynamic nature of the nurse-patient relationship.

While *health* is not specified, it is implied. In her initial work, Orlando focused on illness. Later, she indicated that nursing deals with the individual whenever there is a need for help. Thus, a sense of helplessness replaces the concept of health as the initiator of a need for nursing.

Orlando largely ignores *society*. She deals only with the interaction between a nurse and a patient in an immediate situation and speaks to the importance of individuality. She does make some attempt to discuss the overall nursing system in an institutional setting. However, she does not discuss how the patient is affected by the society in which he lives nor does she use society as a focus of nursing action.

Nursing is, of course the focus of Orlando's work. She speaks of nursing as unique and independent in its concerns for an individual's need for help in an immediate situation. The efforts to meet the individual's need for help are carried out in an interactive situation and in a disciplined manner that requires proper training.

COMPARISON OF ORLANDO'S PROCESS AND THE NURSING PROCESS

Orlando's nursing process may be compared with the nursing process described in Chapter 2. Figure 10-3 helps to guide this comparison.

Certain overall characteristics are similar in both processes. For example, both are interpersonal in nature and require interaction between patient and nurse. The patient is asked for input throughout the process. Both processes also view the patient as a total person. He is not merely a disease process or body part. Orlando does not use the term *holistic*, but she effectively describes a holistic approach. Both processes are also used as a method to provide nursing care and as a means to evaluate that care. Finally, both are deliberate intellectual processes.

The *assessment* phase of the nursing process corresponds to the sharing of the nurse reaction to the patient behavior in Orlando's process. The patient behavior initiates the assessment. The collection of data includes only information relevant to identifying the patient's need for help. An ongoing data base is not useful to the immediate situation of the patient. The nurse's reaction, however, is probably influenced somewhat by her past experiences with the patient.

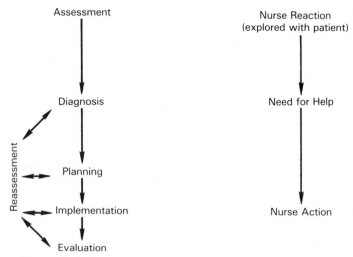

Figure 10-3. Comparison of Orlando's process with the nursing process.

Orlando discusses data collection in her first book, *The Dynamic Nurse-Patient Relationship*. She defines observation as "any information pertaining to the patient that the nurse acquires while she is on duty."[38] Direct data are comprised of "any perception, thought or feeling the nurse has from her own experience of the patient's behavior at any or several moments in time."[39] Indirect data come from sources other than the patient, such as records, other health team members, or the patient's significant others. Both types of data require exploration with the patient to determine their relevance to the specific situation. Both verbal and nonverbal patient behaviors are important. Their consistency or inconsistency is a data piece in itself. This corresponds somewhat with subjective and objective data in the nursing process.

The sharing of the nurse's reaction in Orlando's process has components similar to the analysis in the nursing process. Although the nurse's reaction is automatic, her awareness of it and how she shares it is a deliberate intellectual activity. Orlando's sharing of the reaction, however, is a process of exploration with the patient. The nursing process, on the other hand, makes use of nursing's theoretical base and principles from the physical and behavioral sciences.

The product of the analysis in the nursing process is the *nursing diagnosis*. Exploration of the nurse's reaction with the patient in Orlando's process leads to identification of his need for help. The statement of the nursing diagnosis is a more formal process than that of need. Many nursing diagnoses may be made, given priority ratings, and resolved over time. Since Orlando deals with immediate nurse-patient interaction, only one need is dealt with at a time. Current efforts to develop a taxonomy of nursing diagnosis would be inappropriate in Orlando's theory since each patient encounter is different. Using Orlando's theory, nursing might develop categories of such areas as causes of patient's needs for help. These would, of course, have to be modified to fit the particular patient situation.

The *planning* phase of the nursing process involves writing goals and objectives and deciding upon appropriate nursing action. This corresponds to the nurse's action phase of Orlando's process. Any type of goal beyond the immediate situation is not possible in Orlando's process. Her goal is always relief of the patient's need for help; the objective relates to improvement in the patient's behavior. The nursing process mandates a more formal action of writing and giving priority to goals and objectives.

Both processes require patient participation in determining the appropriate action. In the nursing process this occurs mostly in goal setting. Orlando's process sees the patient as an active participant in determining the actual nurse action. The nursing process, on the other hand, relies more heavily on scientific principles and nursing theories in deciding how the nurse will act.

Implementation involves the final selection and carrying out of the planned action. This is also part of the nurse's action phase of Orlando's process. Both processes mandate that the action be appropriate for the patient as a unique individual. The nursing process expects the nurse to consider all possible effects of the action upon the patient. Orlando's process is concerned only with the effectiveness of the action in resolving the immediate need for help.

Evaluation is inherent in Orlando's action phase of her process. For an action to be deliberative, the nurse must evaluate its effectiveness when it is completed. Failure to do this can result in a series of ineffective actions with failure to meet the patient's need and an increase in the cost of nursing care and materials.

Evaluation in both processes is based on objective criteria. In the nursing process, evaluation asks whether the behaviorally stated objectives were met. In Orlando's process, the nurse observes patient behavior to see whether the patient has been helped. Thus, both processes evaluate in terms of outcomes of care.

Both the nursing process and Orlando's process are described as a series of sequential steps. The steps do not actually occur discretely and in order in either process. As new information becomes available, earlier steps may be repeated. Thus, new assessment data may alter the nursing diagnosis or the plan. Orlando's process is almost a continuous interchange—where patient behavior leads to nurse reaction, which leads to nurse behavior, which leads to patient reaction (see Figures 10–2 and 10–3). Thus, both processes are dynamic and responsive to changes in the patient's situation.

The nursing process used today and Orlando's process have many similarities. They do, however, have important differences. The nursing process is far more formal and has more detailed phases than Orlando's. It requires the nurse to bring her knowledge of scientific principles and nursing theory to guide her behavior. Orlando demands only that the nurse follow the principles she lays down to guide nursing care. Long-term planning is part of the nursing process but is not relevant to Orlando's process. Although both processes call for patient involvement in the process of his care, Orlando's demands this participation more comprehensively.

ORLANDO'S WORK AND THE CHARACTERISTICS OF A THEORY

Can Orlando's work be called a theory of nursing as described in Chapter 1? In the sense of a "vision" of what nursing is, her work certainly qualifies. Does she combine concepts for the purpose of deriving hypotheses about practice? An exploration to see whether Orlando's work meets all of the basic characteristics of a theory helps to answer this question.

Before this is done, a comment on Orlando's use of the term *principle* is appropriate. Principles, as are laws, are truly predictable. They are most useful in the pure sciences. Human beings are too individualistic to be predictable, especially in relation to their behavior. Orlando's principles tell the nurse how to act. They predict only in the general sense that if the nurse uses the principles, the patient's behavior will improve. Thus, *guides for practice* would be a more appropriate term for them than principles.

1. **Theories can interrelate concepts in such a way as to create a different way of looking at a particular phenomenon.** Nursing is the focus of Orlando's work. Her theory views nursing as interacting with an individual in an immediate situation to relieve a sense of helplessness. She does relate concepts into a new and meaningful whole.

2. **Theories must be logical in nature.** Orlando's work does provide a reasonable and sequential process for nursing. Patient behavior initiates the nurse reaction. Exploration of this reaction with the patient leads to identification of a need and of an action to resolve that need. The nurse must react in a carefully prescribed manner to be certain she meets her goal of helping the patient. She must evaluate her action to be certain of its effectiveness. Thus, Orlando provides a logical rather than an intuitive approach to practice.

3. **Theories should be relatively simple yet generalizable.** Although Orlando's theory is simple in nature, it does generalize well to all of nursing practice. The theory remains simple by revolving around the nurse-patient interaction, the basic unit of nursing. This also makes the theory generalizable. This basic unit is applicable re-

gardless of the setting of nursing care or the type of patient receiving care.

4. Theories can be the bases for hypotheses that can be tested. Orlando did derive hypotheses from her theory and tested them. Although her initial study was observational, she tested her ideas in a variety of nursing situations. In her second study, she developed criteria for the nurse's reaction that were specific enough for the development of hypotheses and statistical testing.

5. Theories contribute to and assist in increasing the general body of knowledge within the discipline through the research implemented to validate them. In testing her theory, Orlando added to the general body of nursing knowledge. She was able to test the effectiveness of her process discipline in a nurse's contacts with the patients, staff, and workers she supervises. Her findings showed a positive relationship between use of the process discipline and helpful outcomes of contacts. She also provided support for the idea that the process can be taught in a specified period of time.[40] Although her hypotheses need retesting, they provide a basis for other nurses to develop new theories. Other nursing theorists, such as Orem and Rogers, show consistency with, if not the influence of, aspects of Orlando's work.

6. Theories can be utilized by the practitioners to guide and improve their practice. Orlando has been quite successful in developing a theory useful to practice. Nurses can easily use her principles and process discipline in their interactions with patients and fellow workers. Using her theory, nurses are assured that they will not provide care in a way that is inappropriate for an individual patient. Orlando's theory is more easily applied to practice than that of some of the other nursing theorists. For example, Abdellah's twenty-one nursing problems lend themselves more easily to an educational than a practice setting.[41] However, Orlando's theory does not guide all aspects of nursing practice. Areas for further study include long-term planning, dealing with family and community, and caring for patients who do not recognize that their health is endangered.

7. Theories must be consistent with other validated theories, laws, and principles but will leave open unanswered questions that need to be investigated. Orlando's theory does not conflict with other validated theories if it is viewed in the somewhat limited sense of a nurse-patient interaction. It is most consistent with interaction theory, but systems theory relates to it with difficulty. Orlando does discuss a "system of nursing practice."[42] This encompasses both the nurse-patient interaction and the relationship of nurses among themselves and with others in an organized work setting. She does not, however, view the patient in relation to her subsystem and suprasystem. For this reason, Orlando's theory does not relate well to family theory. The family is mentioned only as a source of indirect data.

Thus, Orlando's work contains many of the characteristics of a theory. Despite her intent, however, it does not provide a comprehensive theory to guide nursing practice. Nonetheless, this deficit does not negate its usefulness in guiding nurse-patient interaction. Nor does it deny its value as a stimulus to other nurses to carry theory development further.

STRENGTHS AND LIMITATIONS

Orlando's theory has much to offer to nursing. The predominant strength of her work is its usefulness in nursing practice. It guides nurses through their interactions with patients. Use of her theory virtually assures that patients will be treated as individuals and that they will have an active and constant input into their own care. The nurse's focus must remain on the patient rather than on the demands of the work setting.

The nurse can keep Orlando in mind while applying the nursing process of today. Use of her theory prevents inaccurate diagnosis or ineffective plans because the nurse has to constantly explore her reactions with the patient. No nurse, following Orlando's principles, could fail to evaluate the care she has given.

Another of Orlando's strengths is her assertion of nursing's independence as a profession and her belief that this independence must be based on a sound theoretical framework. She bases this belief on her definition of nursing function. She believes that this clearly defined function will assist nursing in establishing its independence and in structuring the work setting so that nurses can effectively meet their patients' needs for help. The function of "finding out and meeting the patient's immediate needs for help" is broad enough to encompass nurses practicing in all settings and in all speciality areas.[43] It allows nursing to evolve over time by avoiding a rigid list of nursing activities.

Orlando guides the nurse to evaluate her care in terms of objectively observable patient outcomes. It is not the structure of the setting or the number of nurses on duty that determines effective care. Orlando has found a positive relationship between the use of her process and favorable outcomes of patient behavior. In planning to implement standards for nursing practice, the American Nurses' Association has described patient outcomes as "the ultimate indicators of quality patient care."[44] The immediate and interactive nature of her process does, however, make evaluation a time-consuming process.

Orlando's testing of her theory in the practice setting lends further support to its usefulness. Her first study, published in *The Dynamic Nurse-Patient Relationship,* provided a basis for future work. For a second study, described in *The Discipline and Teaching of the Nursing Process,* she developed specific criteria amenable to statistical testing. Nursing can pursue Orlando's work by retesting and further developing her work.

Although Orlando's ideas contain many of the characteristics of a theory, there are limitations. Her mental health background is probably responsible for the highly interactive nature of her theory. Although this interactive nature is one of the theory's strengths, it also provides limitation in her ideas. Nurses deal extensively with monitoring and controlling the physiological processes of patients to prevent illness and restore health. Orlando scarcely mentions this aspect of the nurse's role. Also the highly interactive nature of Orlando's theory makes it hard to include the highly technical and physical care that nurses give in certain settings such as intensive care units. Her theory does, however, prevent the nurse from forgetting the patient in her efforts to fulfill the technical aspects of her job.

Orlando's theory is also limited by its focus on interaction with an individual, whereas the patient should be viewed as a member of a family and within a community. Often it is vital to deal with the family as a whole to help the patient. Orlando does not deal with these areas.

Long-term care and planning are not applicable to Orlando's focus on the immediate situation. She only views long-term planning as related to adequate staffing within an institution. Orlando herself recognizes this problem. In *The Dynamic Nurse-Patient Relationship* she speculated that "repeated experiences of having been helped undoubtedly culminate over periods of time in greater degrees of improvement."[45] She also identified the cumulative effect of nursing as an area for further study.

In *The Discipline and Teaching of Nursing Process*, Orlando tried to define the entire nursing system. She described this as the "regularly interacting parts of a nursing service."[46] This part of her theory attempts to incorporate nurses' relationships with other nurses and with members of different professions in the job setting. Her theory struggles with the authority derived from the function of the profession and that of the employing institution's commitment to the public. The same process is offered for dealing with others as for working with an individual patient. This part of her process is somewhat confusing. It appears to be more of a description of the administration of nursing services than a theory of nursing practice.

Orlando can be considered a nursing theorist who made a significant contribution to the advancement of nursing practice. She helped nurses to focus on the patient rather than on the disease or institutional demands. The nurse is firmly viewed as the handmaiden of the patient, not of the physician. Nurses must base their practice on logical thinking rather than on intuition. Orlando's nursing process continues to be useful to nurses in their interactions with patients.

SUMMARY

Orlando's nursing process is rooted in the interaction between a nurse and a patient at a specific time and place. A sequence of interchanges involving patient behavior and nurse reaction takes place until the patient's need for help, as he perceives it, is clarified. The nurse, then, decides on an appropriate action to resolve the need in cooperation with the patient. This action is evaluated after it is carried out. If the patient behavior improves, the action was successful and the process is completed. If there is no change or the behavior gets worse, the process recycles with new efforts to clarify the patient's behavior or the appropriate nursing action. Orlando summarizes her process as follows:

> A deliberate nursing process has elements of continuous reflection as the nurse tries to understand the meaning to the patient of the behavior she observes and what he needs from her in order to be helped. Responses comprising this process are stimulated by the nurse's unfolding awareness of the particulars of the individual situation.[47]

NOTES

1. Ida J. Orlando, *The Dynamic Nurse-Patient Relationship: Function, Process and Principles* (New York: G. P. Putnam's Sons, 1961).
2. Ida J. Orlando, *The Discipline and Teaching of Nursing Process* (New York: G. P. Putnam's Sons, 1972).
3. Orlando, *The Dynamic Nurse-Patient Relationship.*
4. Orlando, *The Discipline and Teaching.*
5. Orlando, *The Dynamic Nurse-Patient Relationship*, p. vii.
6. Ibid., p. viii.
7. Orlando, *The Discipline and Teaching.*
8. Orlando, *The Dynamic Nurse-Patient Relationship*, pp. 22–23.
9. Hildegard Peplau, *Interpersonal Relations in Nursing* (New York: G. P. Putnam's Sons, 1952).
10. Bertha Harmer and Virginia Henderson, *Textbook of the Principles and Practice of Nursing*, 5th ed. (New York: Macmillan Publishing Co., Inc., 1955), p. 4.
11. Orlando, *The Dynamic Nurse-Patient Relationship.*
12. Ibid., p. 22.
13. Orlando, *The Discipline and Teaching*, p. 4.
14. Ibid., p. 12.
15. Ida O. Pelletier, "The Patient's Predicament and Nursing Function," *Psychiatric Opinion*, February 1967, p. 28.
16. Orlando, *The Discipline and Teaching*, p. 12.
17. Orlando, *The Dynamic Nurse-Patient Relationship*, p. 5.
18. Martha E. Rogers, "Nursing: A Science of Unitary Man," in *Conceptual Models for Nursing Practice*, 2nd ed., Joan P. Riehl and Callista Roy, eds. (East Norwalk, Conn.: Appleton-Century-Crofts, 1980).
19. Orlando, *The Dynamic Nurse-Patient Relationship*, p. 4.
20. Orlando, *The Discipline and Teaching*, p. 29.
21. Ibid., p. 31.
22. Ibid., p. 24.
23. Orlando, *The Dynamic Nurse-Patient Relationship*, p. 40.
24. Ibid., p. 14.
25. Ibid., p. 37.
26. Ibid., p. 78.
27. Orlando, *The Discipline and Teaching*, p. 25.
28. Orlando, *The Dynamic Nurse-Patient Relationship*, p. 56.
29. Ibid., pp. 35–36.
30. Orlando, *The Discipline and Teaching*, pp. 29–30.
31. Ibid., p. 114.
32. Ibid.
33. Orlando, *The Dynamic Nurse-Patient Relationship*, p. 60.
34. Ibid., p. 67.

35. Ibid., p. 60.
36. Orlando, *The Discipline and Teaching*, p. 16.
37. Orlando, *The Dynamic Nurse-Patient Relationship*, p. 70.
38. Ibid., p. 31.
39. Ibid., p. 32.
40. Orlando, *The Discipline and Teaching*, p. viii.
41. Faye G. Abdellah and others, *Patient-Centered Approaches to Nursing* (New York: Macmillan Publishing Co., Inc., 1960).
42. Orlando, *The Discipline and Teaching*, p. 18.
43. Ibid., p. 20.
44. Congress of Nursing Practice, *A Plan for Implementation of the Standards of Nursing Practice* (Kansas City, Mo.: American Nurses' Association, 1975), p. 16.
45. Orlando, *The Dynamic Nurse-Patient Relationship*, p. 90.
46. Orlando, *The Discipline and Teaching*, p. 18.
47. Orlando, *The Dynamic Nurse-Patient Relationship*, p. 67.

11

MYRA ESTRIN LEVINE

Mary Kathryn Leonard

Myra E. Levine received her nursing education in three institutions: Cook County School of Nursing, Chicago; B.S., University of Chicago; and M.S.N., Wayne State University, Detroit, Michigan. Her nursing experience includes staff nursing, adminstrative and teaching supervision, clinical instruction, and direction of nursing services. She was Chairman of the Department of Clinical Nursing at Cook County School of Nursing. She has also held positions as Associate Professor and Professor of Nursing, College of Nursing, University of Illinois, Chicago; faculty member at Loyola University School of Nursing, Chicago; and Director of Continuing Education, Evanston Hospital, Evanston, Illinois.

Mrs. Levine is the author of a number of articles that have been published in nursing journals and of one book dealing with nursing (see references at end of chapter). In 1965 she presented a paper at the Regional Clinical Conferences sponsored by the American Nurses' Association. This paper, "Trophicogenosis: An Alternative to Nursing Diagnosis," can be found in the American Nurses' Association publication Exploring Progress in Medical-Surgical Nursing Practice, *New York, 1966, vol. 2. In addition, Mrs. Levine has participated in a number of workshops and conferences.*

Gratitude is expressed to Connie Hetrick Esposito for her contribution to this chapter in the first edition.

She is a member of Sigma Theta Tau (Alpha Beta Chapter, Loyola University), a Charter Fellow of the American Academy of Nursing, and an honorary member of the American Mental Health Aid to Israel. She is listed in Who's Who of American Women *and received the Elizabeth Russell Belford Award for Education from Sigma Theta Tau in 1977.*

Within a framework of total patient care, Levine has developed four conservation principles that serve as the basis of her nursing theory. These principles seek to conserve energy, structural integrity, personal integrity, and social integrity. This theory focuses the nurse's intervention on the patient's adaptation and response to illness.*

This chapter will include a discussion of Levine's theory of nursing, its application to the nursing process, and the relationship of the concepts of individual, society/environment, health, and nursing. A case study is included to demonstrate the application of this theory. A brief discussion of the historical basis of this theory is also included.

HISTORICAL BASIS

Nursing practice and health care are continuously changing, and some of the most significant changes occurred prior to the development of Levine's theory of nursing. Many of these changes have occurred in response to, or at least parallel to, significant contributions and discoveries made in the sciences and humanities. Thus a brief discussion of the highlights of this evolution may help the reader to develop a better appreciation for the contribution Levine has made to the practice of nursing.

Nightingale theorized that nursing should focus on providing the individual with a supportive environment to enhance nature's work of healing.[1] At that time, great emphasis was placed on the great healing concept. The basis of this concept was that nature would take its course and healing would occur. Many believed that this was true, but there were still other elements that impacted on sickness and healing. The answer to the missing piece was thought by some to be the germ theory. The germ theory identified a direct relation-

*The terms *intervention* and *patient* are consistent with Levine's terminology.

ship between germs and disease or illness. Although Nightingale never fully accepted the germ theory, nursing followed the lead of medicine and began to focus on disease causation and treatment. Nursing education focused on skill training for the implementation of procedures and treatments.

Research continued and the theory of multiple factors was introduced. This theory had as its premise that illness was the result of a combination of factors rather than just a germ.[2] Maslow's theory of the hierarchy of needs lent support to the theory of multiple factors because Maslow's theory suggested that the healthy individual must sufficiently satisfy increasingly more complex physiological and psychological needs.[3]

The emphasis in nursing changed from focusing solely on physiological needs and skill training to meeting the psychological needs of the patients in addition to the physical needs. This more balanced approach to patient care became known as the concept of total patient care. Lydia Hall is credited with the introduction of this concept.[4]

The importance of the totality (i.e., physiological and psychological aspects) of the person was further elaborated and defined in the concept of holism. The concept of holism, best exemplified by the systems theory premise that the whole is greater than the sum of its parts, and the proposition of a health-illness continuum, which suggests the existence of a sliding scale of health conditions ranging from health to illness, influenced significantly the development of the unified theory of health and disease.[5] Nursing has retained its focus on total patient care. Levine, influenced by the concept of holism and the unified theory of health and disease, developed her own theory of nursing to facilitate the delivery of total patient care to a population of people (patients) who were not at the healthy end of the health-illness continuum.

LEVINE'S THEORY OF NURSING

Levine views nursing as a dynamic, purposeful process. Her definition includes a description of what nursing is, how it accomplishes its purpose, and what its purpose is. She believes nursing is a *discipline*, the basis of which is people's dependence on their relationship with other people.[6] This discipline includes nursing interventions to support or promote the patient's adjustment.[7] Further, she states that the essence of nursing is human interaction.[8]

Assumptions

Levine's theory makes assumptions about: (1) the condition in which the patient enters the health care setting, (2) the responsibilities of the nurse in the situation and as each relates to the nurse-patient interaction, and (3) the functions of the nurse in the situation. These assumptions provide structure and definition to this theory of nursing.

Condition.   Levine has limited the focus of her theory to those patients entering the health care system in a state of illness or altered health.

Responsibilities.   Levine holds the nurse accountable for recognizing the patient's organismic response to an altered health state. Organismic response is change(s) in behavior or change(s) in level of functioning of the body exhibited by the patient adapting or attempting to adapt to the environment. This environment includes his/her illness and the nurse. There are four levels of organismic response identified by Levine. These are: (1) response to fear, (2) inflammatory response, (3) response to stress, and (4) sensory response.[9]

Functions.   The functions of the nurse include: (1) intervening to promote the patient's adaptation to the state of illness, and (2) evaluating the intervention as being supportive or therapeutic. *Supportive nursing interventions* help to maintain the patient's present state of altered health and to prevent further health deterioration. Nursing interventions that promote healing and restoration of health are referred to as *therapeutic interventions*.

Conservation Principles

Levine has identified four conservation principles that serve as the foundation for all nursing interventions. According to her theory, the goal of nursing is to maintain or restore a person to a state of health by conserving energy, structural integrity, personal integrity, and social integrity: (1) *Conservation of energy* refers to balancing energy output and energy input to avoid excessive fatigue, i.e., adequate rest, nutrition, and exercise. (2) *Conservation of structural integrity* refers to maintaining or restoring the structure of the body, i.e., prevention of physical breakdown and the promotion of healing. (3) *Conservation of personal integrity* refers to maintenance or restoration of the patient's sense of identity and self-worth, i.e., acknowledgement of uniqueness. (4) *Conservation of social integrity* refers to the acknowledgment of the patient as a social being. It involves the recognition and presence of human interaction, particularly with the patient's significant others.[10] Conservation in Levine's theory means to keep together or maintain a proper balance.[11] The purpose of the conservation is to maintain the unity and integrity of the patient, and thus the health of the person.

Critical Components

A brief summary of the critical components of Levine's theory of nursing are: (1) the patient is in the predicament of illness, (2) the patient's environment includes the nurse, (3) the nurse must recognize the organismic manifestation of the patient's adaptation to illness, and (4) the nurse must make an intervention in the patient's environment based on the four conservation principles and must evaluate the intervention as therapeutic or supportive.[12]

The following is a simplified example of how Levine's theory could be utilized.

Situation.   Mrs. H. is brought to the emergency room by her husband. She is experiencing severe chest pain, shortness of breath, nausea, and numbness in her left arm. Based on these data (organismic response), the nurse recognizes Mrs. H. is attempting to adjust to an altered state of health. Using the principles of conservation as the theoretical base, the nurse intervenes in Mrs. H.'s environment (see Table 11–1).

The nurse observes Mrs. H.'s response to the nursing interventions to determine how she is adjusting to her altered state of health. Mrs. H.'s chest pain is subsiding and her shortness of breath is relieved with the administration of oxygen via nasal cannula. Mrs. H. is settling into the coronary care unit (CCU) with her husband at

TABLE 11-1

Application of Levine's Theory to a Given
Example

Intervention	Conservation Principle	Therapeutic/ Supportive	Rationale
1. Mrs. H. is put on a stretcher with her head elevated.	1. Energy	1. Supportive	1. Limit the expenditure of energy.
2. Mrs. H. is given an injection of morphine.	2. (a) Energy (b) Structural integrity	2. (a) Supportive (b) Therapeutic	2. (a) To relieve pain and reduce energy expenditure. (b) Decreased pain reduces the oxygen needs of the body, thereby reducing the work load demands on the heart.
3. Mrs. H. is to receive oxygen. She is given a choice of how she prefers to receive it, by nasal cannula or face mask.	3. (a) Structural integrity (b) Personal integrity	3. (a) Supportive/ Therapeutic (b) Supportive	3. (a) Maintain an adequate oxygen supply to reduce labored breathing. (b) Maintain in-dividuality and autonomy.
4. Mrs. H.'s husband accom-panies her to CCU.	4. Social integrity	4. Supportive	4. Provide Mrs. H. with a sup-port system during transfer process.

her side. Based on these and other observations, the nurse decides what further nursing interventions are needed.

LEVINE'S THEORY AND THE FOUR MAJOR CONCEPTS

In the first chapter of this book, the concepts basic to nursing are identified as the human or individual, society/environment, health, and nursing. Levine's theory of nursing relates to each of these concepts.

Levine stresses the need to view the *individual* holistically, which implies that the individual is a complex being. Her definition of nursing is based on the idea that the individual is dependent on his/her relationship with others. The dimensions of this dependence are implied in her delineation of the four conservation principles, i.e., energy needs and expenditures, structural integrity, social integrity, and personal integrity. Individuals are dependent to some extent on others for all aspects of survival: food, safety, recreation, and affiliation. Levine expects the nurse (1) to be aware of the complexities of these interactions, and (2) to support the maintenance or restoration of these relationships when the patient is in an altered state of health. The normal balance is disrupted by the illness, and the patient in an attempt to adjust to the stress of illness may exhibit behavior changes that alter his/her level of functioning. The nurse must assume responsibility in assisting the patient to adapt to these changes in a positive or health-fostering manner.

The *society/environment* implications in Levine's theory are important. The essence of Levine's definition of nursing is human interaction, and her use of the concepts of adaptation and organismic response are highly suggestive of a systems approach. In systems theory, environment is important. Levine also explicitly states that the nurse is part of the patient's environment. Since Levine's theory is individual-oriented, one could assume that the patient's family and/or significant others are also included in the patient's environment. Thus society is viewed broadly as being composed of the environment that the patient experiences at any time. However, the specific environmental context of this theory is the health care system.

One can also assume that Levine's implied definition of *health* is the maintenance of the unity and integrity of the patient. The holistic view of the patient is essential to the application of this theory.

An altered state of health is not restricted to just the impairment of physiological functioning (conservation of structural integrity), but can be viewed as an alteration or need related to any of the four conservation principles. Thus her theory applies only to individuals in an illness state, which restricts the focus of nursing care. Nursing care is directed toward the maintenance or restoration of health. Only in discussing the whole social system does Levine make reference to preventive health practices as being desirable or worth pursuing.[13]

Levine's theory relates to the concept of *nursing* in that it offers an approach to the giving of nursing care. Nursing is viewed as a discipline. A nurse must possess both skills and a theoretical and scientific knowledge base. Levine's theory is heavily grounded in the humanities and sciences; an underlying belief is that people are dependent on their relationships with other people. Nursing care is a process in which interventions are based on the assessment of the patient using the conservation principles, recognizing behavioral changes and/or changes in the level of functioning of the patient in his/her attempt to adapt to illness. Interventions are evaluated in terms of their impact on the health state of the patient.

LEVINE'S THEORY AND THE NURSING PROCESS

Levine's theory for nursing parallels many elements of the nursing process. According to Levine, the nurse must observe the patient, decide on an appropriate intervention, perform it, and then evaluate its usefulness in helping the patient. Also, Levine's theory assumes the nurse and patient will participate together in the patient's care. However, the nursing process described in Chapter 2 emphasizes more mutuality between the patient and the nurse than is implied in Levine's theory.

In Levine's theory, the patient is assumed to be in a dependent position, which may restrict the patient's ability to participate in the data gathering, planning, and/or implementation phases of the nursing process. As a result of this dependent position, the patient is in need of nursing assistance to help in adapting to a state of health. The nurse must assume responsibility for determining the extent to which the patient is able to participate in his/her care. The nursing process, on the other hand, does not necessarily assume the client is in a dependent position.

In the *assessment* phase, the patient is assessed using two methods: interviewing and observation. The focus is on the patient; the family and/or significant others are only considered from the perspective of how they might help or interfere with the patient's well-being. The needs of the family and/or significant others are not considered in relation to the patient. According to Levine, if a family member's needs are going to be dealt with, that person must become the target of the assessment.

In performing the holistic assessment, the nurse uses Levine's four conservation principles as an assessment guide. The nurse is concerned with the patient's balance of energy and maintenance of integrity. Thus, the nurse collects data about the patient's energy sources, i.e., nutrition, sleep-rest, leisure, coping patterns, significant relationships, medications, environment, and expenditures of energy, i.e., the functioning of various body systems, emotional and/or social stresses, and work patterns. In addition, data are collected about the patient's structural integrity, i.e., body defenses and physical body structure; personal integrity (patient's self-system), i.e., uniqueness, values, religious beliefs, and economic resources; and social integrity, i.e., decision-making processes of the patient, the patient's relationships with others, and his/her involvement in social/community affairs.

After the collection of all the data, the nurse critically analyzes the data to obtain a holistic view of the patient. This analysis reflects the patient's balance of strengths and weaknesses in each of the four assessment areas (conservation principles). The analysis also identifies areas needing further data collection. In the analysis, concepts and theories from other disciplines are also considered. Levine's theory has a close kinship to Maslow's hierarchy of needs and Selye's stress theory.[14] A parallel can be drawn between the hierarchy of needs and the conservation principles. Conservation of structural integrity deals with physiologic needs. Energy conservation deals with both physiologic and safety needs. Maslow's belonging and love needs are dealt with through the conservation of personal integrity, and needs for self-esteem are dealt with in the conservation of social integrity.[15] In Selye's stress theory, there is a stressor that stimulates a response as part of the general adaptation syndrome. In Levine's theory, illness is the stressor and the patient is continually trying to adapt to this changed state. This adaptation is manifested in the patient's organismic response, which includes changes in behavior or levels of functioning of the body.

Levine's theory also supports the work and beliefs of Florence Nightingale in relation to her concept of environment (see Chapter 3). Nursing has the responsibility of providing a supportive environment, one that is conducive to health and healing. In Levine's theory, the nurse is part of the patient's environment.

From the analysis, the nurse develops a *nursing diagnosis*. Since the patient is in a state of illness or altered health, the nursing diagnosis will reflect a problem or potential problem related to a deficit or a threatened deficit in one of the four areas of conservation. Levine's theory does not make provision for health promotion needs/teaching. The provision for health promotion is limited to areas directly related to the patient's present problem(s) associated with the illness and/or state of altered health. Therefore, it may be concluded that the nurse utilizing this theory has a time orientation in the present. Thus the nurse is not concerned with future planning except as it relates to the patient's present problem.

In the *planning* phase, which includes goal setting, the nursing process emphasizes the mutuality of this activity between nurse and patient. Levine, however, has not specifically indicated or stressed the need for mutual goal setting. It may be concluded that mutuality is not necessary initially for the application of this theory in the clinical setting. The bases of this assumption are: (1) the dependent position of the patient as a result of the state of illness and/or altered health with need for nursing assistance; and (2) the nurse's responsibility to monitor the patient's condition in order to regulate the balance between nursing intervention and patient participation in care. The nurse, as an individual, may include the patient in this activity based on the nurse's assessment of the patient's ability to participate in the goal-setting activity. In order for these goals to be workable, the nurse states the goal in behavioral terms so it is measurable. The goals reflect an attempt to help the patient adapt and reach a state of health.

Also, in the *planning* phase, the nurse uses the goal (1) to determine the strategies to be used in the plan and (2) to determine the extent to which the plan must be developed to meet the goal. Levine indicated the nurse bases practice on knowledge. Thus, the steps of the nursing plan would be based on principles, laws, concepts, and theories from the sciences and humanities. Also in developing the plan, the nurse considers the patient's ability to participate in the plan of care, and the patient's degree of participation is identified. During the planning phase, the nurse may consult with other health care team members.

As the plan of care is *implemented*, the nurse observes the patient for an organismic response. Data are collected for later use in the evaluation phase. During the implementation phase, the nurse is responsible for the care given to the patient. Levine's theory indicates that (1) the nurse is expected to possess the skill necessary to carry out the nursing interventions, and (2) the nursing interventions are aimed at supporting or promoting the patient's adaptation.

In the *evaluation* phase, the nurse considers the organismic response of the patient to the nursing action. The nurse uses the data collected about the patient's organismic response to determine if the nursing intervention was therapeutic or supportive. If the intervention was therapeutic, the patient is adapting and is progressing toward a state of health.

Levine's theory lends itself to use in the nursing process. However, one must remember that in using Levine's theory, the focus of the process is on one person, the time orientation is the present and/or short-term future, and the patient is in an altered or impaired state of health and in need of nursing intervention.

LEVINE'S WORK AND THE CHARACTERISTICS OF A THEORY

The first characteristic of a theory is that it can interrelate concepts in such a manner as to create a different way of looking at a particular phenomenon. This is true of Levine's ideas about nursing. The concepts of illness, adaptation, nursing interventions, and evaluation of nursing interventions are combined to look at nursing care in a different way (perhaps a more comprehensive view incorporating total patient care) from previous times.

A theory must be logical in nature (characteristic 2). Levine's ideas about nursing are organized in such a way as to be sequential and logical. They can be used to explain the consequences of nursing actions. There are no major contradictions apparent in her ideas.

Levine's ideas are relatively simple and may be partially generalized (characteristic 3). However, in Levine's theory, generalizability is limited by the focus on illness so that the theory is not applicable in all settings where nursing care is delivered today—particularly those settings concerned with health promotion and disease prevention.

A theory is the basis for development of hypotheses that can be tested (characteristic 4). Levine's ideas can be tested. Hypotheses can be derived from them. The principles of conservation are specific enough to be testable. For example, it is possible to test if physiologic structure is being supported or improved, thus testing the principle of conservation of structural integrity. However, more sophisticated research techniques would be needed to test if the patient's social integrity is being supported or improved.

The fifth characteristic is that a theory contributes to and assists in increasing the general body of knowledge within the discipline through the research implemented to validate it. Since Levine's ideas have not yet been widely researched, it is hard to determine if there is a contribution to the general body of knowledge within the discipline.

Chapter 1 indicates the most significant characteristic of a theory is its usefulness to the practitioner (characteristic 6). Levine's ideas can be used by practitioners to guide and improve their practice. These ideas lend themselves to use in practice, particularly in the acute care setting.

The last characteristic of a theory is that it must be consistent with other validated theories, laws, and principles. Levine's ideas seem to be consistent with other theories, laws, and principles, particularly those from the humanities and sciences, and many questions are left unanswered that would be worthy of investigation.

Since Levine's ideas meet five of the seven characteristics of a theory, one might consider them as a framework of nursing.

CONCLUSIONS

Levine's theory for nursing focuses on one person—the patient. In utilizing this theory, the nurse is concerned with the patient's family and/or significant others only to the point that they influence or have an effect on the patient's progress. Thus, the utilization of this theory is limited. This theory could not be used in working with families, groups, or communities.

Levine's theory recognizes nursing as a professional practice based on scientific knowledge and skill. Her theory implies that nursing is considered as an independent practice profession. No mention is made about the relationship of nursing to the other health care professions. This theory does not make provisions for preventive teaching or anticipatory guidance, which are now considered to be nursing functions. These limitations may influence the collaboration with other health care team members. Continuity of care and long-range planning for the patient are limited by the omission of anticipatory guidance and preventive teaching in the area of health promotion. As mentioned before, provisions are made for anticipatory guidance and health teaching only as they relate to the patient's present illness.

Levine's theory for nursing is compatible with the practice of nursing in an acute care setting. The theory emphasizes the dependent position of the patient, the patient's impaired state of health, the patient's limited participation in his/her own care, and the increased responsibility of the nurse in directing and coordinating the patient's care. Thus, one might assume that these conditions are most likely to exist in a critical care unit or in an emergency care area. Levine's theory may offer some limitations when used in areas where the focus is on long-term care and rehabilitation. The time orientation is to the present or short-term future. A present-time orientation limits the attention that can be focused on health promotion and illness prevention. The practice of preventive health care and more specifically health promotion assume an interest in or a concern for anticipating future needs. Thus, in a program or course that is health-oriented and concerned with health promotion with clients in a state of wellness, Levine's theory would be philosophically incompatible.

Levine's theory speaks to the patient's sense of personal integrity, i.e., autonomy and uniqueness. In the illness state, the patient is placed in a dependent position. This placement of the patient may clearly threaten the individual's sense of autonomy. This is a particular area of concern. In this theory, the nurse has the responsibility for determining the patient's ability to participate in the care given and for maintaining the balance between this participation and nursing intervention. If the perceptions of the nurse and the patient about the patient's ability to participate in care do not match, then this mismatch will be an area of conflict. From this placement of the client in a dependent position, one may conclude that the client is not viewed as a member of the health care team. Also, one may question if Levine's theory is not incongruent. If an individual has personal integrity, can the individual be given limited autonomy or be placed in a dependent position?

Finally, Levine's theory reflects the current beliefs about the holistic nature of humanity. However, within the theory there is some obscurity about definitions of the conservation principles, particularly social integrity. The utility of this theory for nursing restricts the practice to an acute care setting, and more specifically, to the critical care or specialty units.

SUMMARY

In Levine's theory of nursing, nursing is human interaction. This is based on the idea that people are dependent on their relationships with others. The nurse has the responsibility to intervene in the patient's situation after recognizing the patient's organismic response. Nursing interventions are supportive (maintain the status quo) or therapeutic (promote healing and restoration). The nurse's interventions are based on the four conservation principles. These are: (1) conservation of energy, (2) conservation of structural integrity, (3) conservation of personal integrity, and (4) conservation of social integrity. These conservation principles provide a guideline for viewing the individual in a holistic manner.

Levine's theory does relate to the concepts of individual, society/environment, health, nursing, and to the nursing process. Its major limitations relate to its focus on the individual in an illness state, and on the dependency of the patient.

NOTES

1. Myra Estrin Levine, *Introduction to Clinical Nursing*, 2nd ed. (Philadelphia: F. A. Davis Co., 1973), pp. 4–5.
2. Ibid., p. 5.
3. A. H. Maslow, *Motivation and Personality* (New York: Harper & Row, Publishers, Inc., 1954).
4. Lydia Hall, "Nursing—What is it?" *Virginia State Nurses' Association*, Winter 1959.
5. Levine, *Introduction to Clinical Nursing*, pp. 6–7.
6. Ibid.
7. Ibid., p. 13.
8. Ibid., p. 1.

9. Myra E. Levine, "The Pursuit of Wholeness," *American Journal of Nursing*, 69, no. 1 (January 1969), 95–96.
10. Levine, *Introduction to Clinical Nursing*, pp. 14–18.
11. Ibid., pp. 13–14.
12. Ibid., pp. 1–3.
13. Ibid., p. 18.
14. Maslow, *Motivation and Personality*; and Hans Selye, *The Stress of Life* (New York: McGraw-Hill Book Company, 1956), pp. 31–33.
15. Marjorie L. Byrne and Lida F. Thompson, *Key Concepts for the Study and Practice of Nursing* (St. Louis, Mo.: The C. V. Mosby Company, 1972), pp. 1–10; and Maslow, *Motivation and Personality*.

ADDITIONAL REFERENCES

HIRSCHFELD, MIRIAM J., "The Cognitively Impaired Older Adult," *American Journal of Nursing*, 76, no. 12 (December 1976), 1981–84.

LEVINE, MYRA E., "Adaptation and Assessment: A Rationale for Nursing Intervention," *American Journal of Nursing*, 66, no. 11 (November 1966), 2450–53.

————, "Holistic Nursing," *Nursing Clinics of North America*, 6, no. 2 (June 1971), 253–64.

————, "The Intransigent Patient," *American Journal of Nursing*, 70, no. 10 (October 1970), 2106–11.

————, "The Four Conservation Principles of Nursing," *Nursing Forum*, 6, no. 1 (1967), 45–59.

NURSING DEVELOPMENT CONFERENCE GROUP, *Concept Formalization in Nursing: Process and Product*. Boston: Little, Brown & Company, 1973.

12

Dorothy E. Johnson

Marie L. Lobo

Dorothy Johnson was born in Savannah, Georgia, in 1919. Her Bachelor of Science in Nursing was from Vanderbilt University, Nashville, Tennessee, and her Masters in Public Health from Harvard. She began publishing her ideas about nursing soon after graduation from Vanderbilt. Most of her teaching career was at the University of California, Los Angeles. She retired as Professor Emeritus, January 1, 1978, and is currently residing in Florida.

Dorothy Johnson has been influencing nursing through her publications since the 1950s.[1] Throughout her career Johnson has stressed the importance of research-based knowledge about the effect of nursing care on clients. Johnson was an early proponent that nursing was a science as well as an art and that nursing had a body of knowledge that reflected both the science and the art. From the beginning, Johnson proposed that the knowledge of the science of nursing that was necessary for effective nursing care included a synthesis of key concepts drawn from basic and applied sciences.[2]

In 1961, Johnson proposed that nursing care facilitated the client's maintenance of a state of equilibrium.[3] Johnson proposed that clients were "stressed" by a stimulus of either an internal or external nature. These stressful stimuli created such disturbances, or "tensions," in the client/patient that a state of disequilibrium occurred. Johnson identified two areas of foci for nursing care based on returning the client to a state of equilibrium. First, nursing care should reduce stimuli that are stressors, and second, "nursing care should provide support of the client's 'natural' defenses and adaptive processes."[4]

In 1968, Johnson first proposed her model of nursing care as the fostering of "the efficient and effective behavioral functioning in the patient to prevent illness."[5] The patient/client is identified as a behavioral system with multiple subsystems. At this point Johnson began to integrate concepts related to systems models into her work. Johnson's integration of systems concepts into her work was further illustrated by her statement of belief that nursing was "concerned with man as an integrated whole and this is the specific knowledge of order we require."[6] Not only did nurses need to care for the "whole" client but the generation of nursing knowledge needed to take a course in the direction of concern with the entire needs of the client.

In the mid to late 1970s, several nurses published conceptualizations of nursing based on Johnson's behavioral systems model. Grubbs, Holaday, Skolny and Riehl, Damus, and Auger are some of the authors who have interpreted Johnson.[7] Roy and Wu and others were sharing their beliefs about nursing at the same time, and Johnson's influence, as their professor, is clearly reflected in their works.[8] In 1980, Johnson published her conceptualization of the "Behavioral System Model for Nursing." This is the first work published by Johnson that explicates her definitions of the behavioral system model.[9] Her evolution in the development of this complex model is clearly demonstrated in the progression of her ideas from works published in the 1950s to her latest available work published in 1980.*

DEFINITION OF NURSING

Johnson developed her behavioral system model for nursing from a philosophical perspective "supported by a rich, sound and rapidly expanding body of empirical and theoretical knowledge."[10] From her early beliefs, which focused on the impaired individual, Johnson

*See note 1 at the end of this chapter.

evolved a much broader definition of nursing. By 1980, she defined nursing as "an external regulatory force which acts to preserve the organization and integration of the patient's behavior at an optimal level under those conditions in which the behavior constitutes a threat to physical or social health, or in which illness is found."[11] Based on this definition, the four goals of nursing are to assist the patient to become a person:[12]

1. Whose behavior is commensurate with social demands.
2. Who is able to modify his behavior in ways that support biologic imperatives.
3. Who is able to benefit to the fullest extent during illness from the physician's knowledge and skill.
4. Whose behavior does not give evidence of unnecessary trauma as a consequence of illness.

ASSUMPTIONS OF THE BEHAVIORAL SYSTEM MODEL

There are several layers of assumptions that Johnson makes in the development of her conceptualization of the behavioral system model. Assumptions are made about the system as a whole as well as about the subsystems. Another set of assumptions deals with the knowledge base necessary to practice nursing.

As with Rogers and Roy, Johnson believes that nurses need to be well grounded in the physical and social sciences.[13] Particular emphasis should be placed on the knowledges in areas from both the physical and social sciences that are found to influence behavior. Thus, Johnson believes it would be equally important to have information available on endocrine influences on behavior as well as on psychological influences on behavior.

In developing assumptions about behavioral systems, Johnson was influenced by Buckley, Chin, and Rapport, early leaders in the development of systems concepts. Johnson cites Chin as the source for her first assumption about systems. In constructing a behavioral system, the assumption is made that there is "organization, interaction, interdependency and integration of the parts and elements (Chin, 1961) of behavior that go to make up the system."[14] It is the interrelated parts that contribute to the development of the whole.

The second assumption about systems also evolves from the work of Chin. A system " 'tends to achieve a balance among the various forces operating within and upon it' (Chin, 1961), and that man strives continually to maintain a behavioral system balance and steady state by more or less automatic adjustments and adaptations to the 'natural' forces impinging upon him."[15] The individual is continually presented with situations in everyday life that require the individual to adapt and adjust. These adjustments are so natural that they occur without conscious effort by the individual.

The third assumption about a behavioral system is that a

> behavioral system, which both requires and results in some degree of regularity and constancy in behavior, is essential to man; that is to say, it is functionally significant in that it serves a useful purpose, both in social life and for the individual.[16]

The patterns of behavior characteristic of the individual have a purpose in the maintenance of homeostasis by the individual. The development of behavioral patterns that are acceptable to both society and the individual foster the individual's ability to adapt to minor changes in the environment.

The final assumption about the behavioral system is that the "system balance reflects adjustments and adaptations that are successful in some way and to some degree."[17] Johnson acknowledges that the achievement of this balance may and will vary from individual to individual. At times this balance may *not* be exhibited as behaviors that are acceptable or meet society's norms. What may be adaptive for the individual in coping with impinging forces may be disruptive to society as a whole. However, most individuals are flexible enough to be in some state of balance that is "functionally efficient and effective" for them.[18]

The integration of these assumptions by the individual provides the behavioral system with the patterns of action to form "an organized and integrated functional unit that determines and limits the interaction between the person and his environment and establishes the relationship of the person to the objects, events and situations in his environment."[19] The function of the behavioral system then is to regulate the individual's response to input from the environment so that the balance of the system can be maintained.

There are four assumptions made about the structure and function of each subsystem. These four assumptions are the "structural elements" common to each of the seven subsystems. The first assumption is "from the form the behavior takes and the consequences it achieves can be inferred what *drive* has been stimulated or what *goal* is being sought."[20] The ultimate goal for each subsystem is expected to be the same for all individuals. However, the methods of achieving the goal may vary depending on culture or other individual variations.

The second assumption is that each individual has a "predisposition to act, with reference to the goal, in certain ways rather than in other ways."[21] This predisposition to act is labeled "set" by Johnson. The concept of "set" implies that despite having only a few alternatives from which to select a behavioral response, the individual will rank those options and chose the option considered most desirable.

The third assumption is that each subsystem has a repertoire of choices or "scope of action" alternatives available from which choices can be made.[22] Johnson subsumes under this assumption that larger behavioral repertoires are available to more adaptable individuals.[23] As life experiences occur, individuals add to the number of alternative actions available to them. However, at some point, the acquisition of new alternatives of behavior decreases as the individual is comfortable with the available repertoire. The point at which the individual loses the desire or ability to acquire new options is not identified by Johnson.

The fourth assumption about the behavioral subsystems is that they produce observable outcomes; that is, the individual's behavior.[24] The observable behaviors allow an outsider—in this case the nurse—to note the actions the individual is taking to reach a goal related to a specified subsystem. The nurse can then evaluate the effectiveness and efficiency of these behaviors in assisting the individual in reaching one of these goals.

In addition, each of the subsystems has three functional requirements. First, each subsystem must be "*protected* from noxious influences with which the system cannot cope."[25] Second, each subsystem must be "*nurtured* through the input of appropriate supplies from the environment."[26] Finally, each subsystem must be "*stimulated* for use to enhance growth and prevent stagnation."[27] As long as the subsystems are meeting these functional requirements, the system and the subsystems are viewed as self-maintaining and self-perpetuating. The internal and external environments of the system need to remain orderly and predictable for the system to maintain homeostasis or remain in balance. The interrelationships of the structural elements of the subsystem are critical for each subsystem to function at a maximum state. The interaction of the structural elements allows the subsystem to maintain a balance that is adaptive to that individual's needs.

An imbalance in a behavioral subsystem produces "tension," which results in disequilibrium. The presence of tension resulting in an unbalanced behavioral system requires the system to increase energy usage to return the system to a state of balance.[28] Nursing is viewed as a part of the external environment that can assist the client to return to a state of equilibrium or balance.

JOHNSON'S BEHAVIORAL SYSTEM MODEL

Johnson believes each individual has patterned, purposeful, repetitive ways of acting that comprise a behavioral system specific to that individual. These actions or behaviors form an "organized and integrated functional unit that determines and limits the interaction between the person and his environment and establishes the relationship of the person to the objects, events and situations in his environment."[29] These behaviors are "orderly, purposeful and predictable . . . [and] sufficiently stable and recurrent to be amenable to description and explanation."[30] Johnson identifies seven subsystems within the behavioral system model. This identification of seven subsystems is at variance with others who have published interpretations of Johnson's model. Johnson states that the seven subsystems identified in her 1980 publication are the only ones to which she subscribes and recognizes they are at variance with Grubb.[31] These seven subsystems were originally identified in Johnson's 1968 paper presented at Vanderbilt University.[32] The seven subsystems are considered to be interrelated, and changes in one subsystem affect all of the subsystems.

Johnson's Seven Behavioral Subsystems

The *attachment or affiliative* subsystem is identified as the first response system to develop in the individual. The optimal functioning of the affiliative subsystem allows "social inclusion, intimacy and the formation and attachment of a strong social bond."[33] Attachment to a significant care giver has been found to be critical for the survival of an infant. As the individual matures, the attachment to the caretaker continues and there are additional attachments to other significant individuals as they enter both the child's and the adult's network. These "significant others" provide the individual with a sense of security.

The second subsystem identified by Johnson is the *dependency* subsystem. Johnson distinguishes the dependency subsystem from the attachment or affiliative subsystem. Dependency behaviors are "succoring" behaviors that precipitate nurturing behaviors from other individuals in the environment. The result of dependency behavior is "approval, attention or recognition and physical assistance."[34] It is difficult to separate the dependency subsystem from the affiliative or attachment subsystem because without someone invested in or attached to the individual to respond to that individual's dependency behaviors, the dependency subsystem has no animate environment in which to function.

The *ingestive* subsystem relates to the behaviors surrounding the intake of food.[35] It is related to the biological system. However, the emphasis for nursing, from Johnson's perspective, is the meanings and structures of the social events surrounding the occasions when food is eaten. Behaviors related to the ingestion of food may relate more to what is socially acceptable in a given culture than to the biological needs of the individual.

The *eliminative* subsystem relates to behaviors surrounding the excretion of waste products from the body.[36] Johnson admits this may be difficult to separate from a biological systems perspective. However, as with behaviors surrounding the ingestion of food, there are socially acceptable behaviors for the time and place for humans to excrete waste. Human cultures have defined different socially acceptable behaviors for excretion of waste, but the existence of such a pattern remains from culture to culture. Individuals who have gained physical control over the eliminative subsystem will control those subsystems rather than behave in a socially unacceptable manner. For example, biological cues are often ignored if the social situation dictates it is objectionable to eliminate wastes at a given time.

The *sexual* subsystem reflects behaviors related to procreation.[37] Both biological and social factors affect behaviors in the sexual subsystem. Again, the behaviors are related to culture and will vary from culture to culture. Behaviors will also vary according to the gender of the individual. The key is that the goal in all societies has the same outcome—behaviors acceptable to society at large.

The *aggressive* subsystem relates to behaviors concerned with protection and self-preservation. Johnson views the aggressive subsystem as one that generates defensive responses from the individual when life or territory is being threatened.[38] The aggressive subsystem does not include those behaviors with a primary purpose of injuring other individuals.

Finally, the *achievement* subsystem provokes behaviors that attempt to control the environment. Intellectual, physical, creative, mechanical, and social skills achievement are some of the areas that Johnson recognizes.[39] Other areas of personal accomplishment or success may also be included in this subsystem.

JOHNSON'S BEHAVIORAL SYSTEM MODEL AND THE FOUR MAJOR CONCEPTS

Johnson views *human beings* as having two major systems, the biological system and the behavioral system. It is the role of medicine to focus on the biological system, whereas nursing's focus is the behavioral system. There is recognition of the reciprocal actions that occur between the biological and behavioral systems when some type of dysfunction occurs in one or the other of the systems.

Society relates to the environment in which an individual exists. According to Johnson, an individual's behavior is influenced by all the events in the environment. Cultural influences on the individual's behavior are viewed as profound. However, it is felt that there are many paths, varying from culture to culture, that influence specific behaviors in a group of people, although the outcome for all of the groups or individuals is the same.

Health is a "purposeful, adaptive response, physically, mentally, emotionally, and socially, to internal and external stimuli in order to maintain stability and comfort."[40] Johnson's behavioral model supports that the individual is attempting to maintain some balance or equilibrium. The individual's goal is to maintain the entire behavioral system efficiently and effectively, but with enough flexibility to return to an acceptable balance if a malfunction disrupts the original balance.

Nursing has a primary goal that is to foster equilibrium within the individual. This allows for the practice of nursing with individuals at any point in the health-illness continuum. Nursing implementations may focus on alterations of a behavior that is not supportive to maintaining equilibrium for the individual. In earlier works, Johnson focused nursing on impaired individuals. By 1980, she says that nursing is concerned with the organized and integrated whole, but that the major focus is on maintaining a balance in the behavioral system when illness occurs in the individual.[41]

JOHNSON'S BEHAVIORAL SYSTEM AND THE NURSING PROCESS

Johnson's behavioral system model easily fits the nursing process model. Grubbs developed an assessment tool based on Johnson's seven subsystems, plus a subsystem she labeled "restorative," which focused on activities of daily living.[42] Activities of daily living are considered to include such areas as patterns of rest, hygiene, and recreation. A diagnosis can be made related to insufficiencies or discrepancies within a subsystem or between subsystems. Planning for the implementation of nursing care should start at the subsystem level with the ultimate goal of effective behavioral functioning of the entire system. Implementations by the nurse present to the client an external force for the manipulation of the subsystem back to the state of equilibrium. Evaluation of the result of this implementation is readily possible if the state of "balance" that is the goal has been defined during the planning phase that occurs before the implementation.

Assessment

In the assessment phase of the nursing process, questions related to specific subsystems are developed. Holaday, Small, and Damus propose that the assessment focus on the subsystem related to the presenting health problem.[43] An assessment based on the behavioral subsystems does not easily permit the nurse to gather detailed information about the biological systems. Assessment questions related to the affiliative subsystem might focus on the presence of a significant other or on the social system of which the individual is a member. In the assessment of the dependency subsystem, attention is placed on understanding how the individual makes needs known to significant others, so the significant others in the environment can assist the individual in meeting those needs. Assessment of the ingestive subsystem would examine patterns of food and fluid intake, including the social environment in which the food and fluid are ingested. The eliminative subsystem generates questions related to patterns of defecation and urination and the social context in which the patterns occur. The sexual subsystem assessment would include information about sexual patterns and behaviors. The aggressive subsystem generates questions about how individuals protect themselves from perceived threats to safety. Finally, the achievement subsystem allows for assessment of how the individual changes the environment to facilitate the accomplishment of goals.

There are many gaps in information about the whole individual if only Johnson's behavioral system model is used to guide the assessment. There is little physiological data on the individual's present or past health status. The exception might be when an impaired health state is demonstrated in the ingestive or eliminative subsystems. Family interaction and patterns are only touched on in the affiliative and dependency subsystems. Basic information relating to education, socioeconomic status, and type of dwelling is tangentially related to most of the subsystems. However, these factors are not clearly identified as an important aspect of any of the subsystems.

Diagnosis

Diagnosis using Johnson's behavioral system model becomes cumbersome. Diagnosis tends to be general to a subsystem rather than specific to a problem. Grubbs has proposed four categories of nursing diagnoses derived from Johnson's behavioral system model.[44]

1. Insufficiency—a state which exists when a particular subsystem is not functioning or developed to its fullest capacity due to inadequacy of functional requirements.
2. Discrepancy—a behavior that does not meet the intended goal. The incongruency usually lies between the action and the goal of the subsystem, although the set and choice may be strongly influencing the ineffective action.
3. Incompatibility—the goals or behaviors of two subsystems in the same situation conflict with each other to the detriment of the individual.
4. Dominance—the behavior in one subsystem is used more

than any other subsystem regardless of the situation or to the detriment of the other subsystems.

It is difficult to evaluate whether these diagnostic classifications are Johnson's or if they are an extension of Johnson's work by Grubbs.

Planning and Implementation

Planning for implementation of the nursing care related to the diagnosis may be difficult because of the lack of client input into the plan. The plan will focus on the nurse's action to modify client behavior. These plans then have a goal, to bring about homeostasis in a subsystem, based on the nurse's assessment of the individual's drive, set, behavioral repertoire, and observable behavior. The plan may include protection, nurturance, or stimulation of the identified subsystem.

Planning and implementation for clients based on Johnson's behavioral system model would focus on maintaining and/or returning an individual's subsystem to a state of equilibrium. Implementation would focus on achieving the goals of nursing.* Although Johnson refers to biological systems in her goals of nursing, they are not included in her behavioral system model and can and do produce incongruities for the planning and implementation of nursing care in relation to a specific diagnosis.

Evaluation

Evaluation is based on the attainment of a goal of balance in the identified subsystems. If base-line data are available for the individual, the nurse may have a goal for the individual to return to the base-line behavior. If the alterations in behavior that are planned do occur, the nurse should be able to observe the return to previous behavior patterns.

There is little or no recognition by either Johnson or Grubbs of the client's input into plans for nursing implementation. They use the term of *nursing intervention*. Holaday's example of implementation also does not contain strong client input.[45] Using Johnson's behavioral system model with the nursing process is a nurse-centered

*See page 197

activity, with the nurse determining the client's needs and the state of behavior appropriate to those needs.

Holaday demonstrates the flexibility available in the use of the Johnson behavioral system model with the nursing process by using a very specific assessment tool to determine appropriate "interventions."[46] Holaday used tests of cognitive development developed by Piaget to determine the level of information to present to a child during a preoperative teaching session.

An example of the use of the nursing process with Johnson's behavioral system model is demonstrated with Johnny Smith, age 6 weeks, brought into the clinic for a routine checkup. He presents with no weight gain since his checkup at age 2 weeks. His mother states she feeds him but he does not seem to eat much. He sleeps 4 to 5 hours between feedings. His mother holds him in her arms without making trunk-to-trunk contact. As the assessment is made the nurse notes that Mrs. Smith never looks at Johnny and never speaks to him. She states he was a planned baby but that she never "realized how much work an infant could be." She says her mother told her she was not a good mother because Johnny is not gaining weight like he should. She states she had not called the nurse when she knew Johnny was not gaining weight because she thought the nurse would think she was a "bad mother" just like her own mother thought she was a "bad mother."

Based on the information available and using the Johnson behavioral system model, assessment would focus on the affiliative and dependency subsystems. The assessment of the affiliative subsystem would focus on the specific behaviors manifested by Johnny to indicate attachment to his mother. The assessment of the dependency subsystem would focus on the specific behaviors manifested by Johnny to cue his mother to his needs. Because of the nature of his problem, a decision is made to use a tool that specifically focuses on parent-infant interaction during a feeding situation. Thus the Nursing Child Assessment Feeding Scale is used during a feeding that takes place at a normal feeding time for Johnny.[47] Johnny cries at the beginning of the feeding and turns toward his mother's hand when she touches his cheek. Mrs. Smith does not speak to Johnny, or in any verbal way acknowledge his hunger. When Johnny slightly chokes on some formula, she does not remove the bottle from his mouth. Mrs. Smith does not describe any of the environment to Johnny, nor does she stroke his body or make eye contact with him. Johnny does not reach out to touch his mother nor does he make any vocalizations. The assessment scale indicates that both mother and baby are not cueing each other at a level where they can respond appropriately.

The diagnoses based on this assessment, using Johnson's behavioral system model, are, "insufficient development of the affiliative subsystem" and "insufficient development of the dependency subsystem." Based on these diagnoses, nursing implementations would focus on increasing Mrs. Smith's awareness of the meaning of Johnny's infrequent cues. By increasing her awareness of the meaning of his cues, she can begin to reinforce them so that he begins to know there is someone in the environment who cares about him, thus fostering his attachment to her. Further assistance needs to be given in assisting Mrs. Smith in communicating with her infant. If further assessment indicates Mrs. Smith is uncomfortable talking with an infant who does not respond with words, it may be suggested that she read to Johnny from a book, thus providing him with needed verbal stimulation. Another implementation may include the nurse placing herself in Johnny's role and "talking" for him to his mother. The nurse may sit, watching Mrs. Smith hold Johnny, and say such things as "I like it when you pat me," "It feels good when you cuddle me," "When I turn my head like this, I'm hungry."

Evaluation of these implementations would be based on two criteria. First, Johnny's weight gains or losses would be carefully assessed. Not gaining weight would place him in a life-threatening situation; therefore it is critical that a pattern of weight gain be initiated. Second, the mother-infant interaction could be reassessed, again using the Nursing Child Assessment Feeding Scale, which would allow for comparison of the first observation with a series of subsequent observations.

JOHNSON'S WORK AND THE CHARACTERISTICS OF A THEORY

Johnson states that she is presenting a model related to subsystems of the human being that have observable behaviors leading to specific outcomes, although the method of attaining the specific outcomes may vary according to the culture of the individual. The characteristics of a theory discussed in Chapter 1 are that theories must (1) interrelate concepts to create a different way of viewing a particular phenomenon, (2) be logical in nature, (3) be relatively simple yet generalizable, (4) be the bases for testable hypotheses, (5) contribute to the general body of knowledge of the discipline, (6) be utilized to guide and improve practice, and (7) be consistent with other validated theories, laws, and principles while allowing the investigation of unanswered questions. Using these as a guide, it is clear that Johnson has indeed developed a model. Johnson's behavioral system model is based on general system concepts. However, the definitions related to the terms used to label her concepts have not been made explicit by Johnson. Grubbs has presented her definitions of Johnson's terms and those are the definitions most often reflected in the literature of other investigators claiming to use Johnson's model.[48]

Johnson does not clearly interrelate her concepts of subsystems comprising the behavioral system model. Thus the logic of her work is difficult to follow. Also the definitions of the concepts are so abstract that they are difficult to use. For example, intimacy is identified as an aspect of the affiliative subsystem, but the concept is not defined or described. An advantage of the abstract definition is that individuals utilizing the model may identify an assessment tool that most specifically fits a problem and use it in their work. There are two major disadvantages. First, the abstract level and multiplicity of definitions make it difficult to compare the same subsystem across studies. Second, the lack of clear definitions for the interrelationships among and between the subsystems makes it difficult to view the entire behavioral system as an entity.

It is difficult to test Johnson's model by the development of hypotheses. Subsystems of the model can be examined, but the lack of definitions and connections of the subsystems makes hypothesis testing difficult.

Johnson's behavioral model can be generalized across the life span and across cultures. However, the focus on the behavioral system may make it difficult for nurses working with physically impaired individuals to utilize the model. Also, Johnson's model is very individual-oriented, so that nurses working with groups of individuals with similar problems would have difficulty using the model. The subsystems in Johnson's behavioral system model are individual-oriented to such an extent that the family can only be considered as the environment in which the individual presents behaviors and not as the focus of care.

Johnson's behavioral system model provides a framework for organizing human behavior. However, it is a different framework than that provided by other nursing theorists, such as Roy or Rogers.[49]

Johnson believes that she is the first person to view "man as a behavioral system." Others have viewed the behavioral subsystem as just one piece of the biopsychosocial human being. Johnson's framework does contribute to the general body of nursing knowledge but needs further development.

Johnson does not clearly define the expected outcomes when one of the subsystems is being affected by nursing implementation. An implicit expectation is made that all humans in all cultures will attain the same outcome—homeostasis. Because of the lack of definitions, the model does not allow for control of the areas of interest, so it is difficult to use the model to guide practice. The authors reportedly using the model to guide practice have not integrated the subsystems to the degree necessary to label this model a theory. In general, the Johnson behavioral system model does not meet the criteria for a theory. However, it must be stressed that Johnson does not suggest that she has developed a theory, although other nurse scholars have identified and utilized Johnson as a theorist.

Johnson's behavioral system model is based on principles of general system theory. Her statements on the multiple modes of attaining the same subsystem goal, regardless of culture, are an example of the principle of "equifinality." As with Rogers, this allows individuals to develop and change through time at unique rates but with the same outcomes at the end of the process: mature, adult behaviors that are culturally acceptable.[50]

Johnson's behavioral system model is not as flexible as Rogers' concept of homeodynamics or Roy's adaptation model.[51] Rogers' concepts are so broadly applicable that nursing care can take place at any level, individual, family, or community. All systems within the human being can be considered for the focus of nursing implementations. With Roy's model, the focus is still at the individual level, but the total human being can be considered. Roy's assumptions include that the human being is a biopsychosocial being.[52] This allows for all of the subsystems of a human being to be included for nursing assessment and implementation.

Johnson's behavioral system model is congruent with many of the nursing models in the belief that the individual is influenced by the environment. Since Nightingale first presented her beliefs about nursing, nurses have been concerned with the individual's relationship with the environment.[53] In practice, nurses often have the necessary control over the environment to promote a healthier state for the individual.

Summary

Although Johnson's behavioral system model has many limitations, she does provide a frame of reference for nurses concerned with specific client behaviors. It must also be noted that Johnson, through her work at the University of California, Los Angeles, has had a profound influence on the development of nursing models and nursing theories. Through her position as a faculty member she influenced Roy, Grubbs, Holaday, and others. As a peer she influenced Riehl, Neuman, Wu, and others, scholars who have generated many ideas about nursing concepts and theories.

Johnson's behavioral system model is a model of nursing care that advocates the fostering of efficient and effective behavioral functioning in the patient to prevent illness. The patient/client is identified as a behavioral system composed of seven behavioral subsystems. The seven behavioral subsystems are affiliative, dependency, ingestive, eliminative, sexual, aggressive, and achievement. Each subsystem is composed of four structural characteristics. These characteristics are drive, set, choices, and observable behaviors. The three functional requirements for each subsystem include: protection from noxious influences, provision for a nurturing environment, and stimulation for growth. An imbalance in any of the behavioral subsystems results in disequilibrium. It is nursing's role to assist the client to return to a state of equilibrium.

NOTES

1. Dorothy E. Johnson, "The Nature of a Science of Nursing," *Nursing Outlook*, 7, no. 5 (May 1959), 291–94; "The Significance of Nursing Care," *American Journal of Nursing*, 61, no. 11 (November 1961), 63–66; "One Conceptual Model of Nursing," paper presented April 25, 1968, Vanderbilt University, Nashville, Tennessee; "Theory in Nursing: Borrowed and Unique," *Nursing Research*, 17, no. 3 (May-June 1968), 206–9; "Development of Theory: A Requisite for Nursing as a Profession," *Nursing Research*, 23, no. 5 (September-October 1974), 372–77; "The Behavioral System Model for Nursing," in *Conceptual Models for Nursing Practice*, 2nd ed., Joan P. Riehl and Callista Roy, eds. (East Norwalk, Conn.: Appleton-Century-Crofts, 1980), 207–16.
2. Johnson, "The Nature of a Science of Nursing," p. 292.
3. Johnson, "The Significance of Nursing Care."
4. Ibid., p. 66.

5. Johnson, "One Conceptual Model of Nursing," p. 2.
6. Johnson, "Theory in Nursing: Borrowed and Unique," p. 207.
7. Judy Grubbs, "The Johnson Behavioral System Model," in *Conceptual Models for Nursing Practice*, Joan P. Riehl and Callista Roy, eds. (New York: Appleton-Century-Crofts, 1974); Bonnie Holaday, "Implementing the Johnson Model for Nursing Practice," in *Conceptual Models for Nursing Practice*; Mary Ann Skolny and Joan P. Riehl, "Hope: Solving Patient and Family Problems by Using a Theoretical Framework," in *Conceptual Models for Nursing Practice*; Karla Damus, "An Application of the Johnson Behavioral System Model for Nursing Practice," in *Conceptual Models for Nursing Practice*; Jeanine R. Auger, *Behavioral Systems and Nursing* (Englewood Cliffs, N. J.: Prentice-Hall, Inc., 1976).
8. Sister Callista Roy, "The Roy Adaptation Model," in *Conceptual Models for Nursing Practice*; and Ruth Wu, *Behavior and Illness* (Englewood Cliffs, N.J.: Prentice-Hall, Inc., 1973).
9. Johnson, "The Behavioral System Model for Nursing."
10. Ibid., p. 207.
11. Ibid., p. 214.
12. Ibid., p. 207.
13. Martha Rogers, *The Theoretical Basis for Nursing* (Philadelphia: F. A. Davis Co., 1970); and Callista Roy, "The Roy Adaptation Model," in *Conceptual Models for Nursing Practice*.
14. Ibid., p. 208.
15. Ibid.
16. Ibid.
17. Ibid.
18. Ibid., p. 209.
19. Ibid.
20. Ibid., p. 210.
21. Ibid., p. 210–11.
22. Ibid., p. 211.
23. Ibid.
24. Ibid.
25. Ibid., p. 212.
26. Ibid.
27. Ibid.
28. Johnson, "One Conceptual Model of Nursing," p. 4.
29. Johnson, "The Behavioral System Model for Nursing," p. 209.
30. Ibid.
31. Ibid., p. 214.
32. Johnson, "One Conceptual Model of Nursing."
33. Johnson, "The Behavioral System Model for Nursing," p 212.
34. Ibid., p. 213.

35. Ibid.
36. Ibid.
37. Ibid.
38. Ibid.
39. Ibid.
40. Ruth Beckman Murray and Judith Proctor Zentner, *Nursing Concepts for Health Promotion* (Englewood Cliffs, N.J.: Prentice-Hall, Inc. 1979), pp. 5–6.
41. Johnson, "One Conceptual Model of Nursing" and "The Behavioral System Model for Nursing."
42. Grubbs, "The Johnson Behavioral System Model."
43. Bonnie Holaday, "Implementing the Johnson Model for Nursing Practice"; Beverly Small, "Nursing Visually Impaired Children with Johnson's Model as a Conceptual Framework," in *Conceptual Models for Nursing Practice*; Karla Damus, "An Application of the Johnson Behavioral System Model for Nursing Practice."
44. Grubbs, "The Johnson Behavioral System Model," pp. 240–41.
45. Holaday, "Implementing the Johnson Model," 1980.
46. Ibid.
47. Kathryn E. Barnard, "Nursing Child Assessment Feeding Scale," University of Washington, Seattle, 1978.
48. Grubbs, "The Johnson Behavioral System Model."
49. Roy, "The Roy Adaptation Model" and Rogers, *The Theoretical Basis of Nursing.*
50. Rogers, *The Theoretical Basis of Nursing.*
51. Ibid.; and Roy, "The Roy Adaptation Model."
52. Roy, "The Roy Adaptation Model."
53. Florence Nightingale, *Notes on Nursing* (Philadelphia: J. B. Lippincott Company, 1859).

ADDITIONAL REFERENCES

HARDY, MARGARET E., "Theories: Components, Development, Evaluation," *Nursing Research*, 23, no. 2 (March-April 1974), 100–107.

JOHNSON, DOROTHY E., "Behavioral System Model for Nursing." Supplemental materials for Nursing Theorists General Session, the Second Annual Nurse Education Conference, December 4–6, 1978.

KAPLAN, ABRAHAM, *The Conduct of Inquiry*, New York: Thomas Y. Crowell Company, Inc., 1964.

NEUMAN, BETTY, "The Betty Neuman Health-Care Systems Model: A Total Person Approach to Patient Problems," in *Conceptual Models for Nursing Practice*, 2nd ed., Joan P. Riehl and Callista Roy, eds. East Norwalk, Conn.: Appleton-Century-Crofts, 1980.

NEWMAN, MARGARET, *Theory Development in Nursing*. Philadelphia: F. A. Davis Co., 1979.

ROGERS, MARTHA E., "Nursing, A Science of Unitary Man," in *Conceptual Models for Nursing Practice*, 2nd ed., Joan P. Riehl and Callista Roy, eds. East Norwalk, Conn.: Appleton-Century-Crofts, 1980.

STEVENS, BARBARA J., *Nursing Theory: Analysis, Application, Evaluation*. Boston: Little, Brown & Company, 1979.

YURA, HELEN, and MARY WALSH, *The Nursing Process*, 3rd ed. East Norwalk, Conn.: Appleton-Century-Crofts, 1978.

13

MARTHA E. ROGERS

Suzanne M. Falco and Marie L. Lobo

Martha E. Rogers was born in Dallas, Texas, May 12, 1914, the eldest of four children. Her family heritage includes many active women suffragists and a strong belief in the necessity of a college education. Before entering the Knoxville General Hospital School of Nursing, she attended the University of Tennessee in Knoxville from 1931 to 1933. She received her diploma in 1936, a B.S. in public health nursing from George Peabody College, Nashville, Tennessee, in 1937; an M.A. in public health nursing supervision from Teachers College, Columbia University, New York, in 1945; and an M.P.H. in 1952 and a Sc.D. in 1954, both from Johns Hopkins University.

Following numerous leadership and staff positions in community health nursing, she moved into higher education as a visiting lecturer and then as a research associate. For twenty-one years, Dr. Rogers was Professor and Head of the Division of Nurse Education at New York University. Since 1975 she has continued to teach at the University and is Professor Emeritus there.

Dr. Rogers has been active in numerous professional organizations, has received many awards and honors, and has published extensively in numerous nursing journals. She has authored several books.

As a humanistic science dedicated to compassionate concern for maintaining and promoting health, preventing illness, and caring for and rehabilitating the sick and disabled, nursing historically has meant service to humanity. Throughout nursing's evolution, from the earliest ages to the present, nurturance of the human race has been an ever-present and central concern.[1] Over the years, the scientific extension of people's centuries-long interest in life and its many manifestations have become integral components of nursing. Thus, the history of humanity is reflected in the evolutionary development of nursing. Consequently, Martha Rogers believes that knowledge of the past is a necessary foundation for the present understanding of nursing, and for evolving the theories and principles that must guide nursing practice.[2]

The concept that human life is valuable did not develop until people had begun to band together into tribes, villages, and towns. Such communal living allowed for sharing of work and responsibility and the provision of mutual support. This more settled life style made it possible for mothers to keep their newborns and care for more children.[3] Thus, partly out of love and partly out of need, human beings began to develop strong feelings about and concern for fellow human beings.

As culture developed and more complex concepts in economic, political, and social structures increased, the value of human life increased. Science, art, and religion brought a growing awareness of one's fellow human beings. The Hebrews developed a monotheistic faith, while the Greeks contributed philosophy, politics, and government. Humanism was becoming strongly entrenched in culture. Following the rise of Christianity, the medieval world was dominated by the Christian religions whose members assumed the responsibility for nursing. With the Dark Ages came a decline in religious, cultural, and political life. The end of this period led to the beginning of modern science.[4]

As modern science evolved, new ideas mushroomed into new discoveries. The nature of the universe was explored. Descartes established the basis of modern philosophy. Einstein's theory of relativity brought a fourth dimension in the coordinate of space-time to man's previously three-dimensional world. Space research has multiplied scientific knowledge and has altered life style. The reality of these evolutionary changes is reflected in man's growing complexity.

As a result of these factors, the rate at which society has been storing up useful knowledge about humanity and the universe has been spiraling upward for the past 10,000 years.[5] This vast store-house of knowledge coupled with a high degree of humanism and value for life has made advancement of nursing through scientific means and theoretical development a reality.

ROGERS'S DEFINITION OF NURSING

Capitalizing on the knowledge base gained from anthropology, sociology, astronomy, religion, philosophy, history, and mythology, Rogers, in 1970, developed a conceptual framework for nursing. Since human beings are at the center of nursing's purpose, this conceptual framework for nursing looks at the total individual and is strongly based in general system theory. *Nursing*, then, is a humanistic and a humanitarian science directed toward describing and explaining the human being in synergistic wholeness and in developing the hypothetical generalizations and predictive principles basic to knowledgeable practice. The science of nursing is a science of humanity—the study of the nature and direction of human development.[6]

BASIC ASSUMPTIONS

Underlying the conceptual framework developed by Rogers are five assumptions about human beings.[7] First, the human being is a unified whole possessing an individual integrity and manifesting characteristics that are more than and different from the sum of the parts. The distinctive properties of the whole are also significantly different from those of its parts. Extensive knowledge of the subsystems is ineffective in enabling one to determine the properties of the living system—the human being. The human being is visible only when particulars disappear from view. Because of this wholeness, the individual's life process is a dynamic course that is continuous, creative, evolutionary, and uncertain, resulting in highly variable and constantly changing patterning.

Second, it is assumed that the individual and the environment are continuously exchanging matter and energy with each other. Environment for any individual is defined as the patterned wholeness of all that is external to a given individual. This constant interchange of materials and energy between the individual and the environment characterizes each of them as open systems.

The third assumption holds that the life process of human beings evolves irreversibly and unidirectionally along a space-time continuum. Consequently, the individual can never go backwards or be something he previously was. At any given point in time, then, the individual is the expression of the totality of events present at that given time.

Identifying individuals and reflecting their wholeness are life's patterns. These patterns allow for self-regulation, rhythmicity, and dynamism. They give unity to diversity and reflect a dynamic and creative universe. Thus, the fourth assumption is that pattern identifies individuals and reflects their innovative wholeness.

Finally, the fifth assumption is that the human being is characterized by the capacity for abstraction and imagery, language and thought, sensation and emotion. Of all the earth's life forms, only the human is a sentient thinking being who perceives and ponders the vastness of the cosmos.

Based on these assumptions are the four building blocks identified by Rogers—energy fields, openness, pattern, and four-dimensionality.[8] A unifying concept for both animate and inanimate environments, *energy fields* have no boundaries; they are indivisible and extend to infinity. Thus, these fields are *open*, allowing exchange with other fields. The interchange between and among energy fields has *pattern*; these patterns are not fixed but change as situations require. The interchanges occur at different points in the *four dimensionality* of space-time. With these building blocks as the base, *unitary humans* are defined as irreducible four-dimensional, negentropic energy fields identified by pattern and manifesting characteristics and behaviors that are different from those of the parts and which cannot be predicted from knowledge of the parts, with the *environment* being an irreducible four-dimensional, negentropic energy field identified by pattern and integral with the human field.[9]

There is a strong parallel between Rogers's basic assumptions and general system theory. According to von Bertalanffy, a system is a set of elements that are interrelated.[10] The interrelated elements in this conceptual model are human beings and their environments. As a living system and energy field, the individual is capable of taking in energy and information from the environment, and releasing energy and information to the environment.[11] Because of this exchange, the individual is an open system—an underlying assumption and building block.

General system theory is a general science of wholeness. It is concerned with the problems of organization, phenomena that are not resolvable to individual events, and dynamic interactions manifested in the difference of the behavior of the parts when isolated. As a result, order and behavior are not understandable by investigation of the respective parts in isolation.[12] Thus, the assumption of wholeness and the building block of pattern result.

The principle of hierarchial order is applicable.[13] The individual as an open system attempts to move toward a higher order by progressive differentiation, as for example, the differentiation of the cells of the zygote to form a human being. Within the order of the universe, the human being is of a higher order than other two-legged animals. Characteristic of this is Rogers's fifth assumption of human beings as sentient thinking beings, and congruent with this is the building block of pattern.

Using these five assumptions and building blocks as a base, the life process in human beings becomes a phenomenon of wholeness, of continuity, of dynamic and creative change. It possesses its own unity. It is inseparable from the environment and occurs in four-dimensionality. Since the individual is the recipient of nursing services, life processes of humanity are the *core* around which nursing revolves. According to Rogers, the science of nursing is directed toward describing the life process of humanity, and toward explaining and predicting the nature and direction of its development.[14]

ROGERS'S THEORY: PRINCIPLES OF HOMEODYNAMICS

Although Rogers offers no theoretical statement, she grounded her *principles of homeodynamics* in the five basic assumptions and four building blocks as discussed above. The principles of homeodynamics are composed of three separate principles—integrality, helicy, and resonancy.[15] By combining the principles of homeodynamics with the concept of humanity from her definition of nursing, a theoretical statement can be postulated. Using the definition that a theory interrelates concepts in such a way as to create a different way of looking at a particular phenomenon, an appropriate theoretical statement might be that nursing is the use of the principles of homeodynamics for the service of humanity.

Integrality

The first principle is that of *integrality*. Because of the inseparability of human beings and their environment, sequential changes in the life process are continuous revisions occurring from the interactions between human beings and their environment. Between the two entities, there is a constant mutual interaction and mutual change whereby simultaneous molding is taking place in both at the same time. Thus, integrality is the continuous, mutual, simultaneous interaction process between human and environmental fields.

Resonancy

The next principle, *resonancy*, speaks to the nature of the change occurring between human and environmental fields. The change in the pattern of human beings and environments is propagated by waves that move from lower frequency longer waves to higher frequency shorter waves. The life process in human beings is a symphony of rhythmical vibrations oscillating at various frequencies. Human beings experience their environments as a resonating wave of complex symmetry uniting them with the rest of the world. Resonancy, then, is the identification of the human field and the environmental field by wave patterns manifesting continuous change from lower frequency longer waves to higher frequency shorter waves.

Helicy

Finally, the principle of *helicy* states that the nature and direction of human and environmental change are continuously innovative, probabilistic, and characterized by the increasing diversity of human field and environmental field pattern emerging out of the continuous, mutual, simultaneous interaction between the human and environmental fields and manifesting nonrepeating rhythmicities. Because the life process is a constantly evolving series of change in which the past has been incorporated and out of which new patterns have emerged, it is a becoming, a dynamic repatterning, a growing complexity, a unidirectional phenomenon, a probabilistic goal-directedness. The concepts of rhythmicality, evolutionary emergence, and the unitary nature of the human-environmental field relationship are encompassed. Therefore, helicy postulates the direction of the change occurring between the human and environmental fields.

Consequently, the principles of homeodynamics are a way of viewing human beings in their wholeness. Changes in the life process of humanity are irreversible, nonrepeatable, rhythmical in nature, and evidence of the growing complexity of pattern. Change proceeds by continuous repatterning of both human and environmental fields by resonating oscillations of lower frequency longer waves to higher frequency shorter waves, and reflects the mutual simultaneous interaction between the two fields at any given point in space-time.

COMPARISON WITH OTHER THEORIES

The principles of homeodynamics are closely aligned to selected principles of general system theory. The homeodynamic principle of helicy can be compared to the principles of equifinality and negentropy. *Equifinality* means that an open system may attain a time-independent state independent of initial conditions and determined only by the system parameters. Thus, the system has a goal.[16] The *negentropic* principle provides that open systems have mechanisms that can slow down or arrest the process of movement toward less efficiency and growth.[17] Environmental exchange can provide support for such mechanisms.

For example, growth and development in the individual are equifinal. The same final state can be reached from different initial states and by means of different pathways. The various phases or stages along the way are maintained for an interval until spontaneous transition toward a higher order evokes new developments. The evolution toward an increase of order and organization at a higher level is made possible by negentropy.[18] Thus, growing complexity and evolutionary emergence are made possible.

Consider the case of identical twins Susie and Joanie. Shortly after their two-month birthday, one of the twins, Susie, spent six weeks in bilateral leg casts to correct a congenital deformity. As a result of this experience, Susie is maintained at a developmental plateau, while Joanie continues to develop along the sequential axis.

Consequently, Susie experiences an altered developmental pattern, the extent of which is depicted in Figure 13-1. At four months, the difference in development between the twins is substantial, whereas at eight months the difference has been greatly reduced. The equifinal state of this development will be achieved despite the increased time required.

Because of the evolutionary nature of this framework, many developmental theories are consistent with it. For example, Erikson's psychosocial stages of development beginning with trust vs. mistrust, and autonomy vs. shame and doubt, through generativity vs. self-absorption and ego integrity vs. despair, profess a forward growth of an increasingly complex individual.[19] Havinghurst's developmental tasks support the same philosophy of growth and development as Erikson.[20] Development is an ongoing process from learning the first basic tasks of walking, eating, and talking to control of bodily functions to adjusting to retirement and/or death of a spouse. Another example is Piaget's concepts of intellectual development.[21] From sensorimotor to preoperational to concrete operational to formal operational thought, a nonreversible growth occurs. Kohlberg validates Piaget's work in his findings that moral development begins when thought processes shift from preoperational to concrete operations.[22] Again, Kohlberg found individuals developed through a series of stages, from a premoral punishment and obedience orientation to a principled morality and a universal ethical principle orienta-

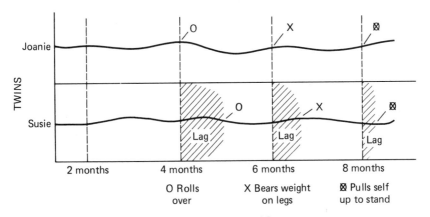

Figure 13-1. Pictorial representation of the altered developmental pattern experienced by one twin, Susie, as a result of leg-casting for 6 weeks following her 2-month birthday.

tion.[23] In all these developmental theories, what has happened in the past in the individual's life will always affect the future.

Biologically, the individual also develops, moving from simple reflex responses to the complex control over fine motor movements. Such progressive differentiation is characteristic of the human organism. Specific biological functions such as the menstrual cycle have an ongoing effect on the body. With the onset of puberty, changes in the body structure such as increased breadth of the hips and breast development begin. Such changes persist past the menopause. Although the functioning of the body before puberty and following menopause may be said to be similar, the persistence of the identified changes mandates that the postmenopausal functioning be viewed differently from prepuberty functioning, thus illustrating the principle of helicy.

Components of Callista Roy's adaptation model may also be viewed as consistent with Rogers's conceptual framework. Roy's model postulates that the individual's physiologic adaptation, self-concept, role function, and relations with others are the results of interactions with the environment. The environment consists of stimuli, status positions, and persons.[24] The physiological adaptation to the environmental stimulus of altitude change such as that experienced by mountain climbers demonstrates the mutual interaction between the individual and the environment. The simultaneous change in the mountain climber and in the altitude is consistent with the principle of integrality.

According to Roy, the individual's adaptation of self-concept is affected by the individuals who become part of the environment.[25] Rogers's principle of helicy postulates that each new mutual interaction will promote continuous innovative changes. For example, a woman who is a wife and mother has developed a self-concept that is consistent with her perceptions of her interactions with husband and children. When that same woman then becomes a college student, interactions with faculty, students, and the college environment will promote changes and adaptations in her self-concept.

This mother/wife/student will have a change in her environment and therefore a change in her interaction with that environment. This is representative of integrality. The new environment of a university will include new faculty, new peers, new books, and new learning experiences in laboratories; and the new environment will cause changes in the old environment—the home—and how the woman interacts with the environment there. At specified points in time the changes caused by the new environment create changes in the life pattern in which she has been functioning.

As the mother/wife/student grows and changes because of her interaction with faculty, peers, and the college environment, she will integrate the material presented and will adapt—emerging from the program as a different woman. This adaptation will affect the rhythms that have related to her former life style. Before entering the program, the mother of the family always cooked the meals; after she enters the program, another member of the family may assume the cooking role, thus changing the rhythms of family functioning. Rogers's principle of helicy can be utilized in the changes of rhythms occurring because of the change in the environment.

Resonancy examines the variations occurring during the life process of the "whole" person. The experiences as a student mandate changes in the wife/mother. Because of the progression in space-time, the wife/mother/student can never return to the wife/mother unaffected by the experience of being a student.

ROGERS'S THEORY AND THE FOUR
MAJOR CONCEPTS

Martha Rogers speaks to the four major concepts. She presents five assumptions about *human beings.* Each human is assumed to be a unified being with individuality. The human is in continuous exchange of energy with the environment. The life processes of a human evolve irreversibly and unidirectionally in space and time. There is pattern to life. Finally, the human is capable of abstraction, imagery, language, thought, sensation, and emotion. Humans are four-dimensional, negentropic energy fields identified by pattern and manifesting characteristics and behaviors that are different from those of the parts and which cannot be predicted from knowledge of the parts.[26]

Environment consists of the totality of patterns existing external to the individual. Both the individual and the environment are considered to be open systems. Environment is a four-dimensional, negentropic energy field identified by pattern and integral with the human field.[27]

Nursing is an art and science that is humanistic and humanitarian. It is directed toward the unitary human and is concerned with the nature and direction of human development.

Health is not specifically addressed and indeed, if viewed as a state, is not appropriate to Rogers's theory. As she speaks clearly of disease and pathology as value terms, it may be inferred that health is also a value term. Values constantly change, and when discussed in terms of the dynamics of the behaviors manifested by the human field, need to be individually defined.[28]

USE OF ROGERS'S PRINCIPLES IN THE NURSING PROCESS

If the profession of nursing is viewed as concerned with unitary human beings, the principles of homeodynamics provide guidelines for predicting the nature and direction of the individual's development as responses to health-related problems are made. Using these guidelines, the professional practice of nursing would then seek to promote symphonic integration of human beings and their environments, to strengthen the coherence and integrity of the human field, and to direct and redirect patterning of the human and environmental fields for the realization of maximum health.[29] These goals would be reflected in the nursing process.

To successfully utilize the principles of homeodynamics, there needs to be a consideration of the nurse and an involvement of both the nurse and the client in the nursing process. If anything or anyone external to the individual is part of the environment, then the nurse would be part of the client's environment. Since the nurse serves as the facilitator of the nursing process, it is vital that she be considered an integral part of the environment. Because of the mutual interaction of the individual and the environment, it is implied that the client is a willing, integral participant in the nursing process. Nursing, then, is working *with* the client, not *to* or *for* the client. This involvement in the nursing process by the nurse demonstrates concern for the total person, rather than one aspect, one problem, or a limited segment of need fulfillment.[30]

In the nursing assessment phase of the nursing process, all facts and opinions about the individual and the environment are collected. Because of our limited measuring devices and data-collection tools, the information collected in the assessment is frequently of an isolate or particulate nature. However, to implement the guidelines, the analysis of the data must be in such a fashion as to reflect wholeness. This may be done by asking several questions and seeking the responses from the collected data.

The first series of questions reflect the principle of integrality. What is the interaction between the person and the environment? How has one adjusted to the other? Are there any maladjustment factors present? Are they able to work together? What factors support or undermine this working relationship? If the individual is in an environment that is not the normal one, how are the two environments different? Based on the differences, what kind of predictions can be made about the individual's interaction with this new environment?

The next series of questions would reflect the principle of resonancy. How has the life process of the individual progressed? What kind of variations have occurred during the course of this life process? What factors have influenced these variations? What role has the environment played in these variations? How would a strange environment affect the individual's life process?

The last series of questions would be influenced by the principle of helicy. What kinds of rhythms are reflected in the collected data? How complex are these rhythms? Are they old established rhythms or new emerging ones? How does the environment support these rhythms? If the individual is in a strange environment, how will these rhythms be affected by the new environment? What sequential stages of development has the individual passed through? What were the effects? How has the environment supported or retarded the progress of the individual? How will a new environment affect this progress? What kinds of goals does the individual have? How have these goals affected development? Where do the individuals wish to go as reflected by their goals? What kinds of new vistas are sought?

To reflect the idea of patterning, additional questions for the principle of helicy would be considered. What kinds of patterns characterize the individual? How have the patterns developed? What kinds of past experience have influenced the development of specified patterns? How has the environment promoted certain patterns? How complex are the patterns? How has time affected the patterns? Although these questions may be answered, it must be remembered that the responses reflect a specific point in space-time. Consequently, the identified patterns are not static but rather ever-changing, reflecting both a change in time and additional new past experiences.

By no means are these questions all-inclusive, but using them as a reference will help provide the nurse with a view of the whole individual. It will identify individual differences and the sequential cross-sectional patterning in the life process. It will also show the total pattern of events for the person at any given point in space-time.[31] The nursing assessment, then, is an assessment of the whole human being and not an assessment of only physical or mental status. It is an assessment of health and health potential for the individual and not an assessment of an illness or a disease process. As a result, the individual is paramount, not the disease.

As a result of the nursing assessment, a conclusion is drawn about the individual. This conclusion is the nursing diagnosis, the second step in the nursing process, and it will reflect the principles of homeodynamics. Rhythms, patterns, complexity, interactions, and life-process variations would become evident. Such a nursing diagnosis would not be consistent with the problem-oriented system for providing care. In the problem-oriented system, a problem would be identified that would be stated as a symptom, finding, or (medical) diagnosis.[32] As such, the problem would reflect a piece of the individual and not the whole human being. Although also imperfect, the nursing diagnoses developed by Kristine Gebbie and Mary Ann Lavin have a greater potential for usefulness within Rogers's framework because they tend to reflect a more unitary view of the individual.[33]

The purpose of the nursing diagnosis is to provide a framework within which the nursing intervention is planned and implemented. Consequently, the thrust of the nursing intervention will depend on the focus of the nursing diagnosis. The focus on integrality will require implementation within the environment as well as within the individual. It can be expected that change in one will cause simultaneous change in the other. Because of the individual's integration with the environment, health problems cannot be separated from the world's social ills. Therefore, these problems cannot be dealt with effectively by means of the commonly accepted transitional, disease-oriented measures.[34] Creativity and imagination become essential.

Resonancy requires that the nursing plan be geared toward supporting or modifying variations in the life process of the whole human being. Because the human life process is a unidirectional phenomenon, the intervention cannot be aimed at returning the individual to a former level of existence; rather, the nurse helps the individual move forward to a higher, more complex level of existence.

Nursing planning in the area of helicy requires an acceptance of individual differences as an expression of evolutionary emergence. The strategies are geared at supporting or modifying rhythms and life goals. To do this requires the informed and active participation of the client in the nursing process. The concept of the unitary human and a recognition of the human being's capacity to feel and to reason will enable the nurse to assist the individual in the resolution of the health problem and in the setting of goals directed toward achieving health.[35] Health will not be achieved by promoting homeostasis and equilibrium, but rather by taking steps to enhance dynamism and complexity within the individual.

Additionally, helicy requires that the nursing plan be geared toward promoting dynamic repatterning of the whole human being. This repatterning includes the individual's relationship to self and to the environment so that the total potential as a human being can be developed. This repatterning is aimed at assisting people to develop patterns of living that coordinate with environmental changes rather than conflict with them.[36] Although the pattern may be altered or maintained, it must be remembered that this is an evolving, ever-changing pattern rather than a static, constant phenomenon.

Regardless of the focus, the aim of the nursing plan is the attainment of an optimum state of health for the individual. This state of health may not be the ideal but will be the maximum health that is potentially possible for the individual.[37] Generally, implementation strategies will seek to strengthen the integrity of the individual-environment relationship and to give direction to humanity's struggle to achieve new levels of well-being. By assisting individuals to mobilize their resources, consciously and unconsciously, their integrity will be heightened.[38]

If attainment of an optimum state of health is the aim of the nursing plan, then it becomes the focus for nursing evaluation, the final phase of the nursing process. Has the integrity of the individual-environment relationship been strengthened? Have resources been mobilized? Has the patterning of the human and environmental fields been directed toward the realization of maximum health potential? Only when the nursing goal of the highest possible health state has been realized can nursing interventions be evaluated as effective.

A schematic representation of the relationship between the principles of homeodynamics and the elements of the nursing process is presented in Table 13-1. As can be seen, there is no absolute distinction between the areas covered by the various principles. Table 13-2 attempts to apply the generalities to the specific situation of Janie who is hospitalized. In no way is either figure designed to be all-inclusive. Rather, they are offered as an attempt to make abstract ideas more concrete and operational.

LIMITATIONS OF ROGERS'S PRINCIPLES OF HOMEODYNAMICS

Although the principles of homeodynamics are consistent with the universally accepted aims and goals of nursing, there are major limitations to the universal implementation of the principles. Many persons will have difficulty understanding the principles. Even though basic assumptions are provided and the principles are defined, the framework remains an abstract phenomenon. Terms have not been sufficiently operationalized to provide for clear understanding.[39] By "operationalizing terms" is meant the description of a set of physical procedures that must be carried out in order to assign to every case a value for the concept.[40] For example, to operationalize the concept of width is to place a tool consisting of the units of inches or centimeters along the edge of the item to be measured and then count the units.

Because of the lack of operatonal definitions, research done to support or verify the principles provides questionable results. Operational definitions are needed for the development of hypotheses that test the theoretical concepts, and for the selection of tools that will adequately measure the concepts involved.[41] Without such definitions just what was confirmed or not confirmed by these studies is in doubt.[42]

At this stage in the development of nursing science, tools that will adequately assess human beings in their totality are nonexistent. Without such tools, the ability to utilize or test the framework successfully is virtually impossible. Furthermore, the inability to adequately utilize or test the framework makes successful nursing implementation difficult. Thus, utilization of principles of homeodynamics in its totality is limited. At best, varying aspects of the principles can be applied to nursing practice in a very limited fashion.

Table 13-1

Relationship of the Principles of Homeodynamics to the Nursing Process

Components of the Nursing Process	Principles of Homeodynamics		
	Integrality	Resonancy	Helicy
Nursing assessment component	Look at the interaction of the individual and the environment—how they work together rather than what they are like in isolation.	Look at the variations occurring during the life process of the whole human being.	Look at the rhythmic life patterns of the individual and the environment. Progression of time of necessity creates changes in the rhythmic life patterns of the whole human being. Look at life goals. Be aware of growing complexity of the whole human being.
Nursing diagnosis component	Reflects integration of the individual and environmental fields.	Reflects the variations in the life process of the whole individual.	Reflect the rhythmic pattern of the individual and environmental fields.
Nursing plan for implementation component	Intervene in the environment as well as in the individual. Change promoted in one area will cause simultaneous change in the other—simultaneous molding.	Support or modify variations in the life process of the whole individual.	Promote dynamic rhythmic repatterning of both the individual and the environment. Accept differences as an expression of evolutionary emergence. Promote dynamism and complexity rather than homeostasis and equilibrium. Support or modify life goals.
Nursing evaluation component	Evaluate changes in the integration that have occurred.	Evaluate the modification made in the variations of the life process of the whole human being.	Evaluate rhythmic repatterning of the individual and the environment. Evaluate goal-directedness. Evaluate relationship of goal to the whole individual.

Table 13-2

Relationship of the Principles of Homeodynamics in the Nursing Process for Janie

Components of the Nursing Process	Principles of Homeodynamics		
	Integrality	Resonancy	Helicy
Nursing assessment component	1. How does Janie see her environment? 2. What kind of differences are there between the hospital and her home? 3. How is she reacting to the changes in her environment? 4. How do her health problem and the environment affect each other?	1. What is Janie's past history? 2. What kinds of deviations from the expected norms have there been? 3. Were these deviations individually or environmentally related? 4. What is the reason for the hospitalization? 5. How will this affect her life?	1. What are Janie's normal behavior patterns and routines? 2. Were the behaviors or routines undergoing a change prior to her admission? 3. What kinds of activities can she perform? 4. What kinds of past experiences has she had? 5. How might those experiences influence her current situation? 6. What is Janie's developmental level? 7. Will the hospital environment support or retard developmental progress? 8. What are Janie's goals?
Nursing diagnosis component	1. What is the nature of the interaction between Janie and the hospital?	1. What is the interference this hospitalization will make in Janie's life?	1. What are the rhythmic patterns that are being exhibited?

Principles of Homeodynamics

Components of the Nursing Process	Integrality	Resonancy	Helicy
Nursing plan for implementation component	1. How can the hospital environment be modified to reduce the differences identified? 2. How can Janie be helped to understand the differences that cannot be eliminated? 3. How can her health potential be improved by manipulating the environment?	1. How can Janie's normal development be promoted? 2. How can the effects of the interferences be minimized?	1. How can Janie's normal behavioral patterns and routines be promoted in the hospital? 2. What kind of modifications can be made to promote her normal behavioral patterns and routines? 3. What kind of provisions can be made to promote her normal growth and development? 4. How can Janie be helped to develop successful rhythmic behavioral patterns within the hospital environment? 5. How can Janie be helped to reach her goals?
Nursing evaluation component	1. Has Janie's behavior changed as a result of environmental modification? 2. What kind of new reactions are now taking place?	1. Is Janie developing normally, based on theories? 2. Has the interference with development been minimized?	1. What kind of rhythmic repatterning has taken place? 2. Is Janie's development being supported? 3. Is she moving toward her goals?

ROGERS'S WORK AND THE
CHARACTERISTICS OF A THEORY

Rogers's principles of homeodynamics are congruent with many of the theory characteristics identified in Chapter 1. For the first characteristic, the theoretical statement that nursing is the use of the principles of homeodynamics for the service of humanity compels one to look at nursing in a very different way. An excellent example is the principle of helicy with its emphasis on pattern and rhythmicity.

For the second characteristic, there is definitely a logical development of the major constructs. This logical development of constructs contributes to the ability to test the framework.

In relation to the third characteristics, the theory is generalizable since it is not dependent on any given setting. However, it is far from simple. New terminology has been created for the theory. This in itself hampers simplicity. In addition, the theory is based on the use of open systems that are inherently complex.

For the fourth and fifth characteristics, research is hampered by the lack of simplicity, operational definitions, and valid instruments to measure outcomes. The complex interrelationships involved in the framework contribute to these difficulties. Efforts to minimize or eliminate these problems need to be continued so that nursing can truly benefit from Rogers's framework.

For the sixth characteristic, Rogers's ideas can be applied to practice. When these ideas are applied to nursing practice, the understanding of the client's behavior takes on new dimensions. This results in alterations in the focus of nursing actions. The case study of Janie presented in this chapter provides an example of the effect on practice.

For the seventh characteristic, Rogers's work is in agreement with other theories. This has been discussed in some detail earlier in this chapter.

SUMMARY

Building on a broad theoretical base from a variety of disciplines, Rogers developed the principles of homeodynamics. Inherent in the principles are five basic assumptions: (1) the human being is a unified whole, possessing individual integrity and manifesting characteristics that are more than and different from the sum of the parts;

(2) the individual and the environment are continuously exchanging matter and energy with each other; (3) the life process of human beings evolves irreversibly and unidirectionally along a space-time continuum; (4) patterns identify human beings and reflect their innovative wholeness; and (5) the individual is characterized by the capacity for abstraction and imagery, language and thought, sensation and emotion. The principles of integrality, helicy, and resonancy are compared to general system theory, developmental theories, and adaptation theories. Ways to utilize the principles in the nursing process are explored. The difficulty in understanding the principles, the lack of operational definitions, and inadequate tools for measurement are the major limitations to the effective utilization of this theory.

NOTES

1. Martha E. Rogers, *The Theoretical Basis of Nursing* (Philadelphia: F. A. Davis Co., 1970), pp. vii, ix.
2. Ibid., p. 4.
3. Ibid., p. 10.
4. Ibid., pp. 12–14.
5. Alvin Toffler, *Future Shock* (New York: Bantam Books, Inc., 1970), p. 30.
6. Martha E. Rogers, "Accountability," Convention address, University of Utah College of Nursing, June 5, 1971, p. 3.
7. Rogers, *The Theoretical Basis of Nursing*, pp. 47–73.
8. Martha E. Rogers, "Science of Unitary Human Beings: A Paradigm for Nursing," paper presented at International Nurse Theorist Conference, Edmonton, Alberta, May 2, 1984.
9. Ibid.
10. Ludwig von Bertalanffy, *General System Theory* (New York: George Braziller, Inc., 1968), p. 38.
11. Mary Elizabeth Hazzard, "An Overview of Systems Theory," *Nursing Clinics of North America*, 6, no. 3 (September 1971), 385.
12. von Bertalanffy, *General System Theory*, p. 37.
13. Ibid., pp. 27–28.
14. Rogers, *The Theoretical Basis of Nursing*, pp. vii, 84–85.
15. Ibid., pp. 97–102; and idem, "Science of Unitary Human Beings."
16. Hazzard, "An Overview of Systems Theory," pp. 389–90.
17. Alvin L. Bertrand, *Social Organization* (Philadelphia: F. A. Davis Co., 1972), p. 99.
18. Hazzard, "An Overview of Systems Theory," p. 390.
19. Erik Erikson, *Childhood and Society*, 2nd ed. (New York: W. W. Norton & Co., Inc., 1963), pp. 247–74.

20. Robert Havinghurst, *Developmental Tasks and Education*, 3rd ed. (New York: David McKay Co., Inc., 1972).

21. Jean Piaget and Rachel Inhelder, *The Psychology of the Child* (New York: Basic Books, Inc., 1969).

22. Lawrence Kohlberg, *Collected Papers on Moral Development and Moral Education* (Cambridge, Mass.: Moral Education and Research Foundation, 1973).

23. Ibid.

24. Callista Roy, "The Roy Adaptation Model," in *Conceptual Models for Nursing Practice*, 2nd ed., Joan P. Riehl and Callista Roy, eds. (East Norwalk, Conn.: Appleton-Century-Crofts, 1980), p. 182.

25. Ibid.

26. Rogers, "Science of Unitary Human Beings."

27. Ibid.

28. Ibid.

29. Rogers, *The Theoretical Basis of Nursing*, p. 122 and idem, "Science of Unitary Human Beings."

30. Helen Yura and Mary B. Walsh, *The Nursing Process* (New York: Appleton-Century-Crofts, 1973), p. 72.

31. Callista Roy, "Rogers' Theoretical Basis of Nursing," in *Conceptual Models for Nursing Practice*, Joan P. Riehl and Callista Roy, eds. (New York: Appleton-Century-Crofts, 1974), pp. 98–99.

32. Rosemarian Berni and Helen Readey, *Problem-Oriented Medical Record Implementation* (St. Louis, Mo.: The C. V. Mosby Company, 1975).

33. Kristine M. Gebbie and Mary Ann Lavin, eds., *Classification of Nursing Diagnoses* (St. Louis, Mo.: The C. V. Mosby Company, 1975).

34. Rogers, *The Theoretical Basis of Nursing*, p. 134.

35. Ibid.

36. Ibid., p. 123.

37. Roy, "Rogers' Theoretical Basis of Nursing," pp. 97, 99.

38. Rogers, *The Theoretical Basis of Nursing*, pp. 134, 139.

39. Imogene King, *Toward a Theory for Nursing* (New York: John Wiley & Sons, Inc., 1971), p. 18.

40. Margaret E. Hardy, "Theories: Components, Development, Evaluation," *Nursing Research*, 23, no. 2 (March-April 1974), 101.

41. Ibid., p. 105.

42. Rogers, *The Theoretical Basis of Nursing*, pp. 103–28.

ADDITIONAL REFERENCE

SAFIER, GWENDOLYN, *Contemporary American Leaders in Nursing*. New York: McGraw-Hill Book Company, 1977.

14

IMOGENE M. KING

Julia B. George

Imogene M. King received her basic nursing education from St. John's Hospital School of Nursing, St. Louis, Missouri. Her Ed.D. is from Teachers College, Columbia University, New York.

King has had experience in nursing as an administrator, an educator, and a practitioner. Her positions in nursing education have included Director, School of Nursing, The Ohio State University, Columbus, Ohio; Professor of Nursing, Loyola University of Chicago, Chicago, Illinois; and Professor, College of Nursing, University of South Florida, Tampa, Florida.

Imogene M. King's *Toward a Theory for Nursing: General Concepts of Human Behavior* was published in 1971 and A *Theory for Nursing: Systems, Concepts, Process* in 1981.[1] These publications grew from King's thoughts about the vast amount of knowledge available to nurses and the difficulty this presents to the individual nurse in choosing the facts and concepts relevant to a given situation.[2] From the early 1960s the rapidity of scientific and technological advances has been having as great an impact on the profession of nursing as on other components of society. Also, as emerging professionals, nurses have been identifying the knowledge base specific to nursing practice and to an expanding role for nurses.

In the preface to *Toward a Theory for Nursing*, King clearly states she was proposing a conceptual framework for nursing and not a nursing theory. As she denoted in the title, her purpose was to help move *toward* a theory for nursing.[3] In contrast, in the preface to *A Theory for Nursing*, she indicates she has expanded and built upon the original framework. In this second publication, she

> presents a conceptual framework by linking concepts essential to understanding nursing as a major system within the health care system . . . offers one approach to developing concepts and applying knowledge in nursing . . . [and] demonstrates strategy for theory construction by presenting a theory of goal attainment derived from the conceptual framework.[4]

King identifies the conceptual framework as an open systems framework and the theory as one of goal attainment. As her extensive documentation indicates, she has drawn from a wide variety of sources in developing the framework and the theory.

Since the theory of goal attainment is derived from the open systems framework, the framework and its assumptions and concepts will be presented first, and then the goal attainment theory will be discussed.

KING'S OPEN SYSTEMS FRAMEWORK

King presents several assumptions that are basic to her conceptual framework. These include the assumptions that "the focus of nursing is the care of human beings," that nursing's goal is "the health of individuals and health care for groups," and that human beings are open systems in constant interaction with their environment.[5]

The conceptual framework is composed of three interacting systems; these are the personal systems, the interpersonal systems, and the social systems. Figure 14–1 presents a schematic diagram of these interacting systems. King summarizes the conceptual framework as follows:

> Individuals comprise one type of system in the environment called personal systems. Individuals interact to form dyads, triads,

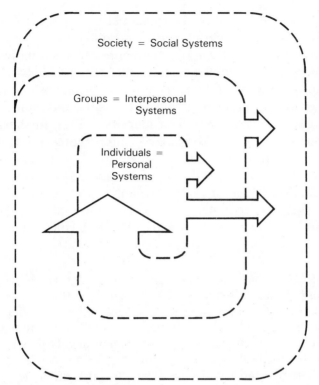

Figure 14-1. Dynamic Interacting systems. Adapted from Imogene M. King, *Toward a Theory for Nursing* (New York: John Wiley & Sons, Inc., 1971), p. 20. Copyright © 1971, by John Wiley & Sons, Inc. Used with permission.

and small and large groups, which comprise another type of system called interpersonal systems. Groups with special interests and needs form organizations, which make up communities and societies and [these] are called social systems.[6]

She then identifies several concepts as relevant for each of these systems.

Personal Systems

Each individual is a personal system. For a personal system the relevant concepts are perception, self, growth and development, body image, space, and time.[7] *Perception* is presented as the major concept of a personal system, the concept that influences all behaviors or to which all other concepts are related. The characteristics of perception are that it is universal, or experienced by all; subjective or personal; and selective for each person, meaning that any given situation will be experienced in a unique manner by each individual involved. Perception is action-oriented in the present and based on the information that is available. Perception is transactions; that is, "individuals enter a situation as active participants, and their existence in the interaction will affect their identity."[8] King further defines perception as "a process of organizing, interpreting, and transforming information from sense data and memory . . . a process of human transactions with environment. It gives meaning to one's experience, represents one's image of reality and influences one's behavior."[9]

The characteristics of *self* are a dynamic individual, an open system, and goal orientation.[10] King accepts Jersild's definition of self:

> The self is a composite of thoughts and feelings which constitute a person's awareness of his individual existence, his conception of who and what he is. A person's self is the sum total of all he can call his. The self includes, among other things, a system of ideas, attitudes, values and commitments. The self is a person's total subjective environment. It is a distinctive center of experience and significance. The self constitutes a person's inner world as distinguished from the outer world consisting of all other people and things. The self is the individual as known to the individual. It is that to which we refer when we say "I."[11]

The characteristics of *growth and development* include cellular, molecular, and behavioral changes in human beings. These changes usually occur in an orderly manner, one that is predictable but has individual variations and is a function of genetic endowment, of meaningful and satisfying experiences, and of an environment conducive to helping individuals move toward maturity.[12] Growth and development can be defined as "the process that takes place in people's lives that helps them move from potential capacity for achievement to self-actualization."[13] Theorists mentioned are Freud, Erikson, Piaget, Gesell, and Havinghurst; but no particular model, theory, or framework of growth and development is specifically selected.[14]

Body image is characterized as very personal and subjective; acquired or learned; dynamic and changing as the person redefines self; and part of each stage of growth and development. "Body image is defined as a person's perceptions of his own body, others' reactions to his appearance, and is a result of others' reactions as well."[15]

Space is characterized as universal because all people have some concept of it; personal or subjective; individual; situational and dependent on the relationships in the situation; dimensional as a function of volumes, area, distance, and time; and transactional or based on the individual's perception of the situation.[16] King's operational definition of space includes that space exists in all directions, is the same everywhere, and is defined by the physical area known as "territory" and by the behaviors of those who occupy it.[17]

Time is characterized as universal or inherent in life processes; relational or dependent on distance and the amount of information occurring; unidirectional or irreversible as it moves from past to future with a continuous flow of events; measurable; and subjective since it is based on perception.[18] King defines time as "a duration between one event and another as uniquely experienced by each human being; it is the relation of one event to another event."[19]

Perception, self, growth and development, body image, space, and time are the concepts of the personal system. When personal systems come in contact with each other, they form interpersonal systems.

Interpersonal Systems

Interpersonal systems are formed by human beings interacting. Two interacting individuals form a dyad, three form a triad, and four or more form small or large groups. As the number of interacting individuals increases, so does the complexity of the interactions.[20] The relevant concepts for interpersonal systems are interaction, communication, transaction, role, and stress.[21]

Interaction is characterized by values; mechanisms for establishing human relationships; being universally experienced; being influenced by perceptions; reciprocity; being mutual or interdependent; containing verbal and nonverbal communication; learning occurring when communication is effective; unidirectionality; irreversibility; dynamism; and having a temporal-spatial dimension.[22] Interactions are defined as the observable behaviors of two or more persons in mutual presence.[23]

Characteristics of *communication* are that it is verbal; nonverbal; situational; perceptual; transactional; irreversible, or moving forward in time; personal; and dynamic.[24] Symbols for verbal communications are provided by language as such communication includes the spoken and written language that transmits ideas from one person to another. A very important aspect of nonverbal behavior is touch. Other aspects of nonverbal behavior are distance, posture, facial expression, physical appearance, and body movements.[25] King defines communication as "a process whereby information is given from one person to another either directly in face-to-face meeting or indirectly through telephone, television, or the written word."[26] It is "the vehicle by which human relations are developed and maintained . . . a fundamental social process in that it facilitates ordered functions of human groups and societies."[27] "All behavior is communication. Communication is the informational component of human interactions."[28]

Transactions, for this conceptual framework, are derived from cognition and perceptions and not from transactional analysis. The characteristics of transactions are that they are unique because each individual has a personal world of reality based on that individual's perceptions; they have temporal and spatial dimensions; and they are experience, or a series of events in time.[29] King defines transactions as "a process of interactions in which human beings communicate with environment to achieve goals that are valued . . . goal-directed human behaviors."[30]

The characteristics of *role* include reciprocity in that a person may be a giver at one time and a taker at another time, with a relationship between two or more individuals who are functioning in two or more roles; learned; social; complex; and situational.[31]

> Several elements give meaning to the concept of role: (1) role is a set of behaviors expected when occupying a position in a social system; (2) rules or procedures define rights and obligations in a position in an organization; (3) role is a relationship with one or more individuals interacting in specific situations for a purpose. Role of a nurse can be defined as an interaction between one or more individuals who come to a nursing situation in which nurses perform functions of professional nursing based on knowledge, skills, and values identified as nursing. Nurses use knowledge, skills and values to identify goals in each situation and to help individuals to achieve goals.[32]

The characteristics of *stress* are that it is dynamic due to open systems being in continuous exchange with the environment; the intensity varies; there is a temporal-spatial dimension that is influenced by past experiences; it is individual, personal, and subjective, a response to life events that is uniquely personal.[33]

Stress is a dynamic state whereby a human being interacts with the environment to maintain balance for growth, development, and performance, which involves an exchange of energy and information between the person and the environment for regulation and control of stressors. . . . Stress is the energy response of an individual to persons, objects and events called stressors. Stress is negative and positive, it is constructive and destructive. It helps people reach the highest level of achievement and at the same time continuously wears them down.[34]

The concepts of interpersonal systems are interaction, communication, transaction, role, and stress. Interpersonal systems join together to form larger systems known as social systems.

Social Systems

A social system is defined as an organized boundary system of social roles, behaviors, and practices developed to maintain values and the mechanisms to regulate the practices and rules.[35]

Examples of social systems include families, religious groups, educational systems, work systems, and peer groups.[36] The concepts relevant to social systems are organization, authority, power, status, and decision making.[37]

King proposes four parameters for *organization*:

(1) human values, behavior patterns, needs, goals and expectations; (2) a natural environment in which material and human resources are essential for achieving goals; (3) employers and employees, or parents and children, who form the groups that collectively interact to achieve goals; (4) technology that facilitates goal attainment.[38]

Organization is characterized by structure that orders positions and activities and relates formal and informal arrangements of individuals and groups to achieve personal and organizational goals; functions that describe the roles, positions, and activities to be performed; goals or outcomes to be achieved; and resources. King defines organization as being "composed of human beings with prescribed roles and positions who use resources to accomplish personal and organizational goals."[39]

The characteristics of *authority* include that it is observable through provisions of order, guidance, and responsibility for actions; universal; essential in formal organizations; reciprocal because it requires cooperation; resides in a holder who must be perceived as legitimate; situational; essential to goal achievement; and associated with power.[40] Assumptions about authority are that it can be said:

(1) to be legitimate and perceived by individuals; (2) to reside in the position held by a person who distributes the sanctions and rewards; (3) to reside in the competence of a person with special knowledge and skills, such as professionals; (4) to reside in the person who uses human relations skills to exercise leadership in a group.[41]

King further defines authority as:

a transactional process characterized by active, reciprocal relations in which members' values, background, and perceptions play a role in defining, validating, and accepting the authority of individuals within an organization. One person influences another, and he [the other] recognizes, accepts, and complies with the authority of that person.[42]

Power is characterized as universal; situational or not a personal attribute; essential in the organization; limited by resources in a situation; dynamic; and goal-directed. Premises about power are that it is potential energy; is essential for order in society; enhances group cohesiveness; resides in positions in an organization; is directly related to authority; is a function of human interactions; and is a function of decision making.[43] King defines power in a variety of ways:

Power is the capacity to use resources in organizations to achieve goals . . . is the process whereby one or more persons influence other persons in a situation . . . is the capacity or ability of a person or a group to achieve goals . . . occurs in all aspects of life and each person has potential power determined by individual resources and the environmental forces encountered. Power is social force that organizes and maintains society. Power is the ability to use and to mobilize resources to achieve goals.[44]

Status is characterized as situational; position dependent; and reversible. King defines status as "the position of an individual in a group or a group in relation to other groups in an organization" and identifies that status is accompanied by "privileges, duties and obligations."[45]

Decision making is characterized as necessary to regulate each person's life and work; universal; individual; personal; subjective; situational; a continuous process; and goal-directed. Decision making in organizations is defined as "a dynamic and systematic process by which goal-directed choice of perceived alternatives is made and acted upon by individuals or groups to answer a question and attain a goal."[46]

The major theses of King's conceptual framework are (1) that "each human being perceives the world as a total person in making transactions with individuals and things in the environment," and (2) that "transactions represent a life situation in which perceiver and thing perceived are encountered and in which each person enters the situation as an active participant and each is changed in the process of these experiences."[47] The concepts and systems of the framework are used as a base to develop a theory of goal attainment.

KING'S THEORY OF GOAL ATTAINMENT

The major elements of this theory are seen "in the interpersonal systems in which two people, who are usually strangers, come together in a health care organization to help and be helped to maintain a state of health that permits functioning in roles."[48] The concepts of the theory are interaction, perception, communication, transaction, self, role, stress, growth and development, time, and space. Although these terms have already been defined as concepts in the conceptual framework, they will be defined again here as part of the theory of goal attainment.

Interaction is defined as "a process of perception and communication between person and environment and between person and person, represented by verbal and nonverbal behaviors that are goal directed."[49] King diagrams interaction as seen in Figure 14-2. Each of the individuals involved in an interaction brings different ideas, attitudes, and perceptions to the exchange. The individuals come together for a purpose and perceive each other; each makes a judgment and takes mental action or decides to act. Then each

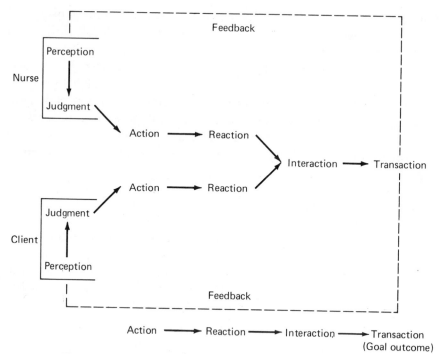

Figure 14-2. Interaction [Adapted from Imogene M. King, *Toward a Theory of Nursing: General Concepts of Human Behavior* (New York: John Wiley & Sons, Inc., 1971), pp. 26, 92. Copyright © 1971 by John Wiley & Sons, Inc. Used with permission.]

reacts to the other and the situation (perception, judgment, action reaction). King indicates that the interaction and transaction are directly observable.[50]

Perception is "each person's representation of reality."[51] The elements of perception are the importing of energy from the environment and organizing it by information; transforming energy; processing information; storing information; and exporting information in the form of overt behaviors.[52]

Communication is defined as "a process whereby information is given from one person to another either directly in face-to-face meetings or indirectly through telephone, television, or the written word."[53] Communication represents, and is involved in, the information component of interaction.

Transaction is defined as "observable behaviors of human beings interacting with their environment."[54] Transactions represent the valuation component of human interactions and involve bargaining, negotiating, and social exchange. When transactions occur between nurses and clients, goals are attained.[55]

Role is defined as "a set of behaviors expected of persons occupying a position in a social system; rules that define rights and obligations in a position; a relationship with one or more individuals interacting in specific situations for a purpose."[56] It is important that roles be understood and interpreted clearly to avoid conflict and confusion.

Stress is "a dynamic state whereby human beings interact with the environment to maintain balance for growth, development and performance . . . an energy response of an individual to persons, objects, and events called stressors."[57] Although stress may be positive or negative, too high a level of stress may decrease an individual's ability to interact and to attain goals.

Growth and development can be defined as the "continuous changes in individuals at the cellular, molecular, and behavioral levels of activities . . . the process that takes place in the life of individuals that helps them move from potential capacity for achievement to self-actualization."[59]

Time is "a sequence of events moving onward to the future . . . a continuous flow of events in successive order that implies a change, a past and a future . . . a duration between one event and another as uniquely experienced by each human being . . . the relation of one event to another."[59]

Space exists "in all directions and is the same everywhere . . . a physical area called territory . . . defined by the behavior of individuals occupying it."[60]

From the theory of goal attainment, King has developed eight predictive propositions, although she indicates that additional propositions may be generated. The eight propositions that she sets forth are as follows:[61]

1. If perceptual accuracy is present in nurse-client interactions, transactions will occur.
2. If nurse and client make transactions, goals will be attained.
3. If goals are attained, satisfactions will occur.
4. If goals are attained, effective nursing care will occur.
5. If transactions are made in nurse-client interactions, growth and development will be enhanced.
6. If role expectations and role performance as perceived by nurse and client are congruent, transactions will occur.

7. If role conflict is experienced by nurse or client or both, stress in nurse-client interactions will occur.
8. If nurses with special knowledge and skills communicate appropriate information to clients, mutual goal setting and goal attainment will occur.

In addition, King specifies internal and external boundary-determining criteria. Internal boundary criteria are derived from the characteristics of the concepts of the theory and speak to the theory itself. External boundary criteria speak to the area in which the theory is applicable. The internal boundary criteria for King's theory of goal attainment are listed below:[62]

1. Nurse and client do not know each other.
2. Nurse is licensed to practice professional nursing.
3. Client is in need of the services provided by the nurse.
4. Nurse and client are in a reciprocal relationship in that the nurse has special knowledge and skills to communicate appropriate information to help client set goals; client has information about self and perceptions of problems or concerns that when communicated to nurse will help in mutual goal setting.
5. Nurse and client are in mutual presence, purposefully interacting to achieve goals.

The external boundary criteria for King's theory of goal attainment are as follows:[63]

1. Interactions in a two-person group.
2. Interactions limited to licensed professional nurse and to client in need of nursing care.
3. Interactions taking place in natural environments.

Thus, King is saying a professional nurse, with special knowledge and skills, and a client in need of nursing, with knowledge of self and perceptions of personal problems, meet as strangers in a natural environment. They interact mutually to identify the problems and to establish and achieve goals. The personal system of the nurse and the personal system of the client meet in the interaction with the interpersonal system of their dyad. Their interpersonal system is influenced by the social systems that surround them.

KING'S THEORY AND THE FOUR
MAJOR CONCEPTS

In discussing her conceptual framework as an introduction to the presentation of her theory of goal attainment, King indicates that the abstract concepts of the framework are human beings, health, environment, and society.[64] Since the theory is presented as a theory for nursing, King also defines nursing. Thus the four major concepts of human beings, health, environment/society, and nursing are defined and discussed by King.

King identifies several assumptions about *human beings*. She describes human beings as social, sentient, rational, perceiving, controlling, purposeful, action-oriented, and time-oriented. From these beliefs about human beings, she has derived the following assumptions that are specific to nurse-client interaction:[65]

> Perceptions of nurse and of client influence the interactive process.
>
> Goals, needs, and values of nurse and client influence the interaction process.
>
> Individuals have a right to knowledge about themselves.
>
> Individuals have a right to participate in decisions that influence their life, their health, and community services.
>
> Health professionals have a responsibility to share information that helps individuals make informed decisions about their health care.
>
> Individuals have a right to accept or to reject health care.
>
> Goals of health professionals and goals of recipients of health care may be incongruent.

King further states that "nurses are concerned with human beings interacting with their environment in ways that lead to self-fulfillment and to maintenance of health."[66] Also, human beings have three fundamental health needs: (1) the need for health information that is usable at the time when it is needed and can be used, (2) the need for care that seeks to prevent illness, and (3) the need for care when human beings are unable to help themselves. She states, "nurses are in a position to assess what people know about their health, what they think about their health, how they feel about it, and how they act to maintain it."[67]

King defines *health* as "dynamic life experiences of a human being, which implies continuous adjustment to stressors in the internal and external environment through optimum use of one's resources to achieve maximum potential for daily living."[68] She discusses health as a functional state, and illness as an interference with that functional state. She then defines illness as "a deviation from normal, that is, an imbalance in a person's biological structure or in his psychological make-up, or a conflict in a person's social relationships."[69]

Environment and *society* are indicated as major concepts in King's framework but are not specifically defined in her work. Society may be viewed as the social systems portion of her open systems framework. Although her definition of health mentions both internal and external environment, the usual implication of the use of environment in A *Theory for Nursing* is that of external environment. Since she presents her material as based on open systems, it is assumed that a definition of external environment may be drawn from general system theory. Systems are considered to have boundaries that separate their internal components from the rest of the world. The external environment for a system is the portion of the world that exists outside of that boundary. Of particular interest as a system's external environment is the part of the world that is in direct exchange of energy and information with the system.[70]

Nursing is defined as "a process of action, reaction, and interaction whereby nurse and client share information about their perceptions in the nursing situation," and as "a process of human interactions between nurse and client whereby each perceives the other and the situation; and through communication, they set goals, explore means, and agree on means to achieve goals."[71] *Action* is defined as a sequence of behaviors involving mental and physical action. The sequence is first mental action to recognize the presenting conditions; then physical action to begin activities related to those conditions; and finally, mental action in an effort to exert control over the situation, combined with physical action seeking to achieve goals.[72] *Reaction* is not specifically defined but might be considered to be included in the sequence of behaviors described in action. *Interaction* has been previously discussed. Although King has altered her definition of nursing from that published in 1971, she has continued to refer to nursing as that which is done by nurses. This weakens her definition.

In addition to the above definition of nursing, King discusses the goal, domain, and function of the professional nurse. The goal of the nurse is "to help individuals maintain their health so they can function in their roles."[73] Nursing's domain includes promoting, maintaining, and restoring health, and caring for the sick, injured, and dying.[74] The function of the professional nurse is to interpret information in what is known as the nursing process to plan, implement, and evaluate nursing care.[75]

THEORY OF GOAL ATTAINMENT AND THE NURSING PROCESS

The basic assumption of the theory of goal attainment—that nurses and clients communicate information, set goals mutually, and then act to attain those goals—is also the basic assumption of the nursing process.

King indicates *assessment* will occur during the interaction of the nurse and client, who are likely to meet as strangers. The nurse brings to this meeting special knowledge and skills, whereas the client brings knowledge of self and perceptions of the problems that are of concern. Assessment, interviewing, and communication skills are needed by the nurse as is the ability to integrate knowledge of natural and behavioral sciences for application to a concrete situation.[77]

All concepts of the theory apply to assessment. Growth and development, knowledge of self and role, and the amount of stress influence perception and, in turn, influence communication, interaction, and transaction. In assessment, the nurse needs to collect data about the client's level of growth and development, view of self, perception of current health status, communication patterns, and role socialization, among other things. Factors influencing the client's perception include the functioning of the client's sensory system, age, development, sex, education, drug and diet history, and understanding of why contact with the health care system is occurring. The perceptions of the nurse are influenced by cultural and socioeconomic background and age of the nurse and the diagnosis of the client.[78] Perception is the basis for gathering and interpreting data, thus the basis for assessment. Communication is necessary to verify the accuracy of perceptions. Without communication, interaction and transaction cannot occur.

The information shared during assessment is used to derive a *nursing diagnosis*, defined by King as a statement that "identifies the disturbances, problems, or concerns about which patients seek help."[79] The implication is that the nurse makes the nursing diagnosis as a result of the mutual sharing with the client during assessment. Stress may be a particularly important concept in relation to nursing diagnosis since stress and disturbance and problem or concern may be closely connected.

After the nursing diagnosis is made, *planning* occurs. King describes planning as setting goals and making decisions about how to achieve these goals. This is part of transaction and again involves mutual exchange with the client. She specifies that clients are requested to participate in decision making about how the goals are to be met.[80] Although King indicates in her assumptions about nurse-client interactions that clients have the right to participate in decisions about their care, she does not say they have the responsibility. Thus, clients are requested to participate, not expected to do so.

Implementation occurs in the activities that seek to meet the goals. Implementation is a continuation of transaction in King's theory.

Evaluation involves descriptions of the outcomes identified as goals are attained. In King's description, evaluation not only speaks to the attainment of the client's goals but also to the effectiveness of nursing care.[81]

Although all of the theory concepts apply throughout the nursing process, communication with perception, interaction, and transaction are vital for goal attainment and must be apparent in each phase. King emphasizes the importance of mutual participation in interaction that focuses on the needs and welfare of the client and of verifying perceptions while planning and activities to achieve goals are carried out together. Although King emphasizes mutuality, she does not limit it to verbal communication, nor does she require the client's active physical participation in actions to achieve goal attainment.

In *A Theory for Nursing*, King presents an application of her theory of goal attainment that she identifies as the use of a goal-oriented nursing record. Her description of this goal-oriented nursing record closely parallels the steps of the nursing process.

KING'S WORK AND THE
CHARACTERISTICS OF A THEORY

King has stated that she has derived a theory of goal attainment from her open system framework of personal, interpersonal, and social systems. How her work compares with the characteristics of a theory presented in Chapter 1 will be discussed below.

1. Theories can interrelate concepts in such a way as to create a different way of looking at a particular phenomenon. King has interrelated the concepts of interaction, perception, communication, transaction, self, role, stress, growth and development, time, and space into a theory of goal attainment. Her theory deals with a nurse-client dyad, a relationship to which each person brings personal perceptions of self, role, and personal levels of growth and development. The nurse and client communicate, first in interaction and then in transaction, to attain mutually set goals. The relationship takes place in space identified by their behaviors and occurs in forward moving time. In particular, the specification of transaction as dealing with mutual goal attainment is a different way of looking at the phenomenon of nurse-client relationships.

2. Theories must be logical in nature. King's theory of goal attainment does describe a logical sequence of events. The concepts are clearly defined. However, a major inconsistency within her writing is the lack of a clear definition of environment, which is identified as a basic concept for the framework from which she derives her theory. In addition, she indicates that nurses are concerned about the health care of groups but defines nursing as occurring in a dyadic relationship. Thus the theory essentially draws on only two of the three systems described in the conceptual framework. The social systems portion of the framework is not clearly connected to the theory of goal attainment. Also, the definition of stress indicates that it is both negative and positive, but discussion of stress always implies that it is negative. Finally, King indicates that the nurse and client are strangers, yet she speaks of their working together for goal attainment and of the importance of health maintenance. Attainment of long-term goals, such as those concerning health maintenance, is not consistent with not knowing each other.

3. Theories should be relatively simple yet generalizable. Although the presentation appears to be complex, King's theory of goal attainment is relatively simple. Ten concepts are identified, defined, and their relationships considered. Even though King indicates many of the concepts are situation-dependent, they are not situation-specific; that is, they are influenced by the situation but may occur in many different situations. The theory of goal attainment is limited in setting only in regard to "natural environments" and, with growth and development as a major concept, is certainly not limited in age. The theory of goal attainment is generalizable to any nursing situation. The emphasis on mutuality would initially appear to limit the theory to dealing with those clients who can verbally interact with the nurse and physically participate in implementations to meet goals. However, King points to observable behaviors and to both verbal and nonverbal communication. Indeed, the comatose individual has observable behaviors in the form of vital signs and does communicate nonverbally. The major limitation in relation to this characteristic is the effort required of the reader to sift through the presentation of a conceptual framework and a theory with repeated definitions to find the basic concepts.

4. Theories can be the bases for hypotheses that can be tested. King presents the following hypotheses that she has derived from her theory of goal attainment:[82]

1. Perceptual accuracy in nurse-patient interactions increases mutual goal setting.
2. Communication increases mutual goal setting between nurses and patients and leads to satisfaction.
3. Satisfactions in nurses and patients increase goal attainment.
4. Goal attainment decreases stress and anxiety in nursing situations.
5. Goal attainment increases patient learning and coping ability in nursing situations.
6. Role conflict experienced by patients, nurses, or both, decreases transaction in nurse-patient interactions.
7. Congruence in role expectations and role performance increases transactions in nurse-patient interactions.

These hypotheses could be used to test the theory.

5. Theories contribute to and assist in increasing the general body of knowledge within the discipline through the research implemented to validate them. King reports the results of a descriptive study conducted to test the theory of goal attainment. The study resulted in a classification system to analyze nurse-patient interactions and identified that goal attainment is facilitated when the nurse and patient have accurate perceptions, adequate communication, and set goals mutually.[83] This is one example of a contribution to the general body of knowledge. The theory of goal attainment needs to be tested further. Such testing will expand the theory's contribution to the discipline.

6. **Theories can be utilized by the practitioners to guide and improve their practice.** As demonstrated in the discussion of nursing process, King's theory of goal attainment can be used to guide and improve practice. Even though this theory in itself can be used as a guide to practice, King has also developed the goal-oriented nursing record in an effort to assist the practice of nursing. She presents the goal-oriented nursing record as an application of the theory of goal attainment in nursing.

7. **Theories must be consistent with other validated theories, laws, and principles but will leave open unanswered questions that need to be investigated.** King's theory of goal attainment is not in apparent conflict with other validated theories, laws, and principles. She has clearly documented the sources on which she has based her characteristics and definitions of concepts, and she states that "the major technique used in developing concepts . . . has been a review of the literature in nursing and related fields to identify characteristics of the concept. From this information, an operational definition of the concept is formulated."[84] Using the review of the literature as a base has helped to avoid being in conflict with others. Also, King shares many similarities with other nursing theorists. As does Peplau, King indicates the nurse and client usually enter the relationship as strangers when the client has a need.[85] King's basic assumptions about human beings as thinking, sentient decision makers who have a right to information and to participate in decisions about themselves has a humanistic base similar to that of Paterson and Zderad.[86] Also the emphasis on the right to participate in decisions is similar to that of Orlando, among others.[87]

Throughout A *Theory for Nursing*, King identifies those theories from other fields that support what she is saying. Although there is no apparent conflict, there are many questions open for exploration. A few of these are discussed in the hypotheses presented earlier in this chapter.

SUMMARY

Imogene King has presented an open systems framework from which she derived a theory of goal attainment. The framework consists of three systems—personal, interpersonal, and social—all of which are in continuous exchange with their environments. The concepts of the personal systems are perception, self, body image, growth and development, time, and space. The concepts of the interpersonal systems are role, interaction, communication, transaction, and stress. Social systems concepts are organization, power, authority, status, decision making, and role.

From these systems, and their abstract concepts of human beings, health, environment, and society, she derives a theory of goal attainment. The major concepts of the theory of goal attainment are interaction, perception, communication, transaction, role, stress, and growth and development. Each of these are defined, and overall propositions and criteria for determining internal and external boundaries of the theory are presented.

Imogene King has developed a theory of goal attainment that is based on a philosophy of human beings and an open systems framework. She presents the results of one descriptive research study to test the theory and proposes an application of the theory in the form of a goal-oriented nursing record.

The theory is useful, testable, and applicable to nursing practice. Although it is not the "perfect theory," it is widely generalizable and not situation-specific. As with her previous writing, Dr. King's work is solidly based in the literature and provides the reader with a rich set of resources for further study.

NOTES

1. Imogene M. King, *Toward a Theory for Nursing: General Concepts of Human Behavior* (New York: John Wiley & Sons, Inc., 1971); and idem, *A Theory for Nursing: Systems, Concepts, Process* (New York: John Wiley & Sons, Inc., 1981).
2. King, *A Theory for Nursing*, p. 9.
3. King, *Toward a Theory*, p. x.
4. King, *A Theory for Nursing*, p. vii.
5. Ibid., p. 10.
6. Ibid., p.141.

7. Ibid., p. 10.
8. Ibid., p. 23.
9. Ibid., p. 24.
10. Ibid., pp. 26–27.
11. A. T. Jersild, *In Search of Self* (New York: Columbia University Teachers College Press, 1952), pp. 9–10.
12. King, *A Theory for Nursing*, pp. 30–31.
13. Ibid., p. 31.
14. Sigmund Freud, *Introductory Lectures on Psychoanalysis*, translated by J. Strachery (New York: W. W. Norton & Co., Inc., 1966); Erik Erikson, *Childhood and Society* (New York: W. W. Norton & Co., Inc., 1950); B. F. Inhelder and Jean Piaget, *The Early Growth of Logic in the Child* (New York: W. W. Norton & Co., Inc., 1964); A. Gesell, *Infant Development* (New York: Harper & Row, Publishers, Inc., 1952); and Robert Havinghurst, *Human Development and Education* (New York: David McKay Co., Inc., 1953).
15. King, *A Theory for Nursing*, p. 33.
16. Ibid., pp. 36–37.
17. Ibid., pp. 37–38.
18. Ibid., pp. 43–44.
19. Ibid., p. 45.
20. Ibid., p. 59.
21. Ibid.
22. Ibid., pp. 84–85.
23. Ibid., p. 85.
24. Ibid., pp. 69, 93.
25. Ibid., pp. 71–72.
26. Ibid., p. 74.
27. Ibid., p. 79.
28. Ibid., p. 80.
29. Ibid., p. 82.
30. Ibid.
31. Ibid., pp. 91–92.
32. Ibid., p. 93.
33. Ibid., p. 96.
34. Ibid., pp. 98–99.
35. Ibid., p. 115.
36. Ibid., p. 113.
37. Ibid., p. 114.
38. Ibid., p. 116.
39. Ibid., p. 119.
40. Ibid., p. 123.
41. Ibid., p. 124.
42. Ibid.

43. Ibid., p. 127.
44. Ibid., pp. 127–28.
45. Ibid., pp. 129–30.
46. Ibid., p. 132.
47. Ibid., pp. 141, 142.
48. Ibid., p. 142.
49. Ibid., p. 145.
50. Ibid., pp. 145–46.
51. Ibid., p. 146.
52. Ibid.
53. Ibid.
54. Ibid., p. 147.
55. Ibid.
56. Ibid.
57. Ibid.
58. Ibid., p. 148.
59. Ibid.
60. Ibid.
61. Ibid., p. 149.
62. Ibid., p. 150.
63. Ibid.
64. Ibid., p. 141.
65. Ibid., pp. 143–44.
66. Ibid., p. 3.
67. Ibid., p. 8.
68. Ibid., p. 5.
69. Ibid.
70. Alvin L. Bertrand, *Social Organization* (Philadelphia: F. A. Davis Co., 1972); and Daniel Katz and Robert Kahn, *The Social Psychology of Organizations* (New York: John Wiley & Sons, Inc., 1966).
71. King, *A Theory for Nursing*, pp. 2, 14.
72. Ibid., p. 60.
73. Ibid., pp. 3–4.
74. Ibid., p. 4.
75. Ibid., p. 9.
76. Ibid., p. 157.
77. Ibid., p. 9.
78. Ibid., p. 24.
79. Ibid., p. 177.
80. Ibid., p. 176.
81. Ibid., p. 177.
82. Ibid., p. 156.
83. Ibid., p. 155.
84. Ibid., p. 22.

85. Hildegard E. Peplau, *Interpersonal Relations in Nursing* (New York: G. P. Putnam's Sons, 1952).

86. Josephine Paterson and Loretta Zderad, *Humanistic Nursing* (New York: John Wiley & Sons, Inc., 1976).

87. Ida Jean Orlando, *The Dynamic Nurse-Patient Relationship: Function, Process and Principles* (New York: G. P. Putnam's Sons, 1961); and idem, *The Discipline and Teaching of Nursing Process* (New York: G. P. Putnam's Sons, 1972).

ADDITIONAL REFERENCES

DAUBENMIRE, M. J., and I. M. KING, "Nursing Process Model: A Systems Approach," *Nursing Outlook*, August 1973, pp. 512–17.

KING, IMOGENE M., "A Conceptual Frame of Reference for Nursing," *Nursing Research*, January–February 1968, pp. 27–31.

_____, "The Health Care System: Nursing Intervention Subsystem," in W. H. Werley et. al., eds., *Health Research: The Systems Approach*. New York: Springer Publishing Co., Inc., 1976.

_____, "Nursing Theory-Problem and Prospect," *Nursing Science*, October 1964, pp. 394–403.

_____, "Planning for Change," *Ohio Nurses Review*, August 1970, pp. 4–7.

15

BETTY NEUMAN

Joanne R. Cross

Betty Neuman was born on a farm in Lowell, Ohio, in 1924. Her first nursing education was completed at People's Hospital School of Nursing in Akron, Ohio, in 1947, and she received her M.S. in Mental Health, Public Health Consultation, from UCLA in 1966. She is presently a candidate for a doctoral degree.

Her major area of practice since 1966 has been in mental health consultation and counseling. A broad background in nursing includes public health, schools, industry, and hospital settings. She also has been involved in family therapy, continuing education, and curriculum consultation. Her teaching experience includes a wide variety of areas such as mental health, consultation and organization, leadership, and counseling. She was closely involved in the community mental health movement during its pioneering days in the late 1960s. It was during her work in organization and planning at UCLA concerning the community mental health movement that she developed her nursing model of the "whole person approach" based on a systems adaptation framework.

Betty Neuman's theoretical approach to nursing is exemplified in a holistic approach to her own life. She has a great zest for life and a keen sense of using time creatively and usefully. She actively maintains a wellness program for herself and participates in volunteer counseling. She continues to act as consultant to uni-

versity schools of nursing who wish to adopt and implement her theoretical framework into their curriculum.[1]

Betty Neuman began developing her health systems model while a lecturer in community health nursing at the University of California, Los Angeles. The model was initially developed in response to graduate nursing students who expressed a need for course content that would expose them to a breadth of nursing problems prior to their focusing on specific nursing problem areas.[2]

The model was published in 1972 as "A Model for Teaching Total Person Approach to Patient Problems," in *Nursing Research*.[3] It was refined and subsequently published in the first edition of *Conceptual Models for Nursing Practice*, 1974, and in the second edition in 1980.[4] The most recent refinement, along with numerous examples for application to curriculum, nursing practice, and administration, is in her 1982 publication, *The Neuman Systems Model: Application to Nursing Education and Practice*.[5]

Although the intent of the Neuman conceptual model was initially in a curricular context, and she asserted that she "had no intention of creating a specific conceptual model for the nursing community,"[6] it is important to note that the works of several other nursing theorists (e.g., Martha Rogers, Dorothea Orem, and Imogene King) were being published at the time of her initial publication.[7] Indeed, it was in the early 1970s that the National League for Nursing (NLN) emphasized the importance of conceptual models for nursing education and that conceptual frameworks became a major emphasis of the NLN criteria for accreditation.[8]

Neuman describes her model as comprehensive and dynamic. It is a multidimensional view of individuals, groups (families), and communities who are in constant interaction with environmental stressors. Essentially the model focuses on the client system's reaction to stress and the factors of reconstitution or adaptation. It is considered an appropriate model not only for nursing but also for all health care professionals.[9]

DEVELOPMENT OF THE MODEL

In developing her model, Neuman was influenced by several theoretical sources, along with her own personal experiences in mental health nursing. Her conceptual approach is the result of a synthesis of knowledge from several sources, including:

de Chardin: Philosophy of wholeness or totality of life.[10]

Cornu: Marxian philosophy of man's oneness with nature.[11]

Gestalt: Interaction of person and environment.[12]

Selye: Stress adaptation and interaction with environment.[13]

von Bertalanffy: General living open system theory.[14]

Caplan: Levels of prevention approach.[15]

Postulating from the above theoretical constructs, interactions in the Neuman model may be summarized as follows:

> Gestalt and field theories emphasize the person's perceptual field as a state of dynamic equilibrium created by a problem, which then results in a disturbance of equilibrium. This disequilibrium is seen as a source of motivation for interaction with the environment. Field and systems theories describe the interrelationship and interdependence of the component parts of the individual or society. Selye indicates that it is the stressors in the environment that produce the stimuli (tension) that cause the individual (whole) to interact with his environment.[16]

Chardin and Cornu suggest that . . .

> the properties of parts are determined partly by the larger wholes within which they exist . . . [and] no one part can be looked at in isolation but must be viewed as part of a whole.[17]

Neuman's model is strongly built on general system theory. She asserts that a conceptual model attempts to represent certain aspects of reality that are basic to theory development. In theory development, one deals with premises, deductions, explanations, predictions, and results, either expected or unexpected. Due to its logical nature, a systems model is useful as it frequently and dramatically represents the nature of a process and leads to an increasingly accurate understanding and prediction.

In comparing a systems model with nursing actions, Neuman postulates that although both are goal-directed, a systems model is general in nature. In contrast, nursing actions have very specific goals for vigorously controlling (or containing) those variables that affect nursing care. Such goals might include general improvement in the client, performance or pattern of behavior change, or a specific improvement in self-care skills. Since nursing is increasingly focusing on primary prevention, Neuman sets forth a description of how primary prevention variables interface with those of secondary and tertiary prevention.

> The intent of the Neuman systems model . . . is to set forth a structure which depicts the parts and the subjects; and their interrelationships for the whole of man, as a complete system. The same fundamental concept could apply to a small group, community, country, or even the whole universe. The Neuman model provides structure, organization, and direction for nursing actions, and is flexible enough to deal adequately with man's infinite complexity.[18]

This health care systems model is a conceptual approach developed at a time when several theoretical approaches used energy as a basis for nursing practice. Although this model was initially developed for use by all health care professionals, Neuman states that nurses can uniquely use it to assist individuals, families, and other groups to attain and maintain maximum levels of total wellness by purposeful interventions. She uses the term *intervention* for the phase of the nursing process described in this book as *implementation*. When discussing her work, the term *intervention* will be used. The interventions are aimed at the reduction of stress factors and adverse conditions that are potential or actual in any given clinical situation.[19]

Basic Assumptions

Neuman has postulated several assumptions that underlie the conceptual framework in the development of her model:[20]

1. Each individual has a basic energy resource structure which contains characteristics both unique and common to all human kind, and is essential to life.
2. Man is a composite of the interrelationships of the four variables (biological, psychological, socio-cultural, and developmental) which are at all times present.
3. Each individual has a *normal line of defense* which is that

person's dynamic state of adaptation (or homeostasis) which has evolved and been maintained over a period of time. This is unique for each individual person's normal state of wellness.

4. Each individual has a *flexible line of defense* which is constantly changing in response to single/multiple variables and stressors (biological, psychological, socio-cultural, developmental).

5. *Stressors* are both universal and known; some are unique to the client. They have potential to disturb equilibrium, thus causing a change in priority of needs at any given moment.

6. The degree of client *reaction to stressors* depends on the resistant factors encountered by the stressors and the interrelationship of variables.

7. Each person has an internal set of resistance factors—*lines of resistance*—whose function is to stabilize and return the client to that person's personal line of defense when/if stressors break through.

8. *Primary prevention* relates to general knowledge applied to client assessment in an attempt to identify stressors before they occur.

9. *Secondary prevention* relates to symptomatology. These are interventions generally initiated after an encounter with a stressor.

10. *Tertiary prevention* relates to the adaptive process as reconstitution begins and moves back toward primary prevention. These are the interventions initiated after treatment.

The Systems Model

The total person framework is basically an open systems model with two components—stress and reaction. The "person"* (represented by a series of concentric circles in Neuman's diagram—see Figure 15-1) is viewed as an open system interacting with the environment. The person or system is capable of intake of extrapersonal/intrapersonal factors from the environment, and interacts with this intake by adjusting to it and adjusting it to the system. Logistically the model appears fairly simple and straightforward.

---

*Person refers to the client system, which can be an individual person, family, other group, or community.

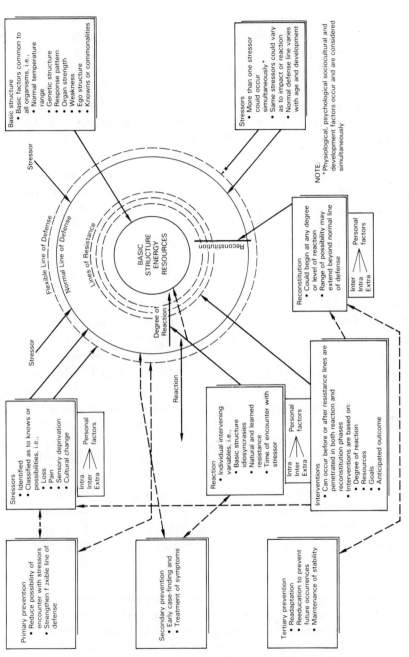

Figure 15-1. The Neuman model: a total person approach to viewing patient problems. [Copyright © 1972, American Journal of Nursing Company. Reproduced, with permission, from *Nursing Research*, May–June, vol. 21, no. 3.]

Note in Figure 15-1 that the series of concentric rings surrounding the basic core structure of human being, family, or community (labeled "basic structure, energy resources") vary in size and distance from the reactor. They represent the *lines of resistance*, the internal factors defending against stressors. The *normal line of defense* is essentially what the person becomes over a lifetime—the normal state of wellness, or steady state—and is composed of biological-psychological-sociocultural-developmental skills that the system uses to deal with stressors. This line of defense is considered to be dynamic since it relates to the way a system is stabilized over time. The *flexible line of defense* (outer broken line) is "accordianlike" in function. It is also dynamic and can be altered rapidly over a short period of time. Its effectiveness can be reduced by such changes as loss of sleep, malnutrition, or any alterations in activities of daily living.

Stressors

Stressors impinge on the system's flexible line of defense where they generate varying degrees of reaction/response. The flexible line of defense, made up of an interaction/adjustment process, is the buffer against these stressors. Influencing factors on this flexible line of defense are the basic biological-psychological-sociocultural-developmental characteristics, which interact simultaneously at any given time. It is important to view the total person (system) in this multidimensional aspect rather than in relation to just one of these variables at a time. The wholeness concept is based on the interrelationship of these variables, which will determine the amount and outcome of the resistance applied by the system to any given stressor.

More than one stressor can occur at a time. The number of stressors influences to some extent the system's reaction. Neuman classifies stressors into the following categories, with examples of the influencing variables:[21]

1. *Extrapersonal*—forces which occur outside the system.
   e.g. unemployment (outside force) influenced by peer acceptability (socio-cultural force), personal feelings about present and past unemployment (psychological), ability to perform the job (biological/developmental/psychological).
2. *Interpersonal*—forces occurring between one or more individuals.

e.g. parent-child role expectations, forces between individuals that are influenced by local child-rearing practices
(socio-cultural), age and development of both child and parents (biological and developmental) and feelings about the
role (psychological).

3. *Intrapersonal*—forces that occur within the individual.
   e.g. anger: an internal force within the individual whose
   expression is influenced by age (developmental), peer group
   acceptability (socio-cultural), physical abilities (biological), and
   past experiences coping with anger (psychological).

Other factors will also influence the system's reaction to a
stressor. What is noxious to one may not be to another. It is important
to consider the number and strength of the stressors, the length of
the encounter with them, and their specific meaning to this system.
Therefore, careful assessment of the impact and meaning of stressors
to the system as well as knowledge of past coping skills are important
for adequate nursing intervention.

Reaction

Primary prevention can begin at any point at which a stressor
is either suspected or identified. If a reaction has not occurred, the
intervention would enter at the primary level. The goal of primary
intervention is to prevent the stressor from penetrating the normal
line of defense or to lessen the degree of reaction by reducing the
possibility of encounter with stressors and by strengthening the line
of defense.

If primary prevention is not possible and reaction has occurred,
intervention would begin at the level of *secondary prevention*. At this
level, the goal is treatment of existing symptoms to lead to reconstitution. Secondary prevention deals mainly with early case finding,
early treatment of symptoms, and attempts to strengthen the internal lines of resistance to reduce reaction. Nursing intervention at this
level can begin at any point where stress reaction is recognized. It
may progress beyond or below the usual level of wellness or line of
defense.

Tertiary prevention is the intervention that follows the active
treatment plan when reconstitution or some reasonable degree of
stabilization has occurred. The goal of the tertiary phase is to main-

tain this adaptation by strengthening the lines of resistance, thus preventing future occurrences. This goal is primarily accomplished by the use of re-educative measures and by optimum utilization of the system's total resources, including the internal and external environments.

These levels of intervention are interrelated and are said to be circular in nature. This circularity lends itself especially to similarities in primary and tertiary prevention. For example, primary prevention emphasizes the avoidance of specific stressors that are hazardous, and tertiary prevention seeks to desensitize the system to these hazardous stressors.

Neuman views the model as multidimensional; that is, there must be consideration of all variables affecting the system and the "proper ranking of need priority at any given point."[22] She continues:

> Although this model is relatively new and untested, it may well prove to be a reliable system for unifying various health-related theories and thus help to clarify relationships of variables in nursing care. Based on this assumption, role definition at various levels of nursing practice could be classified.[23]

NEUMAN'S THEORY AND THE FOUR MAJOR CONCEPTS

The Neuman model will be viewed in terms of congruency and consistency with the four concepts of individual/human, society/environment, health/wellness, and nursing.

Individual/Human

The focus of the Neuman model is based on the philosophy that each human is a "total person" as a client system and that this person is multidimensional, a composite of biological, psychological, sociocultural, and developmental variables. Other variables include basic survival core characteristics possessed in common with other human beings, such as normal temperature range, genetic response patterns, ego structure, and various strengths and weaknesses of the physical body. The dynamic interaction of these variables and core characteristics along with the lines of normal defense and flexible resistance, combined with multiple stressors, provide the essence of the "total person approach." The model is based in part on general system theory, in which the whole is different from and more than the sum of its parts. Thus the concept of "wholeness" or totality is integral to Neuman's model. She states:

> We must now emphatically refuse to deal with single components but instead relate to the concept of wholeness. We need to think and act systematically. Systems thinking enables us to effectively handle all parts of a system simultaneously in an interrelated manner, thus avoiding the fragmented, isolated nature of past functions in nursing.[24]

The entire system than is bound by the *available* environment and its constraints, whether they be man, nursing, family, or community, as shown in Figure 15–2.

Society/Environment

Basic to the Neuman model is the concept that humans are in constant interaction with their environment. This is the fundamental phenomenon of her conceptual model. She defines environment as

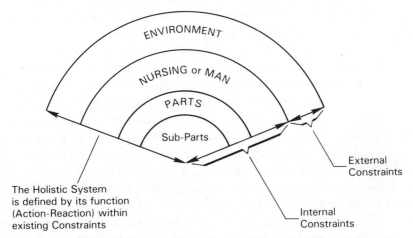

Figure 15-2. Nursing and/or man in the holistic system. [From Betty Neuman, *The Neuman Systems Model: Application to Nursing Education and Practice* (Norwalk, Conn.: Appleton-Century-Crofts, 1982), p. 12. Used with permission.]

those internal and external forces surrounding humans at any given point in time, and states:

> Consideration of environment is critical since it varies as to needs, drives, perceptions and goals of all living organisms. The environment is that viable arena which has relevance to the life space of an organism. Environment has been conceptualized as all factors affecting and affected by the system.[25]

In relation to environment, Neuman specifically notes similarities between her model and the field of Gestalt theories when she speaks of the occurrence of stressors and the reaction to stressors and to the organisms itself. These stressors (intra-, inter-, and extrapersonal), a prominent subsystem of her model, comprise the environment in which the client system operates.

Health/Wellness

A total person definition of wellness can be derived from the Neuman model. Mayer states that "the assumption of this model can lead one to see wellness as a dynamic composite of physical, psychological, socio-cultural, and developmental balance that is flexible yet retains an unbroken ability to resist disequilibrium."[26]

In her initial writings, Neuman stated that a person retains "varying degrees of harmony and balance" between the internal and external environments through a process of interaction and adjustment.[27] Terms used were *wellness, variation from wellness,* and *stability of the client system.*[28] Wellness was equated with stability of the normal line of defense, and illness appeared to be "variances of wellness."[29] In later writings, Neuman stated that "man is an interacting open system in his total interface with his environment and is at all times either in a dynamic state of wellness or ill health in varying degrees. Health, therefore, is reflected in the level of wellness."[30] In addition, she states that "if man's total needs are met, he is in the state of optimal wellness. Conversely, a reduced state of wellness is the result of a need not met."[31]

Neuman continues to mention levels of wellness, which suggests she views health in a continuum rather than as a dichotomy of wellness and illness. It also suggests she holds a linear view rather than a holistic view, although her diagram and model attempt a view of holism.[32] In any event, nursing has as its goal those acts that conserve energy, whether the client system moves toward the wellness state or toward the illness state. Neuman illustrates this phenomenon in the paradigm shown in Figure 15–3.

Other concepts included in her writings are defined in terms of "systems terminology," such as:

Wellness: State of saturation; of inertness free of disruptive needs.[33]

Illness: State of insufficiency; disruptive needs are yet to be satisfied.[34]

Neuman's term *reconsitution* also needs to be addressed in relation to the concept of health. It can be inferred from her model that reconstitution can be equated with moving from "variances from wellness" to desired wellness levels and client stability. Again, reconstitution is viewed holistically as multidimensional in that the biological-psychological-sociocultural-developmental components are affected by intra-inter-extrapersonal variables.

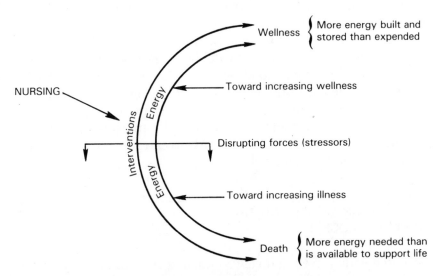

Figure 15–3. Wellness-illness based on the systems concept. [Adapted from Betty Neuman, *The Neuman Systems Model: Applications to Nursing Education and Practice* (Norwalk, Conn.: Appleton-Century-Crofts, 1982), p. 11. Used with permission.]

Nursing

In general, Neuman views nursing as a "unique profession" that concerns itself with all the variables affecting human response to stressors, with a primary concern for the total person. "The primary goal of nursing is the retention and attainment of the client system stability."[35]

She defines the parameters of nursing more clearly when she states that nursing assists individuals, families, and groups to attain and maintain a maximum of total wellness by purposeful interventions aimed at reduction of stress factors and adverse conditions that affect optimal functioning in any given patient situation.[36]

As Mayer points out, nursing's purpose is to deliberately intervene where there is variance from wellness, and purposive nursing interventions are designed to produce positive changes. These changes or results should be measured according to an accepted model, theory, or wellness definition.[37] In order to facilitate movement toward the positive end of a wellness-illness continuum, the nurse needs both a philosophy and an operational model. Neuman has operationalized her model into the nursing process by providing an assessment/intervention tool for use by practitioners. This tool is displayed in Table 15-1.

The assessment/intervention tool (Table 15-1) includes the various aspects of Neuman's model but is flexible enough to allow for the inclusion of any additional data deemed necessary. Factors influencing the use of the tool would be the client, client situation, the practitioner, and the agency involved in the assessment. In Neuman's work, the tool is accompanied by an explanatory section that includes specific rationales, charts to categorize data, and plans for interventions at all levels.

THE NEUMAN MODEL AND THE NURSING PROCESS

As noted earlier, Neuman viewed nursing as a "unique profession" that is "concerned with all the variables affecting the system's response to stressors. The central concern of nursing is the 'total person' or system, while the primary goal is to retain/attain client stability."[38]

Table 15-1

An Assessment/Intervention Tool

A. Intake Summary
1. Name _____
   Age _____
   Sex _____
   Marital _____
2. Referral source and related information.

B. Stressors as Perceived by Patient
   (If Patient is incapacitated, secure data from family or other resources.)
   1. What do you consider your major problem, stress area, or areas of concern? (Identify problem areas)
   2. How do present circumstances differ from your usual pattern of living? (Identify life-style patterns)
   3. Have you ever experienced a similar problem? If so, what was that problem and how did you handle it? Were you successful? (Identify past coping patterns)
   4. What do you anticipate for yourself in the future as a consequence of your present situation? (Identify perceptual factors i.e., reality versus distortions-expectations, present and possible future coping patterns)
   5. What are you doing and what can you do to help yourself? (Identify perceptual factors, i.e., reality versus distortions-expectations, present and possible future coping patterns)
   6. What do you expect care givers, family, friends, or others to do for you? (Identify perceptual factors, i.e., reality versus distortions-expectations, present and possible future coping patterns)

C. Stressors as Perceived by Care Giver
   1. What do you consider to be the major problem, stress area, or areas of concern? (Identify problem areas)
   2. How do present circumstances seem to differ from the patient's usual pattern of living? (Identify life-style patterns)
   3. Has the patient ever experienced a similar situation? If so, how would you evaluate what the patient did? How successful do you think it was? (Identify past coping patterns)
   4. What do you anticipate for the future as a consequence of the patient's present situation? (Identify perceptual factors, i.e., reality versus distortions-expectations, present and possible future coping patterns)
   5. What can the patient do to help himself? (Identify perceptual factors, i.e., reality versus distortions-expectations, present and possible future coping patterns)
   6. What do you **think** the patient expects from care givers, family, friends, or other resources? (Identify perceptual factors, i.e., reality versus distortions-expectations, present and possible future coping patterns)

Summary of Impressions
Note any discrepancies or distortions between the patient's perception and that of the care giver related to the situation.

D. Intrapersonal Factors
   1. Physical (Examples: degree of mobility, range of body function)

(continued)

271

Table 15–1
(Continued)

2. Psycho-sociocultural (Examples: attitudes, values, expectations, behavior patterns, and nature of coping patterns)
3. Developmental (Examples: age, degree of normalcy, factors related to present situation)

E. Interpersonal Factors

Resources and relationship of family, friends, or care givers that either influence or could influence Area D.

F. Extrapersonal Factors

Resources and relationship of community facilities, finances, employment, or other areas which either influence or could influence Areas D and E.

G. Formulation of the Problem

Identify and rank the priority of needs based on the total data obtained from the patient's perception, the care giver's perception, and/or other resources, i.e., laboratory reports, other care givers, or agencies.

With this format, reassessment is a continuous process and is related to the effectiveness of intervention based upon the stated goals. Effective reassessment would include the following as they relate to the total patient situation:

1. Changes in nature of stressors and priority assignments
2. Changes in intrapersonal factors
3. Changes in interpersonal factors
4. Changes in extrapersonal factors

In reassessment it is important to note the change of priority of goals in relation to the primary, secondary, and tertiary prevention categories. An assessment tool of this nature should offer a current, progressive, and comprehensive analysis of the patient's total circumstances or relationships of the four variables (physiologic, psychologic, sociocultural, and developmental).

Source: From Betty Neuman, *The Neuman Systems Model: Application to Nursing Education and Practice* (East Norwalk, Conn.: Appleton-Century-Crofts, 1982), pp. 27–28. Used with permission.

This view is reflected in the way Neuman has systematized the nursing process into the three categories of nursing diagnosis, nursing goals, and nursing outcomes. Table 15–2 briefly summarizes this process. At first glance, it would appear that Neuman had ignored or given less emphasis to the assessment and implementation phases of the nursing process. However, she frequently refers to assessment and intervention in relation to stressors and to the three levels of prevention. An assessment tool (Table 15–1) was included in her second revision of the model with an explanation of how to utilize the tool.[39] In developing this tool, Neuman considered three underlying principles:[40]

1. Good assessment requires knowledge of all the factors influencing a client's perceptual field.
2. The meaning a stressor has to the client is validated by the client as well as the care-giver.
3. Factors in the care-giver's perceptual field that influence the assessment of the client's situation should become apparent.

Table 15–2

Nursing Process According to Betty Neuman

Category		Description of Process
Nursing diagnosis	1.	Based on acquisition of appropriate data base, the diagnosis identifies, assesses, classifies, and evaluates the dynamic interaction of the bio-psycho-sociocultural-developmental variables.
	2.	Variances from wellness (needs/problems) are determined by correlations and constraints through synthesis of theory and data base.
	3.	Broad hypothetical interventions are determined; i.e., maintain flexible line of defense.
Nursing goals	1.	Nurse/client system negotiates for prescriptive change.
	2.	Nurse intervention strategies postulated to retain, attain, and maintain client system stability.
Nursing outcomes	1.	Nursing intervention using one or more prevention modes.
	2.	Confirmation of prescriptive change or reformulation of nursing goals.
	3.	Short-term goal outcomes influence determination of intermediate/long-term goals.
	4.	Client outcome validates nursing process.

Table 15–3 lists the theoretical issues involved in the three levels of prevention. Although not inclusive, it offers operational possibilities for the nursing practitioner and provides a view of the relationships between the levels of prevention and other major concepts in Neuman's model.

TABLE 15-3

Levels of Prevention—Theoretical Issues and Considerations

Primary Prevention	Secondary Prevention	Tertiary Prevention
STRESSORS[a] Mainly covert.	STRESSORS[a] Mainly overt or known.	STRESSORS[a] Mainly overt or residual—covert factors also a possibility.
REACTION Hypothetical. Potential.	REACTION Identified by symptomatology or known factors.	REACTION Hypothetical or known—residual symptoms or factors.
ASSESSMENT[b] Based on patient assessment, experience, and theory. Data should include: 1. Risks or possible hazards to the patient based on patient/nurse assessment. 2. Meaning of the experience to the patient. 3. Life-style factors. 4. Coping patterns (past-present-possible). 5. Individual differences. 6. Other.	ASSESSMENT[b] Determine nature and degree of reaction. Determine internal/external resources available to resist the reaction. Rationale for goals—with collaborative goal setting with the patient when possible.	ASSESSMENT[b] Degree of stability following treatment; possible further reconstitution level assessed. Possible regression factors.

[a] Stressors—Include biological-psychological-sociocultural-developmental factors.

[b] Assessment—Includes the relationship of the four variables (biological-psychological-sociocultural-developmental).

Table 15-3
(Continued)

Primary Prevention	Secondary Prevention	Tertiary Prevention
NURSING GOALS	NURSING GOALS	NURSING GOALS
1. Classify stressors as to client/client system stability. Prevent stressor invasion.	1. Following stressor invasion, protect basic structure.	1. During reconstitution, attain/maintain maximum level of wellness and stability.
2. Negotiate with client for desired prescriptive change.	2. Negotiate with client for desired prescriptive change.	2. Negotiate with client for desired prescriptive change.
3. Provide information to maintain or strengthen existing client/client system strengths.	3. Mobilize and maximize internal/external resources toward stability and energy conservation.	3. Educate, re-educate, and/or reorient as needed.
4. Support positive coping and functioning.	4. Facilitate purposeful manipulation of stressors and reactions to stressors.	4. Support client/client system in appropriate goal directedness and efforts to change.
5. Desensitize existing or possible noxious stressors.	5. Motivate, educate, and involve client and client systems in health care goals.	5. Coordinate and integrate health service resources.
6. Motivate toward wellness.	6. Facilitate appropriate treatment/intervention measures.	6. Provide primary and/or secondary prevention/intervention as needed.
7. Coordinate/integrate interdisciplinary theories and epidemiologic input.	7. Support positive reaction toward illness.	
8. Educate/re-educate.	8. Promote advocacy by coordination/integration.	
	9. Provide primary prevention/intervention as required.	

(continued)

Table 15-3
(Continued)

Primary Prevention	Secondary Prevention	Tertiary Prevention
NURSING INTERVENTIONS Major goal: To strengthen flexible line of defense.	NURSING INTERVENTIONS Major goal: To protect basic structure and facilitate wellness/reconstitution. Based on the following:	NURSING INTERVENTIONS Major goal: To attain/maintain maximum wellness level.
Strengthen resistance to the hazard by: 1. Education. 2. Desensitization. 3. Avoidance of hazard. 4. Strengthen individual resistance factors. 5. Use stress as a positive intervention strategy.	1. Ranking of priority of needs related to symptoms. 2. Patient strengths and weaknesses as related to the four variables. 3. Shift of priorities needed as the patient responds to treatment or as the nature of stressors change. (Primary prevention needs may occur simultaneously with treatment or secondary prevention.) 4. Need to deal with maladaptive processes. 5. Optimum use of internal/external resources, i.e., conservation of energy, noise reduction, and financial aid.	Might include: 1. Motivation. 2. Re-education. 3. Behavior modification. 4. Reality orientation. 5. Progressive goal setting. 6. Optimal use of appropriate available resources. 7. Maintenance of a reasonable adaptive level of functioning.
Intervention should: Prevent invasion of stressors.	Intervention should: Reduce the degree of reaction to stressors.	Intervention should: Support internal/external resources for reconstitution.

Adapted from Betty Neuman, *The Neuman Systems Model* (Norwalk, Conn.: Appleton-Century-Crofts, 1982), pp. 17, 23, 24, 25, 26. Used with permission.

The Neuman model was one of the first systems that explicated a tool (Table 15-1) that is intended to assist the practitioner in applying the model and bridging theory and practice. Neuman designed a specific format of the nursing process to facilitate the use of her systems model and to incorporate the process into the categories she identified as nursing diagnosis, nursing goals, and nursing outcomes. Within the Neuman format the essential elements are explicitly defined and in actuality contain the five-phase process defined in Chapter 2 of this book. Tables 15-4 and 15-5 demonstrate the correlation between Neuman's categorization and the nursing process as utilized in this book.

NEUMAN'S WORK AND THE CHARACTERISTICS OF A THEORY

In nursing literature, the terms *theoretical models, conceptual frameworks,* and *theories* are frequently used interchangeably. Although there are crucial differences between theories and frameworks and usually separate criteria to analyze them, for the purpose of this book the phenomena related to the Neuman model will be compared to the characteristics of a theory provided in Chapter 1.

1. Theories can interrelate concepts in such a way as to create a different way of looking at a particular phenomenon. The Neuman model represents a timely focus on nursing interest in the total person approach to the interaction of environment and health. The emphasis on wellness and primary prevention is unique to this framework.

The interrelationships between the concepts of person, health, nursing, and society/environment are repeatedly mentioned throughout the Neuman model and are considered to be basically adequate according to the criteria. The concepts and definition statements concerning primary, secondary, and tertiary prevention "provide the required general linkages among the concepts of the model."[41]

However, some concept areas need clarification of their definitions and further explanation. Examples include the meaning of internal and external environments and their relation to stressors with the human person. Another area is the specific meaning of wellness—or "variances" thereof—and ensuing "levels of wellness." The concept of reconstitution is neither defined nor explored as to definitive meaning.

Table 15-4

Nursing Process Format for the Neuman Model

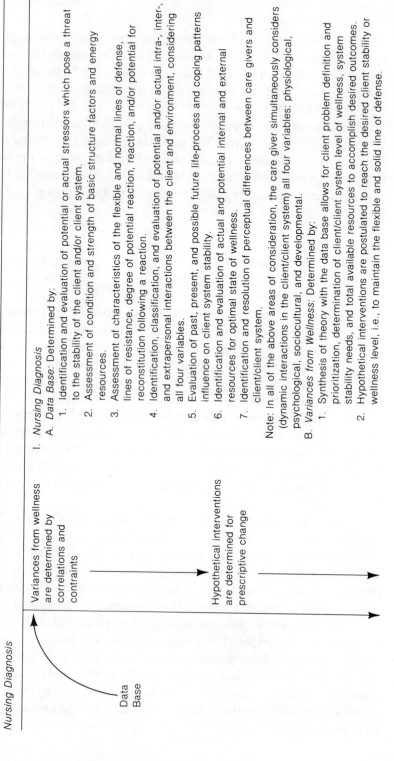

Nursing Diagnosis

Data Base → Variances from wellness are determined by correlations and contraints

Hypothetical interventions are determined for prescriptive change

I. *Nursing Diagnosis*
   A. *Data Base:* Determined by:
      1. Identification and evaluation of potential or actual stressors which pose a threat to the stability of the client and/or client system.
      2. Assessment of condition and strength of basic structure factors and energy resources.
      3. Assessment of characteristics of the flexible and normal lines of defense, lines of resistance, degree of potential reaction, reaction, and/or potential for reconstitution following a reaction.
      4. Identification, classification, and evaluation of potential and/or actual intra-, inter-, and extrapersonal interactions between the client and environment, considering all four variables.
      5. Evaluation of past, present, and possible future life-process and coping patterns influence on client system stability.
      6. Identification and evaluation of actual and potential internal and external resources for optimal state of wellness.
      7. Identification and resolution of perceptual differences between care givers and client/client system.

   Note: In all of the above areas of consideration, the care giver simultaneously considers (dynamic interactions in the client/client system) all four variables: physiological, psychological, sociocultural, and developmental.

   B. *Variances from Wellness:* Determined by:
      1. Synthesis of theory with the data base allows for client problem definition and prioritization, determination of client/client system level of wellness, system stability needs, and total available resources to accomplish desired outcomes.
      2. Hypothetical interventions are postulated to reach the desired client stability or wellness level, i.e., to maintain the flexible and solid line of defense.

278

Nursing Goals

II. *Nursing Goals:* Determined by:
1. Negotiation with the client for desired prescriptive change to correct variances from wellness, based on classified needs and resources identified in the nursing diagnosis.
2. Appropriate intervention strategies are postulated for retention, attainment, and/or maintenance of client system stability as desired outcome goals.

Nursing Outcomes

III. *Nursing Outcomes:* Determined by:
1. Nursing intervention accomplished through use of one or more of the following three prevention modes: (1) primary prevention (action to retain system stability), (2) secondary prevention (action to attain system stability), (3) tertiary prevention (action to maintain system stability), usually following secondary prevention/ intervention.
2. Evaluation of outcome goals following intervention either confirms outcome goals or serves as a basis for reformulation of subsequent nursing goals.
3. Intermediate and long-range goals for subsequent nursing action are structured in relation to short-term goal outcomes.
4. Client outcome validates the nursing process.

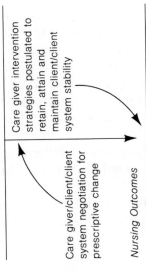

Care giver intervention strategies postulated to retain, attain and maintain client/client system stability

Care giver/client/client system negotiation for prescriptive change

Confirmation of prescriptive change or reformulation of nursing goals

Short-term goal outcomes influenced intermediate/ long-range goal determination

Nursing intervention using one or more prevention modes.

Client outcome validates nursing process

Source: From Betty Neuman, *The Human Systems Model: Application to Nursing Education and Practice* (East Norwalk, Conn.: Appleton-Century-Crofts, 1982), pp. 22–23. Used with permission.

Table 15-5
Comparison of Nursing Processes

Chapter 2 Nursing Process	Neuman Nursing Process

1. *Assessment* phase
Analysis
	1. *Nursing Diagnosis*
	  A. Accurate data base.
	  B. Synthesize theory; define problem and "variance from wellness"; prioritize needs.

2. *Nursing Diagnosis* phase
3. *Planning* phase
  Goals
  Objectives
	C. Hypothetical intervention postulated.
	2. *Nursing Goals*
	  A. Mutual negotiation with client for prescriptive change to correct problem.
	  B. Appropriate intervention strategies planned (retain, attain, maintain client stability).

4. *Implementation* phase	3. *Nursing Outcomes*
	  A. Nursing intervention (using one or more modes of prevention).
	  B. Confirmation of change (or reformulate goals).

5. *Evaluation* phase	C. Short-term goals influence long-term goals for subsequent nursing action. D. Client outcome validates nursing process.

2. Theories must be logical in nature. Neuman's model in general presents itself as logically consistent. It provides a logical sequence in the process of nursing wherein emphasis on the importance of accurate data assessment is basic to the sequential steps of the nursing process as previously defined. However, there are other philosophical issues that are not supported in the model. One such issue involves the theoretical component wherein Neuman considers the person as an open system. There is little to support this contention in her theory other than the statement that "man adjusts to the environment and it to him," because the primary focus is on man who is "capable of intake from the environment."[42] Nowhere is the concept of feedback addressed as man's output into the environment, which is necessary for open systems theory. This would tend to view man as a closed system.[43]

In the logical translation of the Neuman model, there appear to be incompatible elements since the model reflects both mechanistic and organismic views of the relationship of "person" to the environment. Humans as beings reacting to a stimulus in the environment is a view held by the mechanistic theorists. This is essentially a stress-adaptation theory. Because the person is a reactive being, then any activity is primarily the result of external forces.

On the other hand, the organismic view is one of holism where the person is an active organism in continuous interaction with the environment. This view emphasizes the whole person, not any one component or discrete part. This "world view" incorporates Neuman's use of Gestalt, field, and other philosophies that support the unity of the person.[44] However, Neuman presents her model as essentially an organismic view. Therefore some redefining of terms incorporating a more dynamic view of stress is needed to translate this model to a more logical consistency.

3. **Theories should be relatively simple yet generalizable.** Given the abstract nature of most conceptual models, Neuman's model is fairly simple and straightforward in approach. The terms used are easily identifiable and for the most part have definitions that are broadly accepted. The multiple use of the model in many and varied nursing situations (practice, curriculum, and administration) is testimony in itself of its broad use.[45] The potential use of this model by other health care disciplines also attests to its generalizability for use in practice.

One potential drawback in relation to simplicity is the diagrammed model (Figure 15–1) since it presents over thirty-five variables, which tends to become awesome to the viewer. Like many systems models, it becomes overly complex when it specifies so many components and so many relationships. This makes it difficult to manage the model or to evaluate effects of the model on nursing practice. In the main, the model identifies the components without specifying the *nature* of the relationships between them, which causes some difficulty in the functional use of the model.[46] Thus, at this point, it lends itself to "reductionism" rather than "holism."

4. **Theories can be the bases for hypotheses that can be tested.** Neuman's model, due to its high level and breadth of abstraction, lends itself to theory development, although no testable hypotheses have yet been generated.[47] One area for future consideration as a beginning testable theory might be the concept of prevention as intervention, subsequent to basic concept refinement in the Neuman model. Other areas for research have been developed and suggested both by Neuman and by Fawcett.[48]

5. **Theories contribute to and assist in increasing the general**

body of knowledge within the discipline through the research implemented to validate them. The multidimensional nature of the model produces a framework that is attractive to many health care professionals in varied health care settings. Decidedly the model has provided clear, comprehensive guidelines for both nursing education and practice in a variety of settings, and perhaps this is its primary contribution to nursing knowledge. Although the concepts within the guidelines are clearly explicated, and many applications of the theory have been published, no research studies explicitly derived from this model have been published to date. This is necessary if validity is to be established.[49]

6. **Theories can be utilized by the practitioners to guide and improve their practice.** One of the most significant attributes of the Neuman model is the assessment/intervention tool together with comprehensive guidelines for its use with the nursing process. These guidelines have provided a practical resource for many nursing practitioners and have been used extensively in a variety of settings in nursing practice, education, and administration. As Neuman points out, this multidimensional model may indeed in the future provide the "unifying" force tying together various health-related theories and behaviors, thus assisting in clarifying the relationship of variables within nursing practice.

With the current emphasis on self-help, primary prevention, and increasing consumer awareness of the importance of health promotion, health care workers are moving into the arena of wellness-focused care. This is especially true of the nurse moving from illness-oriented activities to wellness-oriented settings such as clinics and ambulatory care settings. Thus, the Neuman model is very congruent with today's health care philosophies and offers some direction in wellness settings.

7. **Theories must be consistent with other validated theories, laws, and principles but will leave open unanswered questions that need to be investigated.** In general, there is no direct conflict with other theories. There is, however, a lack of specificity in systems concepts such as "feedback" and the exact nature of the total system "boundaries," which are indirectly addressed throughout the model. The solving of problems in these areas could be facilitated with greater exploration and clarification of definitions. Caplan's theory of the three levels of prevention as intervention leaves an interesting area to be explored.[50] Indeed, Neuman also suggests an area to be ex-

plored is how to recognize and deal with the impact of environmental forces on the nursing profession in order to develop a holistic nursing posture.[51]

SUMMARY AND CONCLUSIONS

Conceptual models are imperative to the development of nursing as a profession. Neuman's total person approach to health care is one such model that should be considered. In essence, she presents an approach to viewing the person's perception of the stressors affecting the "parts" of the whole individual in constant interaction with the environment. It is a multidimensional, total unit approach, one that can be used to describe an individual, a group, or an entire community. Inasmuch as the model emphasizes the total person, it transcends the nursing model to become a health care model, applicable to all health care disciplines.[52]

Although Neuman describes nursing as a "unique" profession, this is not clearly documented in her writings. As Venable points out, "the lack of a unique role for nursing is not necessarily seen as a detriment but rather as a call for reexamination of traditionally defined roles assigned to health care workers in general."[53]

Even though the model is interdisciplinary, it certainly has universal applicability to nursing. One of its greatest strengths is the clear directions it gives for interventions through primary, secondary, and tertiary prevention. Although society's expectation of the nursing role is tied very specifically to certain behavior in various levels of prevention (i.e., primary: community health; secondary: acute care; and tertiary: limited settings), in actuality all three levels are important aspects of care in all nursing settings. Primary and tertiary prevention will have more social congruence as society becomes increasingly aware of the emerging role of the nurse as a nucleus of the health care system.

Another strength of this model is its flexibility as a stimulus-response system model. This flexibility has lent itself to use in a variety of nursing settings as documented in Neuman's text.

The model is relatively new but has great potential for laying the groundwork for the formation of a theory, and for testing interrelationships between nursing theory, nursing research, and nursing practice.[54]

NOTES

1. Betty Neuman, "Family Intervention Using the Betty Neuman Health Care Systems Model," in *Family Health: A Theoretical Approach to Nursing Care,* Imelda Clements and Florence B. Roberts, eds. (New York: John Wiley & Sons, Inc., 1983), pp. 239–40.

2. Betty M. Neuman and Rae Jeanne Young, "A Model for Teaching Total Person Approach to Patient Problems," *Nursing Research,* 21 (May–June 1972), 264–69.

3. Ibid.

4. Betty Neuman, "The Betty Neuman Health-Care Systems Model: A Total Person Approach to Patient Problems," in Joan P. Riehl and Callista Roy, eds., *Conceptual Models for Nursing Practice* (East Norwalk, Conn.: Appleton-Century-Crofts, 1974 and 1980).

5. Betty Neuman, *The Neuman Systems Model: Application to Nursing Education and Practice* (East Norwalk, Conn.: Appleton-Century-Crofts, 1982).

6. Jacqueline Fawcett and others, "A Framework for Analysis and Evaluation of the Neuman Systems Model," in Betty Neuman, *The Neuman Systems Model: Application to Nursing Education and Practice* (East Norwalk, Conn.: Appleton-Century-Crofts, 1982), p. 36.

7. Martha E. Rogers, *An Introduction to the Theoretical Basis of Nursing* (Philadelphia: F. A. Davis Co., 1970); Dorothea Orem, *Nursing: Concepts of Practice* (New York: McGraw-Hill Book Company, 1971); and Imogene M. King, *Toward a Theory for Nursing* (New York: John Wiley & Sons, Inc., 1971).

8. C. J. Peterson, "Questions Frequently Asked about the Development of a Conceptual Framework," *Journal of Nursing Education,* April 1977.

9. Neuman, *The Neuman Systems Model,* p. 16.

10. P. T. de Chardin, *The Phenomenon of Man* (London: Collins, 1955), pp. 109–12.

11. A. Cornu, *The Origins of Marxist Thought* (Springfield, Ill.: Charles C. Thomas, Publisher, 1957), pp. 12–17.

12. M. Edelson, *Sociotherapy and Psychotherapy* (Chicago: University of Chicago Press, 1970), pp. 225–31.

13. Hans Selye, *The Physiology and Pathology of Exposure to Stress* (Montreal: ACTA, Inc., 1950), pp. 12–13.

14. Ludwig von Bertalanffy, *General System Theory* (New York: George Braziller, Inc., 1968).

15. Gerald Caplan, *Principles of Preventive Psychiatry* (New York: Basic Books, Inc., 1964).

16. Ruth B. Craddock and Martha K. Stanhope, "The Neuman Health-Care Systems Model: Recommended Adaptation," in Joan P. Riehl

and Callista Roy, eds., *Conceptual Models for Nursing Practice* 2nd ed. (East Norwalk, Conn.: Appleton-Century-Crofts, 1980), p. 159.

17. Neuman, *The Neuman System Model*, p. 14.
18. Ibid., p. 11.
19. Ibid.
20. Ibid., pp. 12–14.
21. Janet F. Venable, "The Neuman Health-Care Systems Model: An Analysis," in Joan P. Riehl and Callista Roy, eds., *Conceptual Models for Nursing Practice*, 2nd ed. (East Norwalk, Conn.: Appleton-Century-Crofts, 1980), p. 136.
22. Neuman, *The Neuman Systems Model*, p. 16.
23. Ibid.
24. Ibid., p. 1.
25. Ibid., p. 9.
26. Marlene G. Mayer, *A Systematic Approach to the Nursing Care Plan*, 2nd ed. (East Norwalk, Conn.: Appleton-Century-Crofts, 1978), p. 3.
27. Fawcett and others, "A Framework for Analysis," p. 37.
28. Ibid.
29. Ibid.
30. Neuman, *The Neuman Systems Model*, p. 9.
31. Ibid.
32. Ann L. Whell, "Congruence between Existing Theories of Family Functioning and Nursing Theories," *Advances in Nursing Science*, 3 (1980), pp. 59–67.
33. Neuman, *The Neuman Systems Model*, p. 10.
34. Ibid.
35. Fawcett and others, "A Framework for Analysis," p. 37.
36. Neuman, *The Neuman Systems Model*, p. 11.
37. Mayer, *A Systematic Approach*, p. 2.
38. Fawcett and others, "A Framework for Analysis," p. 37.
39. Neuman, "The Betty Neuman Health-Care Systems Model," in Riehl and Roy, *Conceptual Models*, 2nd. ed. 1980, pp. 127–31.
40. Ibid., p. 125.
41. Fawcett and others, "A Framework for Analysis," p. 39.
42. Ibid.
43. Ibid.
44. Ibid., p. 40.
45. Neuman, *The Neuman Systems Model*.
46. Barbara Stevens, *Nursing Theory: Analysis, Application and Evaluation* (Boston: Little, Brown & Co., 1979), pp. 212–13.
47. Fawcett and others, "A Framework for Analysis," p. 41.
48. Ibid.; and Neuman, *The Neuman Systems Model*.
49. Fawcett and others, "A Framework for Analysis," p. 41.

50. Caplan, *Principles of Preventive Psychiatry.*
51. Neuman, *The Neuman Systems Model,* p. 21.
52. Venable, "The Neuman Health-Care Systems Model," p. 140.
53. Ibid., p. 141.
54. Marion K. Hoffman, "From Model to Theory Construction," in Betty Neuman, *The Neuman Systems Model: Application to Nursing Education and Practice* (East Norwalk, Conn.: Appleton-Century-Crofts, 1982), p. 48.

16

JOSEPHINE E. PATERSON AND LORETTA T. ZDERAD

Susan G. Praeger and Christina R. Hogarth

Josephine E. Paterson and Loretta T. Zderad have written a book entitled Humanistic Nursing.[1] *Josephine Paterson is a clinical nurse specialist at the Northport Veterans Administration Medical Center at Northport, New York. She is a graduate of Lenox Hill Hospital School of Nursing and St. John's University. She received her master's degree from Johns Hopkins School of Hygiene and Public Health, Baltimore, Maryland. Her Doctor of Nurse Science is from Boston University School of Nursing, Boston, Massachusetts, where she specialized in mental health and psychiatric nursing. Dr. Paterson has conceptualized and taught humanistic nursing to graduate students, faculty, and staff in a variety of settings. She is also currently on the faculty of the State University of New York at Stonybrook.*

Loretta T. Zderad is presently the Associate Chief for Nursing Education at the Northport Veterans Administration Medical Center, Northport, New York. She is a graduate of St. Bernard's Hospital School of Nursing and of Loyola University. She received her Master of Science degree from Catholic University, Washington, D.C. and a Doctor of Philosophy from Georgetown University, Washington, D.C. She has taught in several universities and has led groups on humanistic nursing. Dr. Zderad also serves on the faculty of the State University of New York at Stonybrook.

Josephine E. Paterson and Loretta T. Zderad have described what they call a "humanistic nursing practice" theory in several publications and presentations. It is a practice theory because they believe that the theory of a science of nursing develops from the lived experiences of the nurse and the nursed* in the practice of nursing. Theory, then, becomes a response to the phenomenological experience. R. D. Laing is quoted as saying that "theory is the articulated vision of experience."[2] This means that theory becomes the philosophical perspective that is derived from the nurse's existential encounter in the health care world.

Humanistic nursing is an expression of the humanistic psychology, or third force, movement. The movement is often called the "third force" in psychology because it was seen as an alternative response to the two dominant psychological views. Freudian psychology was seen as being limited in its orientation toward the sick personality, and behavorial psychology was seen as being too mechanistically oriented.[3] The humanistic orientation tries to take a broader view of the potential of human beings, and rather than trying to supplant other views, it is aimed toward supplementing them.[4]

There is no simple way to define the essence of humanistic psychology because it is concerned with the phenomenological experiences of individuals—the exploration of human experiences. Thus, although humanistic psychologists might present their own particular view of humanistic psychology, they can also appreciate the views and unique wording used by others. Paterson and Zderad have been influenced by the writings of existentialists and humanistic psychologists as seen in their emphasis on the nature of dialogue and the importance of the perceptual field. Their work, *Humanistic Nursing*, was conceptualized while they were in Northport and most of their efforts have been with the staff there.[5]

HUMANISTIC NURSING THEORY AND
THE FOUR MAJOR CONCEPTS

Human Beings

In humanistic nursing practice theory, human beings are viewed from an existential framework of becoming through choices. "Man

Nursed is used as a noun throughout this chapter, meaning the recipient(s) of nursing.

is an individual being necessarily related to other men in time and space. As every man is beholden to other men for his birth and development, interdependence is inherent in the human situation, . . . [and] human existence is coexistence."[6] It is through relationships with others that the human being becomes; this, in turn, allows for each person's unique individuality to become actualized.

Health

Health is described as more than the absence of disease. Individuals have the potential for well-being, but also for *more-being*. Well-being implies a steady state, whereas more-being refers to being in the process of becoming all that is humanly possible.[7]

Nursing

Nursing, then, is seen within the human context. It is a nurturing response of one person to another in a time of need that aims toward the development of well-being and more-being. Nursing works toward this aim by helping to increase the possibility of making responsible choices, since this is how human beings are able to become. "The nursing situation is a particular kind of human situation in which the interhuman relating is purposely directed toward nurturing the well-being or more-being of a person with perceived needs related to the health-illness quality of living."[8] If viewed in terms of the human situation, nursing focuses on the individual's unique being and striving toward becoming. Nursing focuses on the whole and looks beyond the categorizations of the parts. When a person is ill and the body is manifesting certain changes, these changes influence the person's world and the experience of being in the world. The client's perspective of the world is an important consideration in nursing.

> Nursing implies a special kind of meeting of human persons. It occurs in response to a perceived need related to the health-illness quality of the human condition. Within that domain, which is shared by other health professions, nursing is directed toward the goal of nurturing well-being and more-being (human potential). Nursing, therefore does not involve a merely fortuitous encounter but rather one in which there is purposeful call and response. In this vein, humanistic nursing may be considered as a special kind of lived dialogue.[9]

Nursing is seen as a unique blend of theory and methodology. The theory may be articulated from the open framework that is derived from the human situation. This framework can be used to suggest the possible dimensions of humanistic nursing practice. Theory cannot exist without the practice of nursing, for it depends on the experience of nursing and on the reflecting of that experience. The elements of the framework for humanistic nursing, as stated by Paterson and Zderad, may be described as follows:

> Incarnate men (patient and nurse) meeting (being and becoming) in a goal-directed (nurturing well-being and more-being) intersubjective transaction (being with and doing with) occurring in time and space (as measured and as lived by patient and nurse) in a world of men and things.[10]

In order to utilize this framework for a nursing practice theory, the authors have suggested three concepts that together provide the basis (or components) of nursing. These concepts are dialogue, community, and phenomenologic nursology.

Dialogue.   Nursing is a lived dialogue. It is the nurse-nursed relating creatively. Humans need nursing. Nurses need to nurse. Nursing is an intersubjective experience in which there is real sharing. Involved in this dialogue are meeting, relating, presence, and a call and response.[11]

Meeting is the coming together of human beings and is characterized by the expectation that there will be a nurse and a nursed. Factors that influence this meeting are feelings that are aroused by the anticipation of the meeting, the amount of control that the nurse and/or client has in coming together, the uniqueness of the nurse and the client, and the decision for disclosure and enclosure with the other.

Relating refers to the process of nurse-nursed "doing" with each other; it means being with the other. Two ways of relating are described that distinguish the human situation, that is, we are able to relate as subject to object as well as subject to subject. "Both types of relationships are essential for genuine human existence."[12] Subject-object relating refers to how human beings use objects and know others through abstractions, conceptualizations, categorizing, labeling, etc. Subject-subject relating occurs when two persons are open to each other as fully human. The "I-Thou" relationship described by Martin Buber provides the opportunity to develop this unique potential.[13]

> Through the scientific objective approach, that is, subject-object relating, it is possible to gain certain knowledge about a person; through intersubjective, that is, subject-subject relating, it is possible to know a person in his unique individuality. Thus, both subject-subject and subject-object relationships are essential to the clinical nursing process. Both are integral elements of humanistic nursing.[14]

Presence is the quality of being open, receptive, ready, and available to another person in a reciprocal manner. Presence necessitates being open to the whole of the nursing experience; this is behavior that is difficult to achieve when the nurse at times is required to focus on specific details of the client's body or behavior. "Man is an embodied being, and the nurse, in nurturing the patient's well-being and more-being, must relate to him and his body in their mysterious interrelatedness."[15]

Call and response is an indication of the complex nature of the lived dialogue. Call and response are transactional, sequential, and simultaneous. Nurses and clients call and respond to each other, and this occurs both verbally and nonverbally.

It is through nursing acts that the dialogue of nursing is lived. The meaning of those acts to the nurse and to the client may differ and may act as a potential catalyst for effecting change in the dialogue.

When considering nursing as a lived dialogue, it is necessary to take into account the situation in which it occurs—the real world of other human beings and things within a framework of time and space.

Community. The phenomenon of community is the second component critical to humanistic nursing practice theory. It is two or more persons striving together, living-dying all at once. To understand community is to recognize and value uniqueness. Humanistic nursing leads to community; it occurs within a community and is affected by community. It is through the intersubjective sharing of meaning in community that human beings are comforted and nurtured. Community is the experience of persons, and it is through community, persons relating to others, that it is possible to become.[16]

Phenomenologic nursology.   Nursing, its practice and theory, would not be complete without a methodology. This methodology has been presented as phenomenologic nursology. There are five phases in this phenomenologic approach to nursing, as discussed below.

1. *Preparation of the nurse knower for coming to know.* The nurse is ever prepared and striving to be open and caring. This involves learning to take risks, being open to experiences—to one's own view of the world and to another's perceptual framework. In order to achieve this, the nurse needs to be exposed to a wide range of experiences. Nurses can be prepared for this by immersing themselves in studies in the humanities where different views about the nature of being are expressed. Individual experiences, as a person and a nurse, are valid and important. The wider the range of experiences that the nurse has, the wider the possibility for knowing. Relating the experiences of human beings in literature and the other arts to the nurse's experience with persons will open the way for knowing individuals in the nursing situation. Self-knowledge, the "authenticity with self," is important to knowing and can be facilitated through clinical supervision and/or different forms of personal growth therapy.[17]

2. *Nurse knowing the other intuitively.* This phase is the merging of the self with the rhythmic spirit of the other. Intuitive knowing of the other requires getting "inside" the other, into the rhythm of the other's experience, which results in a special, difficult to express, knowledge of the other. Intuitive knowing presumes the I-Thou relationship described by Buber.[18]

3. *Nurse knowing the other scientifically.* This phase implies a separateness from what is known. It requires taking the all-at-once phenomena known intuitively and looking at them, mulling it over, analyzing, sorting out, comparing, contrasting, relating, interpreting, giving a name to, and categorizing it.[19] This is taking the I-Thou and reflecting it as an "it." Paterson says, "The challenge of communicating a lived nursing reality demands authenticity with the self and rigorous effort in the selection of words, phrases, and precise grammar."[20]

4. *Nurse complementarily synthesizing known others.* This phase involves relating, comparing, and contrasting what occurs in nursing situations to enlarge one's understanding of nursing. Buber has said that "the area of contrasting, carried out properly and adequate-

ly, leads to the grasp of the principle."[21] The nurse compares and synthesizes multiple known realities and arrives at an expanded view. The nurse allows a dialogue between the realities and permits differences.

5. *Succession within the nurse from the many to the paradoxical one.* The fifth phase evolves from the descriptive process of a lived phenomenon. It is the articulated vision of experience that becomes expressed in a coherent whole. This phase is the process of refining the intuitive grasp achieved before, struggling with the known realities, and making an intuitive leap toward truth, thus forming a new hypothetical construct. Since the multiple realities and known truths are part of the knower—the nurse, the new truth is really an expression of the knower in abstract or conceptual terms beyond the individual data. It is a truth beyond the synthesis of the whole. So, the paradox rests in the fact that the nurse starts with a general notion, an intuitive grasp; then studies it, compares, contrasts, and synthesizes it in order to arrive at a truth that is uniquely personal but has meaning for all—thus, a descriptive theoretical construct of nursing.

PHENOMENOLOGIC NURSOLOGY AND THE NURSING PROCESS

Phenomenologic nursology as developed by Paterson and Zderad is a methodology for understanding and describing nursing situations. It is a method of inquiry, as is the problem-solving approach of the nursing process. Phenomenologic nursology is a method of seeking to understand the nurse-nursed experience so that the nurse can be with the nursed in a human and therefore healing manner. The nursing process assumes the presence of a nursing problem that the nurse and client will solve together. Phenomenologic nursology assumes a perceived health need by an individual who is involved in interaction with a health care provider.

Phenomenology is a descriptive process. Theory development begins with description, and in the case of phenomenological development, the process is a "progressive intellectual intuition by which one isolates and identifies the essence."[22] Phenomenology is not concerned specifically with facts; it assumes that facts exist. Rather it is concerned with the nature of the facts and what they mean to the individual. Phenomenology describes phenomena but does not attempt to explain or predict their occurrence.

Nursing process and nursology are similar in many aspects. Both methodologies utilize assessment, analysis, diagnosis, planning, implementation, and evaluation.

The first step of the nursing process is *assessment*. Assessment includes a collection of subjective and objective data about an individual obtained through observation, interaction with the client, and information from other sources such as laboratory studies. Phenomenologic nursology includes subjective and objective data but expands the assessment to two pre-assessment phases. These are: (1) preparation of the nurse knower for coming to know, and (2) knowing the other intuitively.

1. *Preparation of the nurse knower for coming to know.* This phase can be seen as a prerequisite similar to but distinct from the nursing process wherein nurses are educated in the humanities and sciences before beginning nursing practice in the clinical situation. The nursing process assumes that the individual undertaking the process is educated in the bio-psycho-spiritual needs of the individual. Phenomenologic nursology makes these same assumptions but also assumes that the nurse has a sensitivity to and knowledge of the human condition as well as self-knowledge. The humanistic theory and practice of nursing require that the practitioner be able to subjectively experience the other. As mentioned earlier, the nursing student can be helped to understand another's situation by studying the humanities and fine arts. Experiencing life events, through literature, drama, and the arts, enriches the student's understanding of human experiences such as love, joy, loneliness, suffering, and death. The use of guided imagery and other exercises are also useful in developing empathy, the ability to experience the other. The development of self-awareness of authenticity is important if the nurse expects to encounter others in dialogue and with presence.

2. *Nurse knowing the other intuitively.* This phase can be seen as occurring prior to the assessment phase of the nursing process, even though intuition is indeed a kind of initial assessment. This phase is characterized by a "taking in" of the nursed in the human situation, the empathic encounter, the beginning of the I-Thou relationship wherein the nurse understands the other's experience all-at-once. It is an intuitive grasp of the other's situation.[23] The use of intui-

tion is a significant aspect of assessment. Although intuition is not a new tool in nursing, its respectability has often been denied. In the effort to establish itself as a profession, nursing has been utilizing an increasingly scientific, objective approach to the study of nursing and the individuals who utilize nursing services. The humanistic nurse, however, believes that the subjective experience of human beings is as valid as the objective experience that can be measured.

The assessment and early analysis phases of the nursing process can be compared to the *nurse knowing the other scientifically*. This phase includes the more familiar method of looking at a phenomenon from many aspects: comparing, classifying, looking for themes in relationships and among the parts. Dividing persons into biological, psychological, social, and spiritual parts is an example of classifying data. It is important to understand, in the phenomenologic method of nursology, that the call comes first, followed by intuition, then assessment, and then analysis. In the problem-solving method, a problem statement by the nursed is followed by scientific data collection organized by parts, and intuition is not included in the assessment or analysis.

The later stages of analysis in the nursing process are quite similar to the phase in nursology called *nurse complementarily synthesizing known others*. During the analysis portion of the nursing process, as described earlier, the nurse compares the data with other known realities such as developmental stages, Maslow's hierarchy of needs,[24] and physiologic principles. In nursology, the nurse compares "multiple known realities" with the data and the experience of the nursed.[25] In other words, the nurse examines the data and experience of the nursed in light of scientific and subjective knowledge and then compares, contrasts, and ultimately synthesizes to an expanded view.[26] Comparisons do occur in the phenomenologic method, but the purpose of the comparisons is directed toward identifying relationships and patterns with much consideration given to opposites and polarities.[27] The phenomenologist synthesizes opposites and patterns into a larger concept, whereas the problem solver chooses a pattern and decides whether it is a problem or not.

Diagnosis refers to the step of the nursing process wherein the nurse makes a problem statement. The nurse collects data regarding the client's stated need, then analyzes the data by classifying it, comparing it to known theory and principles, and finally arriving at a conclusion that is a statement of the problem. *Succession within the nurse from the many to the paradoxical one* can be compared to the stage of identifying a diagnosis. After synthesizing the ideas, data, and experience, a conclusion is reached that is broader than the classifications and reflects the experience of the nursed as well as the nurse's initial intuitive grasp of the nursed. This conclusion has meaning for all. The conclusion or truth is really the formation of a concept as Paterson and Zderad intended it, not the formation of a diagnosis or patient problem, although the conclusion can be a diagnosis.

The *planning* and *implementation* phases of the nursing process describe a goal or outcome to be reached by the client with steps (objectives) to be accomplished toward the goal. Specific nurse and client actions are spelled out in detail. Phenomenologic nursology does not describe the formation of a goal-directed nursing care plan. Humanistic nursing is concerned with being with another who is in need. The goal of more-being or well-being is accomplished through dialogue. In the dialogue between nurse and nursed, there is the *meeting* and the *presence* of the nurse for the other, and the *call* and *response* between the nurse and the nursed, the I-Thou relationship. This is the therapeutic relationship. Paterson and Zderad say that this relationship takes place in the nursing situation in the real world; however, they do not elaborate on incorporating the "doing" aspects of nursing into the dialogue. The theory evolved from the authors' psychiatric nursing practice and experience where the "doing" is the relationship.

The *evaluation* phase of the nursing process is deciding whether the client's behavior has changed as measured by the goals and objectives. The behavior change results from the actions of the nurse and client. The humanistic nurse expects a change in the nursed's perspective of their experience. For example, humanistic nursing is a being-with another who is grieving, rather than utilizing a series of strategies designed to assist a person toward resolution of grief work. Being-with a person who is grieving in an I-Thou relationship expands the individual's humanness or more-being so that sadness may be shared with another. This may result in the nursed feeling more able to continue with life's demands. An outcome of nursing process, in contrast, would be that the client demonstrates an activity that indicates grieving is progressing, for instance, returning to school.

PATERSON AND ZDERAD'S WORK
AND THE CHARACTERISTICS OF A
THEORY

Paterson and Zderad say that nursing is a "lived dialogue" between the nurse and the nursed, one that is "directed toward the goal of nurturing well-being and more-being," and nursing takes place "in a world of men and things [society]".[28] The authors have inter-related the four concepts of human beings, health, nursing, and society so that a different way of looking at the phenomenon of nursing (characteristic 1) has been created for utilizing the existential philosophy and the phenomenological methodology. Nursing is described as an intersubjective transaction that is a new and different description of nursing. Theories describe, explain, or predict phenomena. Humanistic nursing theory is descriptive; the phenomenological approach is a descriptive method.

Humanistic nursing theory is logical (characteristic 2) because Paterson and Zderad provide a framework and methodology for nursing practice. Also, the ideas and concepts fit together in a meaningful way.

Humanistic nursing theory is not simple; indeed it is somewhat difficult to grasp unless the nurse is familiar with existential philosophy and phenomenology. The theory focuses on the dialogue between the nurse and nursed as a unique encounter between two people. Knowledge gained by repeated study of this encounter will provide a generalizable concept (characteristic 3). In fact, the final step of nursology is the expression of a concept. Thus the theory is generalizable.

Paterson and Zderad's theory provides a basis for hypotheses that can be tested (characterisic 4). The authors describe several replications of the methodology in their book.[29] Since it is testable, phenomenologic nursology is an excellent medium for concept and theory development (characteristic 5).

Humanistic nursing theory, including phenomenologic nursology, can certainly be utilized by nurses to guide and improve practice (characteristic 6). Although nurses may find the concepts new at first, a study of humanistic psychology and existential philosophy will facilitate an understanding of the concepts and an appreciation of human potential.

Humanistic nursing theory is consistent with existentialism, humanistic psychology, and phenomenology upon which it is based (characteristic 7). Because the theory is descriptive and generalizable, it can be applied in any nursing situation and leaves the nursing situation always open for examination.

STRENGTHS AND LIMITATIONS

There are several notable strengths of this theory. The methodology is well developed and the concepts are fully described within the parameters of existential philosophy, phenomenology, and nursing as the authors perceive it. This theory broadens the possibilities for explaining and describing nursing. The subjective study of human beings and nursing using this phenomenological method is a valid approach, one that enhances knowledge in the very human endeavor of nursing. An important contribution of this theory is that the methodology leads to concept formation that is the basis of theory and the springboard of new inquiry. The theory provides a unique, unusual approach to the study of nursing.

On the other hand, Paterson and Zderad's humanistic nursing theory is limited for several reasons. The primary limitation is that the nurse must be well read in the humanities, particularly philosophy, in order to understand the language and the existential tone. Also an inconsistency exists in that humanism implies a concern for all human beings, whereas this theory may be difficult to understand for those not educated in phenomenology and existentialism. Another difficulty may occur for new practitioners regarding the functional aspects of nursing. Nursology refers to the interaction between two people and does not address how to integrate dialogue with tasks. Since it is essentially descriptive, humanistic nursing theory provides challenges for quantitative validation that some may view as a limitation, although this is of limited concern to a humanistic nurse or philosopher. A final limitation is that nursology refers to the subjective interaction between two individuals and does not discuss the subjective encounter with a group of clients or with the family. The methodology does provide the framework for exploring and developing this kind of human nursing situation.

NOTES

1. Josephine Paterson and Loretta Zderad, *Humanistic Nursing* (New York: John Wiley & Sons, Inc., 1976. Copyright © 1976 by John Wiley & Sons, Inc.)

2. Loretta T. Zderad, "From Here-and-Now to Theory: Reflections on 'How'," *Theory Development: What, Why, How?* (New York: National League for Nursing, 1978), p. 45.

3. Abraham H. Maslow, *Toward a Psychology of Being*, 2nd ed. (New York: Van Nostrand Reinhold Company, 1968), pp. iii–v.

4. J. F. T. Bugental, "The Third Force in Psychology," *Humanistic Psychology: A Sourcebook*, D. Welch, G. Tate, and F. Richards, eds. (Buffalo, N. Y.: Prometheus Books, 1978), p. 16.

5. Paterson and Zderad, *Humanistic Nursing*.

6. Ibid., p. 16.

7. Josephine Paterson and Loretta Zderad, "Humanistic Nursing," presentation at the 2nd Annual Nurse Educator Conference, New York, N. Y., December 4–6, 1978.

8. Paterson and Zderad, *Humanistic Nursing*, p. 19.

9. Ibid., p. 26.

10. Ibid., p. 23.

11. Paterson and Zderad, "Humanistic Nursing."

12. Paterson and Zderad, *Humanistic Nursing*, p. 29.

13. Martin Buber, *I and Thou*, 2nd ed. (New York: Charles Scribner's Sons, 1958), pp. 3–34.

14. Paterson and Zderad, *Humanistic Nursing*, p. 30.

15. Ibid., p. 32.

16. Paterson and Zderad, "Humanistic Nursing"; and Susan G. Praeger, *Humanistic Nursing Education: Considerations and Proposals*, dissertation project (University of Northern Colorado, 1980), pp. 18–24.

17. Paterson and Zderad, *Humanistic Nursing*, pp. 63–66.

18. Buber, *I and Thou*, pp. 3–34.

19. Paterson and Zderad, *Humanistic Nursing*, p. 79.

20. Ibid., pp. 79–80.

21. Ibid., p. 80.

22. Thomas Owens, *Phenomenology and Intersubjectivity* (The Hague, Netherlands: Martinus Nijhoff, 1970), p. 6.

23. Paterson and Zderad, *Humanistic Nursing*, p. 78.

24. Abraham Maslow, *Motivation and Personality* (New York: Harper & Row, Publishers, 1954).

25. Paterson and Zderad, *Humanistic Nursing*, p. 80.

26. Carolyn Oiler, "The Phenomenological Approach to Nursing Research," *Nursing Research*, 31 (May–June 1982), p. 180.

27. Paterson and Zderad, *Humanistic Nursing*, p. 23.

28. Ibid., pp. 103–29.

29. Ibid.

17

SISTER CALLISTA ROY

Julia Gallagher Galbreath

Sister Callista Roy (1939–   ) is the Chairman of the Depart-ment of Nursing at Mount Saint Mary's College in Los Angeles. She is a fellow of the American Academy of Nursing and a member of Sigma Theta Tau. Unfolding of the Roy adaptation model as a conceptual framework for nursing began during her graduate study at the University of California in 1964. Roy credits Dorothy E. Johnson as having a strong influence in stimulating her crea-tive processes. In 1968, fellow faculty at Mount Saint Mary's Col-lege voted unanimously to adopt the adaptation framework as the philosophical basis of the nursing curriculum. Roy, again, credits Johnson for encouraging her to publish her work. Resulting publica-tions include the first and second editions of Introduction to Nurs-ing: An Adaptation Model.[1]

ELEMENTS OF ROY'S ADAPTATION MODEL

There are five elements in Roy's adaptation model. These elements are the person, the goal of nursing, nursing activities, health, and the environment.[2] Let us consider the definitions of these elements, their application to the nursing process, and their characteristics as the theory.

The Person

Roy states that the recipient of nursing care may be the individual, a family, a group, a community, or a society. Each is considered as an adaptive system. The idea of an adaptive system combines the concepts of adaptation and of a system.

First, consider the concept of system as applied to an individual. Persons, as living systems, are in constant interaction with their environments. Between the system and the environment occurs an exchange of information, matter, and energy. This characteristic of a living system is called openness. Dunn, a system theorist, calls our attention to the smallest unit of life, the cell. The cell is a living open system. The cell has its inner and outer worlds. From its outer world it must draw forth the substances it needs to survive. Within itself the cell must maintain order over its vast numbers of molecules.[3] These system qualities are also held by the person. The constant interaction of persons with their environment is characterized by both internal and external change. Within this changing world persons must maintain their own integrity; that is, each person must adapt. Hence, the person is viewed as an adaptive system.

Figure 17–1 is utilized by Roy to represent the adaptive system of a person. The adaptive system has input coming from the external

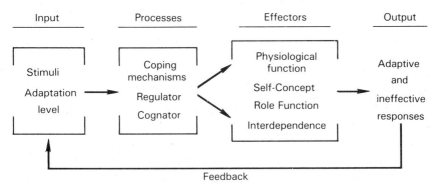

Figure 17–1. The person as an adaptive system. [From Sister Callista Roy, *Introduction to Nursing: An Adaptation Model*, 2nd ed. (Englewood Cliffs, N.J.: Prentice-Hall, Inc., 1984), p. 30. Used with permission.]

environment as well as input coming internally from itself. Roy identifies inputs as stimuli. Examples of external stimuli might be the temperature, an electrical current, or a sound. Examples of internal stimuli are the partial pressure of oxygen in the body, the presence of pain, or the movements of an unborn child.

Outputs of the person as a system are the behaviors of the person. Output behaviors can be both external and internal. Thus, these behaviors may be observed, measured, or subjectively reported. Output behaviors become feedback to the system. Roy has categorized outputs of the system as either adaptive responses or ineffective responses. *Adaptive responses* are those that promote the integrity of the person in terms of survival, growth, reproduction, and mastery. *Ineffective responses* do not support these goals.[4]

Roy has utilized the term *coping mechanisms* to describe the control processes of the person as an adaptive system. Some coping mechanisms are inherited or genetic, such as the white blood cell defense system against bacteria seeking to invade the body. Other mechanisms are learned, such as the use of antiseptics to cleanse a wound. Roy presents a unique nursing science concept of control mechanisms. These mechanisms are called the *regulator* and the *cognator*. Roy's model considers the regulator and cognator mechanisms as subsystems of the person as a system.[5]

The *regulator subsystem* has the system components of input, internal process, and output. Input stimuli may originate externally or internally to the person. The transmitters of the regulator system are chemical, neural, or endocrine in nature. Autonomic reflexes, which are neural responses originating in the brain stem and spinal cord, are generated as output behaviors of the regulator subsystem. Target organs and tissues under endocrine control also produce regulator output behaviors. Finally, Roy presents psychomotor responses originating from the central nervous system as regulator subsystem behaviors.[6] Many physiological processes can be viewed as regulator subsystem behaviors. For example, several regulatory feedback mechanisms of respiration have been identified. One of these is increased carbon dioxide, the end product of metabolism, which stimulates chemoreceptors in the medulla to increase the respiratory rate. Strong stimulation of these centers can increase ventilation six- to sevenfold.[7]

An example of a regulator process is when a noxious external stimulus is visualized and transmitted via the optic nerve to higher brain centers and then to lower brain autonomic centers. The sympathetic neurons from these origins have multiple visceral effects, including increased blood pressure and increased heart rate. Roy's schematic representation of the regulator processes is seen in Figure 17–2.

The other control subsystem original to the Roy model is the *cognator subsystem.* Stimuli to the cognator subsystem are also both external and internal in origin. Output behavior of the regulator subsystem can be feedback stimuli to the cognator subsystem. Cognator control processes are related to the higher brain functions of perceptual/information processing, judgment, and emotion. Perceptual/information processing is related to the internal process of selective attention, coding, and memory. Learning is correlated to the processes of imitation, reinforcement, and insight. Problem solving and decision making are the internal processes related to judgment; and finally, emotion has the processes of defense to seek relief, affective appraisal, and attachment.[8] A schematic presentation by Roy of the cognator subsystem is presented in Figure 17–3.

In maintaining the integrity of the person, the regulator and cognator are postulated as frequently acting together. Let us take an example.

Example.   A decrease in the oxygen supply to Albert Smith's heart muscle stimulates pain receptors that transmit the message of pain along sympathetic afferent nerve fibers to his central nervous system. The autonomic centers of his lower brain then stimulate the sympathetic efferent nerve fibers, and there is an increase in heart and respiratory rates. The result is an increase in the oxygen supply to the heart muscle. This can be viewed as regulator subsystem action.

The cognator subsystem also receives the internal pain stimuli as input. Mr. Smith has learned from past experiences that the left chest and arm pain is related to his heart. His judgment is activated in deciding what action to take. He decides to go inside to air conditioning, to sit with his legs elevated, and to take slow, deep breaths. He also decides not to call for emergency help. Certainly, he believes an adaptive response secondary to these actions will occur. However, he may be increasingly alert for further regulator subsystem output behaviors that might change his decision. This represents the cognator process of selective attention and coding. Following the episode of pain, Mr. Smith may attempt to gain further insight into the cause of the episode. He may decide that the 90° weather was causal and remember to limit his activities during extreme heat. In this example,

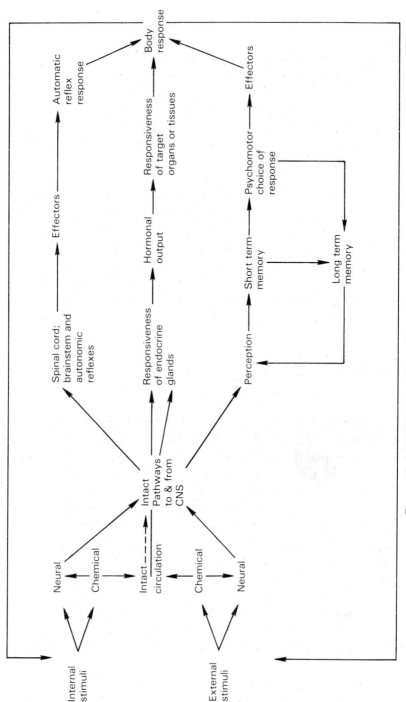

Figure 17-2. The Regulator. [From Sister Callista Roy and Dorothy McLeod, "Theory of the Person as an Adaptive System," in Sister Callista Roy and Sharon L., Roberts, *Theory Construction in Nursing: An Adaptation Model* (Englewood Cliffs, N.J.: Prentice-Hall, Inc., 1984), p. 61. Used with permission.]

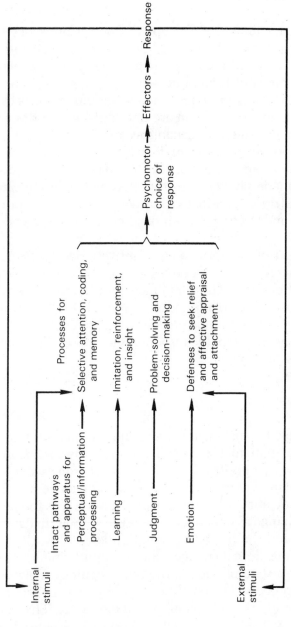

Figure 17-3. The Cognator. [From Sister Callista Roy and Dorothy McLeod, "The Theory of the Person as an Adaptive System," in Sister Callista Roy and Sharon L. Roberts, *Theory Construction in Nursing: An Adaptation Model* (Englewood Cliffs, N.J.: Prentice-Hall, Inc., 1981, p. 64. Used with permission.]

Mr. Smith utilized the cognator subsystem processes of perception, learning, and judgment.

Roy does not limit the concept of control processes to the regulator and cognator subsystems. Many coping mechanisms are known, says Roy, and others are yet to be discovered to explain the complex phenomena of human behavior.[9]

Further guidelines to understanding the internal processes of the person as an adaptive system are developed in the Roy model. The regulator and cognator mechanisms are viewed as acting with the four effector or adaptive modes of *physiological function, self-concept, role function,* and *interdependence.*[10] The adaptive mode of physiological function has been further subdivided into the areas of oxygenation, nutrition, elimination, activity and rest, skin integrity, the senses, fluid and electrolytes, neurological function, and endocrine function.[11]

The concept of the above four adaptive modes came early in Roy's work in an effort to answer the question, How do people adapt to the changes they incur? These four modes are the channels through which the person adapts to internal and external changes. Response to change by the person may be processed predominately in a single adaptive mode. More often, the response is processed simultaneously in more than one mode.

Goal of Nursing

Roy defines the goal of nursing as the promotion of adaptive responses in relation to the four adaptive modes.[12] *Adaptive responses* are those that positively affect health. Helson's work is cited by Roy as useful in understanding the concept of adaptation in relation to the holistic qualities of the person. Helson views the person's adaptation to change as dependent upon the stimuli that are input for the person and the person's adaptation level.[13]

Internal and external changes, that is, input stimuli, interface with the person's state of coping, the other significant element in the adaptation process. The condition of the person or the individual's state of coping is that person's *adaptation level.* The person's adaptation level will determine whether a positive response to internal or external sitmuli will be elicited. The person's adaptation level is determined by focal, contextual, and residual stimuli. The stimuli immediately confronting the person are the *focal stimuli*. *Contextual stimuli* are all other stimuli of the person's internal and external world that influence the situation and are observable, measurable, or subjectively reported by the person. *Residual stimuli* are those make-up characteristics of the person that are present and relevant to the situation but are elusive or difficult to measure objectively.[14]

In the example of the person experiencing chest pain, the stimulus immediately confronting Mr. Smith, the focal stimulus, is the deficit of oxygen supply to his heart muscle. The contextual stimuli include the 90° temperature, the sensation of pain, Mr. Smith's age, weight, blood sugar level, and degree of coronary artery patency. The residual stimuli include his history of cigarette smoking and work-related stress.

The degree of change facing the person is equated to the focal stimulus. If the person's adaptation level is viewed as a line, the zone of adaptation is the distance above and below that line that sets the limit of the person's adaptation capacity. When the total stimuli (focal, contextual, and residual) fall within the person's zone of adaptation, an adaptive response or output results. However, when the total stimuli fall outside the individual's zone of adaptation, ineffective output behavior or responses occur.[15] Figure 17–4 depicts this conceptualization.

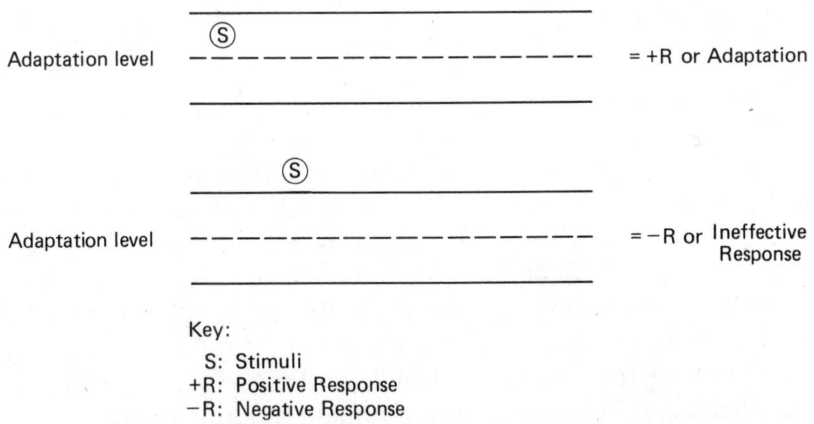

Adaptation level   ⓢ — — — — — — — — — — — — — = +R or Adaptation

Adaptation level   ⓢ — — — — — — — — — — — — — — — = −R or Ineffective Response

Key:
  S: Stimuli
+R: Positive Response
−R: Negative Response

Figure 17–4. Adaptation level. [From Sister Callista Roy, *Introduction to Nursing: An Adaptation Model*, 2nd ed. (Englewood Cliffs, N.J.: Prentice-Hall, Inc., 1984), p. 38. Used with permission.]

In the example of Mr. Smith, the total stimuli had fallen outside his adaptation zone. The resulting deficit of oxygen to his heart, indicated by chest pain, was an ineffective response. This response became feedback to the system and a focal stimulus. Mr. Smith utilized the cognator mechanism to adjust the total stimuli by going indoors to a cooler room and decreasing his oxygen needs by sitting down and elevating his legs. After the adjustment of the stimuli, the oxygen needs of his heart muscle were met, and the pain stopped.

A person's ability to cope varies with the state of the person at different points in time. For example, the person who has suffered major trauma has a narrowed zone of adaptation and may not survive exposure to a bacterial infection. That same person prior to the injury may have tolerated exposure to the same bacteria without developing any symptoms of illness.

Nursing Activities

Nurses act by manipulating the focal, contextual, or residual stimuli impinging on the person so that adaptive responses are promoted. Recall that adaptive responses are those that positively affect health.[16] Additionally, nurses act to expand the person's adaptation level so that coping ability is expanded and the person can tolerate a wider range of stimuli. Plans that broaden the person's adaptation level correlate with the ideas of health promotion currently found in the literature.[17]

Health

Previously, the Roy model defined health as a continuum from death to high-level wellness. This is no longer utilized in the present model. Instead, Roy presently defines health as "a state or process of being or becoming an integrated and whole person."[18] The integrity of the person is expressed as the ability to meet the goals of survival, growth, reproduction, and mastery.[19] The nurse using Roy's model utilizes the concept of health as the goal point for the person's behavior. When a disproportionate amount of the person's energy is utilized in coping, less energy is available to meet the goals of survival, growth, reproduction, and mastery. Energy freed from ineffective behavior becomes available for promotion of health. Roy states that this conceptualization of health implies a humanistic philosophy of valuing the creative powers of the person and the dimension of purpose in life.[20]

Environment

In the Roy model, people exist in a relationship open to the internal and external stimuli that impinge on them. The environment is, therefore, considered as the internal and external stimuli relative to the person. Roy defines the environment as "all conditions, circumstances, and influences surrounding and affecting the development and behavior of persons or groups."[21]

THE NURSING PROCESS

The Roy adaptation model offers guidelines to the nurse in developing the nursing process. The elements of the Roy nursing process include first and second level assessment, diagnosis, goal setting, intervention, and evaluation.[22] If first and second level assessments are considered subparts of the same element, the five elements of Roy's nursing process parallel the five phases of the nursing process identified in Chapter 2.

First Level Assessment

First level assessment is considered the gathering of output behaviors of the person as an adaptive system in relation to each of the four adaptive modes: physiological function, self-concept, role function, and interdependence. First level assessment is referred to as *behavioral assessment*. Especially significant are data collected about behaviors reflecting regulator or cognator subsystem activity within the four adaptive modes. The behaviors observed are evaluated in terms of whether they promote the integrity of the person. The nurse considers if the behaviors support the goals of survival, growth, reproduction, and mastery; or more simply, Do the behaviors support the health of the person? The nurse identifies ineffective responses as well as adaptive responses that require nurse support.[23]

Second Level Assessment
and Diagnosis

With this preliminary work completed, the nurse moves to second level assessment. Second level assessment consists of the collection of data about the focal, contextual, and residual stimuli impinging on the person. Analysis of the data results in a statement of the problem or a nursing diagnosis.[24]

Roy describes three methods of making a nursing diagnosis.[25] One method is to utilize a typology of diagnoses developed by Roy and related to the four adaptive modes. Table 17-1 is a list of common adaptation problems using this typology. In applying this method of diagnosis to the example of Mr. Smith, the diagnosis would be: "Hypoxia."

The second method is to make a diagnosis by stating the observed behavior along with the most influencing stimuli. Using this method, a diagnosis for Mr. Smith could be stated as: "Chest pain caused by a deficit of oxygen to the heart muscle associated with an overexposure to hot weather."

The third method summarizes behaviors in one or more adaptive modes related to the same stimuli. For example, if the person experiencing chest pain is a farmer, working outside in hot weather is necessary for success in his work. In this case, an appropriate diagnosis might be: "Role failure associated with limited physical (myocardial) ability to work in hot weather."

On the other hand, a nursing diagnosis using any of the above methods can also be a statement of adaptive behaviors that the nurse wishes to support. For example, if Mr. Smith is seeking help through vocational counseling to adapt to his physical limitation, the nurse may diagnose a need to support this behavior. In this case, an appropriate diagnosis would be: "Adaptation to role failure by seeking an alternative career."

Goal Setting

The next step of the nursing process is goal setting. Goals are written as statements of end point behaviors that the person should achieve.[26] Goals, whenever possible, are set mutually with the person. Mutual goal setting respects the privileges and rights of the person. When the person is unable to give input into goal setting, legal

Table 17-1.

Working Typology of Common Adaptation
Problems (Revised)

A. Physiologic Mode	B. Self-Concept Mode	C. Role Function Mode	D. Interdependence Mode

1. *Oxygenation*
   Hypoxia
   Shock
   Overload
2. *Nutrition*
   Malnutrition
   Nausea
   Vomiting
3. *Elimination*
   Constipation
   Diarrhea
   Flatulence
   Incontinence
   Urinary retention
4. *Activity and rest*
   Inadequate physical
   activity
   Potential disuse
   consequences
   Inadequate rest
   Insomnia
   Sleep deprivation
   Excessive rest
5. *Skin integrity*
   Itching
   Dry skin
   Pressure sores
	1. *Physical self*
	   Decreased sexual
	   self-concept
	   Aggressive sexual
	   behavior
	   Loss
	2. *Personal self*
	   Anxiety
	   Powerlessness
	   Guilt
	   Low self-esteem
		Role transition
		Role distance
		Role conflict
		Role failure
			Separation anxiety
			Loneliness

Source: Sister Callista Roy, *Introduction to Nursing: An Adaptation Model*, 2nd ed. (Englewood Cliffs, N.J.: Prentice-Hall, Inc., 1984), p. 56. Used with permission.

and ethical principles should be utilized to guide the nurse's goal setting.

Intervention

Nursing interventions are planned with the purpose of altering or manipulating the focal, contextual, or residual stimuli that are inputs of the person as an adaptive system. When possible, the focal stimuli pressing the individual beyond the personal zone of adaptation are altered so an adaptive response is made. Interventions may also focus on broadening the person's coping ability, or adaptation zone, so that the total stimuli fall within that person's ability to adapt.[27]

Evaluation

The nursing process is completed by the evaluation. Goal behaviors are compared to the person's output behaviors, and movement toward or away from goal achievement is determined. Readjustments to goals and interventions are made, based on evaluation data.[28]

The Roy Nursing Process Applied to Nursing in a Recovery Room

The Roy model can be applied to nursing assessment and intervention within various clinical situations. In the following case study, the Roy model will be applied to a person during the period of immediate recovery from surgery and anesthesia.

First level assessment focuses on the physiological mode behaviors during the first hour of recovery time after a person experiences surgery and general anesthesia. Applying the Roy model, significant behaviors can be conceptualized as regulator output behaviors. Increased sympathetic or parasympathetic system activity can signal regulator system activity. Regulator output behaviors that vary from base-line values determined for the person may be the first warning of an ineffective response to postoperative stimuli. Key base-line values are the person's presurgery measures of heart rate, blood pressure, and respiratory rate. Immediately upon observation of changes from the base-line, second level assessment is done. Goals are set with the basic survival of the person as a priority. Interventions are taken so that focal and contextual stimuli are altered and adaptation is promoted. The evaluation of goal achievement is made, and further actions are taken as necessary.

Situation.   Mrs. Reed is received from surgery after a major abdominal operation. Before surgery, her base-line vital signs were: heart rate, 80 beats per minute; blood pressure, 120/80 mm Hg; and respiratory rate, 16 per minute. After 45 minutes in recovery, her vital signs are: heart rate, 150 beats per minute; blood pressure, 90/60 mm Hg; respiratory rate, 32 per minute. Increased regulator output behavior is signaled by sympathetic nervous system stimulation of the heart in response to decreased blood pressure. The nurse decides that an ineffective response is occurring for Mrs. Reed. Therefore second level assessment is done.

The focal stimulus is a decrease of arterial blood pressure secondary to an unknown underlying cause. The contextual stimuli are: age 45 years, cool extremities, poor nail blanching, no food or drink for 12 hours, intravenous infusion (IV) of dextrose 5 percent in water with lactated Ringer's solution at 100 cc per hour. Also, contextual stimuli include 200 cc of IV fluids infused during surgery, 10 cc of urine excreted during the first 45 minutes in recovery, 1½ hours of general anesthesia, estimated blood loss of 500 cc during surgery, no operative site bleeding, and level of consciousness slow to respond to tactile stimuli after 45 minutes in recovery. The residual stimuli include history of renal infections.

The nursing diagnosis of a decreased arterial blood pressure secondary to fluid volume deficit is made. A fluid volume loss is suggested both by the contextual data and by the changes in the base-line heart rate, blood pressure, and urine output. The nurse then intervenes by altering contextual stimuli so that an adaptive response is promoted. The goal of a circulatory volume adequate to maintain a blood pressure of plus or minus 20 mm Hg of base-line levels within 15 minutes is set. The nurse plans and then takes the following intervention steps. The IV rate is increased to 300 cc per hour. The foot of the bed is elevated to increase venous return. Forty percent oxygen is given by mask. Mrs. Reed is verbally and tactilely stimulated and told to take slow deep breaths. The nurse prepares vasopressor medications for immediate use and applies an external continuous blood pressure cuff for constant blood pressure monitoring. The nurse also consults with other team members as to Mrs. Reed's clinical presentation.

A constant evaluation as to the effectiveness of the nursing actions is made. The nurse holds Mrs. Reed in recovery until the behavior goal of adequate circulating volume is met. Evaluation criteria would include urine output greater than 30 cc per hour, mental alertness, rapid nail bed blanching, blood pressure plus or minus 20 mm Hg of presurgery levels, pulse plus or minus 20 beats per minute of base-line, and respirations plus or minus 5 per minute of presurgery levels.

ROY'S WORK AND
CHARACTERISTICS OF A THEORY

The characteristics of a theory are presented in Chapter 1. The Roy model will be considered in relation to each of these characteristics.

First, the Roy model does interrelate concepts in such a way as to present a new view of a phenomenon being studied. Applying this model to the nursing care of persons, the nurse takes a unique way of looking at the person. The person is viewed as an adaptive system in constant interaction with the internal and external environment. This approach utilizes a broad perspective rather than a view of the person in isolation from the environment. Hence, assessment includes both the output behaviors of the person and the environmental stimuli that influence that person. Maintaining health in life is related both to the person's coping abilities and to the total of internal and external changes. The person's ability to adapt to the changes encountered is based on whether the total stimuli fall within that person's adaptation zone. This is the most abstract idea presented in the Roy model. Its purpose is to conceptually and systematically present the relationship between change, both internal and external, and the range or potential of an individual to cope with change. Ineffective responses versus adaptive responses are the opposing outcomes for the person.

Second, the elements of the Roy model flow logically. Discussion throughout the work returns to the defined underlying concepts. None of the concepts appear contrary to each other. However, although Roy states that the recipient of nursing care can be an individual, group, community, or society, the discussion and the examples provided relate primarily to individuals. The theory would be enhanced by the addition of further discussion of groups, communities, and societies as recipients of nursing care.

Third, the Roy model meets the criterion of relative simplicity yet generalizability. The Roy model has five basic concepts. The idea of a living system is a familiar concept. The generalizability of the work is demonstrated by the use of the model as a basis of the nursing curriculum at Mount Saint Mary's College in Los Angeles.

Fourth, hypotheses may be generated from the model. Because of the abstract nature of the zone of adaptation concept, the question of "What percentage of nurses would draw the same conclusions when applying this concept within a particular nursing situation?" arises. Of course, this is asking how reliable is the concept. Basically the nurse must draw this conclusion from comparing the person's response behavior to Roy's definition of adaptation. Recall that adaptation promotes the integrity of the person in relation to the personal goals of survival, growth, reproduction, and mastery.[29] Although this definition appears to be a valid one, it is indeed broad. Development of criteria for identification of adaptive versus ineffective behaviors within the four adaptive modes would be a worthy pursuit.

It would be unfair to fail to mention that the key to development of criteria for judging an adaptive versus an ineffective behavior may already be present in the model. This may be the result of further development of the concepts of the regulator and cognator mechanisms. Recall that regulator and cognator mechanisms are the internal control processes of the person in coping with change. These concepts are unique to nursing science and have been developed exclusively by Roy. Furthermore, according to Roy, behaviors that indicate the activation of regulator or cognator control processes concurrently indicate a person/system active in the process of adapting to change. Also, behaviors identified as failures of the regulator or cognator control processes immediately signal ineffective responses to change. Hence, by knowing the regulator and cognator behaviors related to a particular adaptive mode, the nurse can firmly make a judgment that attempts at adaptation are occurring for the person. Additional behaviors indicating failure of these control processes specifically indicate that an adaptation problem exists and further assessment and intervention are required. To date, Roy has developed preliminary criteria for identification of behaviors related to these processes within the four adaptive modes. This work would not mean treading on totally untouched territory.

As to the fifth and sixth characteristics, perhaps the most important aspect of a theory is its usefulness in practice. How does application of the Roy model guide and improve the work of the practitioner? A major strength of the model is that it guides nurses to utilize observation and interviewing skills in doing an individualized assessment of each person. Behavior related to the four adaptive modes is collected during first level assessment. In considering all the adaptive modes—physiological function, self-concept, role function, and interdependence—the nurse is likely to have a comprehensive view of the person.

The concepts of the model are applicable within the many practice settings of nursing. The use of the model may demand a change in the allocation of time and resources. Painstaking application of the model would require significant input of time and effort. The benefit to the client of complete assessment and interventions in areas of concern, however, justifies the effort and allocation of resources. Even in practice settings requiring quick action, the elements of the model are still compatible with quality care. Especially useful is the second level assessment guide to identification of focal, contextual, and residual stimuli. The development by Roy of a typology of nursing diagnoses of common adaptation problems is an exciting outflow of the model. This may be especially useful in nurse-to-nurse communication. Basically, goals of nursing care are more likely to be achieved when all nurses involved in the case are using the same words to mean the same things.

The model, because it encourages identification of the focal, contextual, and residual stimuli within a situation, immediately indicates the course of nursing action. Nursing actions are geared to altering these stimuli. This aspect of the model helps the practitioner to get down to specifics in decisions as to what actions to take. In another way, practitioners can see the importance of their actions in influencing the adaptation of the person. For example, the nurse can view nursing actions such as maintaining bed rest or relieving pain or fears as significant in maintaining an adaptive response for the person.

In relation to the seventh characteristic—consistency with other validated theories, etc.—many laws and principles that attempt to explain the regulatory processes of the person have been pursued by other scientists. The work of physiologists, especially endocrine studies by Selye, comes to mind.[30] The body of work in this area would involve the organizing of many known ideas for the other sciences into this unique nursing perspective. Hence, the Roy model is open to incorporation of other validated theories, laws, and principles, yet leaves us with unanswered questions.

SUMMARY

The Roy model consists of the five elements of person, goal of nursing, nursing activities, health, and environment. Persons are viewed as living adaptive systems whose behaviors may be classified as adaptive responses or ineffective responses. These behaviors are derived from the regulator and cognator mechanisms. These mechanisms work within the four adaptive modes of physiological function, self-concept, role function, and interdependence. The goal of nursing is to promote adaptive responses in relation to the four adaptive modes, utilizing information about the person's adaptation level, and focal, contextual, and residual stimuli. Nursing activities involve the manipulation of these stimuli to promote adaptive responses. Health is a process of becoming integrated and able to meet the goals of survival, growth, reproduction, and mastery. The environment consists of the person's internal and external stimuli.

These elements are utilized in a nursing process that consists of first and second level assessments, diagnosis, goal setting, intervention, and evaluation. First level assessment, or behavioral assessment, deals with the four adaptive modes, whereas second level assessment focuses on the three areas of stimuli. Diagnosis consists of stating the problem. Goals are set in relation to the problem and are written in behavioral terms. Interventions are planned to manipulate the stimuli, and evaluation compares the person's output behaviors with the desired behaviors established in the goals.

Roy's model is seen as applicable in the nursing process presented in Chapter 2. The characteristics of a theory are also met. There is need for continued research that centers on hypotheses generated by the model.

NOTES

1. Sister Callista Roy, *Introduction to Nursing: An Adaptation Model* (Englewood Cliffs, N. J.: Prentice-Hall, Inc., 1976); and idem 2nd ed., 1984.
2. Roy, *Introduction to Nursing*, 2nd ed., p. 28.

3. Halbert L. Dunn, *High Level Wellness* (Arlington, Va.: R. W. Beatty, 1971).
4. Roy, *Introduction to Nursing*, 2nd ed., p. 28.
5. Ibid., p. 31.
6. Ibid.
7. Arthur C. Guyton, *Basic Human Physiology: Normal Function and Mechanisms of Disease* (Philadelphia: W. B. Saunders Company, 1971), p. 353.
8. Roy, *Introduction to Nursing*, 2nd ed., p. 33.
9. Ibid., pp. 30–31.
10. Ibid., p. 28.
11. Ibid., p. 89.
12. Ibid., p. 12.
13. Harry Helson, *Adaptation Level Theory* (New York: Harper & Row, Publishers, Inc., 1966); and Roy, *Introduction to Nursing*, 2nd ed., pp. 37–38.
14. Roy, *Introduction to Nursing*, 2nd ed., pp. 52–54.
15. Ibid., p. 37
16. Ibid., p. 28.
17. Ibid., p. 38.
18. Ibid., p. 39
19. Ibid., p. 38.
20. Ibid., p. 36.
21. Ibid., p. 39.
22. Ibid., pp. 42–63.
23. Ibid., pp. 45–51.
24. Ibid., p. 38.
25. Ibid., pp. 55–57.
26. Ibid., p. 59.
27. Ibid., pp. 59–60.
28. Ibid., p. 61.
29. Ibid., p. 28.
30. Hans Selye, *The Stress of Life* (New York: McGraw-Hill Book Company, 1956).

18

NURSING THEORIES AND THE NURSING PROCESS

Marjorie Stanton

The focus of this chapter is on the professional nurse's use of nursing theories/models as a framework to guide nursing practice through use in the nursing process. As professional nurses, we need to test those theories that we believe useful to practice. If nurses deliberately use the same theories/models in a variety of nursing situations, then it becomes possible to analyze the results and contribute to the body of nursing knowledge.

It is possible that a combination of these theories/models can be used so that the practicing nurse can identify new relationships and new ideas for testing. It is also possible that as we consistently use nursing theories/models in practice, we can identify those with which we as professionals feel most confident. We may also find that certain ones work better in selected situations than others. By keeping accurate records and by communicating our successes and failures to others, the practice of nursing becomes more scientific and rational.

A REVIEW OF THE FIFTEEN THEORIES

Using various nursing theories/models, the focus of nursing practice will differ. Florence Nightingale focused on changing and manipulating the environment in order to put the patient in the best possible conditions for nature to act. She also emphasized the point that nurses should alleviate and prevent unnecessary suffering and pain. Nightingale's notions about nursing laid the groundwork for and influenced other nursing theorists (see Chapter 3).

Hildegard Peplau presents nursing as therapeutic interactions between the nurse and patient in order to clarify the patient's problems and to set mutually acceptable goals to solve those problems. Conflict may occur if the nurse and patient cannot come to agreement about the goals; however, both the patient and nurse should grow from this experience (see Chapter 4). Peplau identifies four phases in the relationship: orientation, identification, exploitation, and resolution. Her influence on the notion of nursing as interpersonal in nature is pervasive.

Virginia Henderson views nursing as doing for patients what they cannot do for themselves, and she identifies fourteen components of nursing care that need to be considered (see Chapter 5). Her view of nursing seems to foster dependence initially, although her goal is to make the patient independent. The influence of Henderson is seen in the writings of later nursing theorists.

Ernestine Wiedenbach strongly believes that the nurse's individual philosophy lends credence to nursing care. She believes that nurses help to meet the individual's need for help. Wiedenbach also believes nursing to be a deliberative action, as does Orlando (see Chapter 6).

Lydia Hall's notion of nursing centers around three components: care, core, and cure. Care represents nurturance and is exclusive to nursing. Core involves the therapeutic use of self and emphasizes the use of reflection. Cure focuses on nursing related to the physician's orders. Hall views the three components as interrelated, with one component taking precedence over the other two at varying points during the patient's course of progress. Hall's focus is primarily on the ill adult during the recovery stage (see Chapter 7).

Dorothea Orem's theory of nursing (see Chapter 8) consists of three theoretical constructs: self-care, self-care deficit, and nursing systems. The self-care construct is divided into the three self-care requisites of universal self-care, developmental self-care, and health deviation self-care. The self-care deficit construct is the core of Orem's general theory of nursing because it identifies when nursing is needed. The nursing systems construct is divided into the wholly compensatory, partly compensatory, and supportive-educative nursing systems.

Orem's theoretical construct of self-care deficit has some similarity to Henderson's general concept of nursing.

Faye Abdellah focuses on the nurse rather than on the patient. She provides a means for categorizing patient needs under twenty-one common nursing problems relative to caring for patients (see Chapter 9). There is some similarity to Henderson's fourteen components of basic nursing care.

Ida Jean Orlando advances to some extent Henderson's theory of nursing since she believes that the nurse helps patients meet a perceived need that the patients cannot meet for themselves. Orlando (see Chapter 10) believes that nurses provide direct assistance to meet an immediate need for help in order to avoid or to alleviate distress and/or helplessness. She emphasizes the need to evaluate care based on observable outcomes. Orlando indicates that nursing actions can be automatic (those chosen for reasons other than the immediate need for help) or deliberative (those resulting from validating the need for help, exploring the meaning of the need, and validating the effectiveness of actions taken to meet the need).

Myra Levine sees nursing as human interaction: the dependency of individuals on one another. She uses four conservation principles to describe nursing interventions: conservation of energy, conservation of structural integrity, conservation of personal integrity, and conservation of social integrity. She believes this provides a way to view people holistically. Levine uses the concept of organismic response to illness, which indicates to what extent adaptation is taking place (see Chapter 11).

Dorothy E. Johnson has developed a behavioral system model for nursing that has seven subsystems. These subsystems are: attachment or affiliative, dependency, ingestive, eliminative, sexual, aggressive, and achievement. These seven subsystems need nurturance and stimulation for growth, and they also need protection from noxious influences (see Chapter 12). Nursing problems occur when there are difficulties in the structure or function of the system or a subsystem and when behavioral functioning falls below what is considered desirable. The goal of nursing is to keep the behavioral system in balance and to maintain stability in the system. Nursing focuses on the person who is ill or is threatened with illness; and medicine, using the biological system model, focuses on the illness itself.

Martha Rogers developed the principles of homeodynamics, which focus on the wholeness of human beings and their integration with their environment. The movement of human beings toward maximum health is the purpose of nursing. Rogers believes that the science of nursing is the science of unitary human beings (see Chapter 13).

Imogene King has developed a theory of goal attainment from an open systems framework that integrates personal systems, interpersonal systems, and social systems. The interpersonal systems provide the major emphasis in this theory of goal attainment. Nurse-client interactions are the essential component in goal setting and in identifying the means of goal achievement. King views human beings as the focus of nursing and as open systems interacting with the environment (see Chapter 14).

Betty Neuman presents a health-care systems model that focuses on the whole person and that person's reaction to stress. Her model can be used in illness or wellness. She focuses on three components in her model—man, environment, and stress—and relies on the nurse's understanding and knowledge of these components to carry out the purpose of her model (see Chapter 15).

Josephine Paterson and Loretta Zderad have developed a humanistic nursing practice theory based on their belief that nursing is an existential experience. Nursing is viewed as a lived dialogue that involves the coming together of the nurse and the person to be nursed. The essential characteristic of nursing is nurturance. Humanistic nursing cannot take place without the authentic commitment of the nurse to being with and doing with the client. Humanistic nursing also presupposes responsible choices (see Chapter 16).

Sister Callista Roy's major emphasis is on the person as an adaptive system. To further describe the client of nursing, four adaptive modes are used: physiological needs, self-concept, role functioning, and interdependence. The person has two major internal processor subsystems, the regulator and the cognator, which are seen as mechanisms for adapting or coping. The goal of nursing is to promote adaptive responses (see Chapter 17).

COMPARISON OF THE THEORIES/MODELS

A review of the theories presented indicates that there are similarities and differences among them. Most of the theorists were influenced by each other in their advancement of nursing knowledge. This fact is valuable and useful to the students of professional nursing practice. The concept of looking specifically at the environment in relation to patients/clients was initiated by Nightingale and was considered later by Johnson, King, Neuman, Orem, Roy, and Rogers; but was not specifically considered by Henderson, Abdellah, Peplau, and Orlando. The concept of dependency and its role in nursing was identified by Henderson and was also used by Orlando, Orem, and Levine. Independence is a focus in the theories/models of Peplau, Rogers, Hall, and King. Adaptation is considered in the theories/models of Nightingale, King, Levine, Rogers, and Roy; however, where Roy views adaptation as health-producing, Rogers's concept of adaptation would be viewed as not being conducive to health. Peplau, Levine, Paterson and Zderad, and King emphasize interpersonal/interactive concepts in their writings, although these concepts are not overlooked by other theorists, e.g., Hall and Orlando. Systems theory is used specifically by Rogers, King, Roy, Johnson, and Neuman. The theories/models of Henderson, Orlando, Hall, and Levine seem primarily useful in the care of the ill, whereas those of Nightingale, Peplau, Wiedenbach, Orem, King, Rogers, and Roy are useful for caring for the well and the ill. Abdellah's ideas seem more consistent with the technical aspects of nursing care, whereas the others' ideas do not.

One way of looking at the differences among the nurse theorists is to explore the variety of ways they characterized nursing actions. A quick summary of the theorists presented identifies at least three different forms of nursing actions: (1) assuming responsibility for the person until he/she is ready to assume responsibility for self; (2) changing or manipulating the environment to facilitate health; and (3) helping the person toward some goal. The reader may be able to identify other similarities and differences.

Practitioners of nursing need to use the theories/models that are most useful in a given situation. As stated earlier, a combination of theories/models can be considered, and if used consistently, should be analyzed by the user as to their effectiveness. By using various nursing theories/models, the focus and consequences of nursing practice may differ, as discussed in the following example.

Consider the following situation: Mrs. Mary James is a sixty-eight-year-old woman recovering from a stroke that occurred three days ago. She has weakness of the left side of her body. She is left-handed and requires retraining in the following areas: balancing while standing, climbing stairs, self-feeding, bladder control, and personal hygiene activities including dressing. She is in a hospital room with four other patients and is in the bed nearest the door. There is one window in the room. Before her hospitalization for the stroke, Mrs. James maintained her own home, was quite independent, volunteered one day a week at the local hospital, and was active in the local garden club.

Table 18-1 provides a brief overview of the direction a nurse might take using the various nursing theories/models as a framework to guide nursing practice through use in the nursing process. You will note that although each theorist moves Mrs. James to some point of independence, the methods are different due to different orientations. A fully developed nursing process using any one of the theories/models as a framework would provide much more detailed and specific information about Mrs. James than is given in this table. However, the brief overview in Table 18-1 does give the reader an idea of how the process might differ if a particular theory were used. It is not intended to be an all-inclusive discussion on nursing care for Mrs. James.

The consistent use of selected nursing theories/models in nursing practice provides a way to validate and test these theories/models. The transmission of such knowledge by practicing nurses and nurse researchers adds to the unique body of knowledge necessary to a profession.

The systematic use of nursing theories/models provides a structure and discipline for nursing practice. It also provides a framework for teaching professional nursing students how to base practice on knowledge.

Table 18-1

Overview of Theories/Models and Nursing Process

Theorist	Assessment	Nursing Diagnosis	Planning	Implementation	Evaluation
Nightingale	Focus is on environment of patient. What in environment is contributing to disability or illness of Mrs. James? What are inhibiting factors, i.e., position of bedside table; lack of flowers; too far from window; slippery, cold floor; lack of space (four-bed room); too many people in room?	Relates to environment or what is lacking in the environment as a condition to restore health, i.e., crowded, restricted environment that inhibits movement toward independence and health.	Focus is on identifying those areas of the environment needing modification or change to provide Mrs. James with the best possible conditions for nature to restore or improve health; i.e., remove restrictions, maximize use of right hand, provide sunlight and ventilation, etc.	Carries out the actions necessary to change or manipulate the environment to provide optimum conditions for restoration or improvement of health. Move Mrs. James to room with two beds for more space but with companionship; provide chair near the window; place bedside table and things needed by Mrs. James on right side of bed; provide warm, sturdy slippers or shoes; place other patient in room on Mrs. James's right; provide flowers.	Relates to how well the changes in or manipulation of the environment worked to effect optimal conditions for restoration or improvement of health, i.e., able to move about room with some assistance. Sits by window and talks to patient in room. Uses right hand to feed self and care for other needs. Arranges flowers in room. Taking an interest in what is happening inside and outside the room.

(continued)

Table 18-1
(Continued)

Theorist	Assessment	Nursing Diagnosis	Planning	Implementation	Evaluation
Peplau	Focus is on the orientation phase—Mrs. James has an expressed need for help. The nurse, family, and Mrs. James work together to clarify the problems: Mrs. James' loss of independence, her fear about what has happened to her, how will she cope, how will her family cope.	Relates to the identification of the health problem or deficit by the nurse and Mrs. James, i.e., inability to cope with dependent role caused by diminished function of left side of body.	Focus is on the nurse and Mrs. James setting mutual goals for Mrs. James to become more independent through the development of the interpersonal relationship. Mrs. James should feel comfortable in discussing how she will become more independent. This is likened to the identification phase.	Carries out plans mutually agreed upon by nurse and Mrs. James. However, Mrs. James is in control in asking for what she needs; i.e., "I don't need to be fed. Teach me to feed myself. I'm ready." The nurse helps Mrs. James to recognize and explore her feelings when she becomes frustrated in her attempts to feed herself. This can be likened to the exploitation phase.	Relates to how well Mrs. James progressed through orientation, identification, and exploitation phases. Have the needs been met? When the answer is yes, terminating the relationship (resolution phase) begins.
Henderson	Focus is on assessing Mrs. James's ability relative to the 14 components of basic nursing care; i.e., Mrs. James is left-handed with left-	Relates to deficits in the ability of Mrs. James to function in each of the 14 components. Takes into consideration strength, will, and	Focus is on identifying those areas of the 14 components that Mrs. James cannot do for self and which therefore the nurse must do or	Carries out the plan to initially feed Mrs. James while teaching her to use her right hand to feed herself.	Relates to how soon and how well Mrs. James is able to feed herself with her right hand; i.e., for the first three days she needed to

326

	sided weakness (relates to component #2—"eat and drink adequately").	knowledge, i.e., inability to feed self due to left-handed weakness (relates to component #2).	assist in doing, i.e., feed Mrs. James until she is able to feed self with right hand. This should lead to independence on the part of Mrs. James.	be fed; by fourth day, held utensils and fed self with assistance; by seventh day, was able to feed self if food was bite-size.
Wiedenbach	Focus is on the nurse's perception and awareness of the situation; i.e., "Mrs. James must feel so helpless since she is unable to feed herself."	Relates to the situation perceived, i.e., "feeling of helplessness."	Focus is on the nurse and Mrs. James's plan to reduce Mrs. James's feeling of helplessness by teaching her how to eat with her right hand, with food prepared in bite-size pieces.	Carries out the plan of teaching after confirming it with Mrs. James. "I'll assist you in using your right hand until you can feed yourself. I'll stay with you until you learn how to feed yourself with your right hand."	Relates to validating that Mrs. James feels less helpless when she can use her right hand for feeding herself.
Hall	Focus is on increasing Mrs. James's self-awareness through observation and reflection. Helps Mrs. James hear herself; i.e., "I'm a sick woman. I can't take care of myself. I can't even dress or feed my-	Statement of Mrs. James's need or problem. Mrs. James is in control; i.e., "I need to learn to take care of myself. I need to learn to use my right hand to feed and dress myself. I need to think about my-	Focus is on setting goals and priorities with Mrs. James, i.e., needs to learn to care for self: 1. Learn to use right hand to feed and dress self. 2. Walk by self to bathroom.	Carries out plans with Mrs. James. Intimate bodily care is given; i.e., help her to feed self and begin to use right hand; assist her to dress until she learns to dress self; support and listen to her.	Relates to Mrs. James's progress toward goals; i.e., able to feed self with right hand, able to dress self with assistance, able to walk to bathroom with assistance, able to state, "I think I'll be

(continued)

327

Table 18-1
(Continued)

Theorist	Assessment	Nursing Diagnosis	Planning	Implementation	Evaluation
	self. Everyone is looking at me.'" Biological data are also being collected; i.e., cannot grasp or hold with left hand.	self for awhile and not worry about others.'"	3. Improve self-concept.		able to take care of myself."
Orem	Focus is on appraising the situation: determining why a person needs care; considering life history and life style; considering the physician's perspective and Mrs. James' perspective; —i.e., Mrs. James needs help because she has left-sided weakness, is left-handed, and cannot feed herself or walk without assistance.	Relating to the partly compensatory system; i.e., inability to feed self without assistance, inability to walk without assistance, ability to learn alternate methods of self-care relating to deficits identified.	Focus is on improving the self-care abilities of Mrs. James relative to eating, walking, and other deficits in activities of daily living. Identify Mrs. James's strengths, such as previous independent life style. Reach agreements with Mrs. James and family about role each will play.	Carries out the plan to assist Mrs. James in the performance of self-care tasks, i.e., learning to feed herself and using a walker to assist in walking.	Relates to monitoring progress of Mrs. James with regard to self-care activities and making adjustments and recommendations as necessary.

Abdellah	Focus is on each of the 21 nursing problems to collect data about Mrs. James; i.e., #7—"to facilitate maintenance of elimination." Mrs. James has not had a bowel movement in two days, has difficulty moving about, does not like fruits and vegetables.	Problems with elimination possibly due to insufficient exercise and lack of roughage in diet.	Focus is on facilitating the maintenance of elimination; i.e., assisting Mrs. James to walk at least 15 minutes twice daily and move about in bed. Also speak to dietician regarding diet of grain cereals, sliced fruit or finger fruits, etc.	Carries out the nursing activities to assist Mrs. James to change position in bed. Encourage Mrs. James to eat diet prescribed; assist in feeding and praise her for trying fruits and vegetables.	Relates to the resolution of Mrs. James' elimination problems. Is elimination achieved and maintained?
Orlando	Focus is on collecting data relative to the immediate situation; i.e., Mrs. James has left side weakness. What are the factors identified in this situation, i.e., inability to feed self, difficulty in balancing? The nurse also clarifies own reaction to Mrs. James.	Relates to identifying Mrs. James's needs that she cannot meet by self. This is validated with her; i.e., Mrs. James needs to be taught to use her right hand to feed and bathe self.	Focus is on planning with Mrs. James and mutually setting goals; i.e., clarifying with Mrs. James that she indeed needs to learn to use her right hand in order to feed and bathe self.	Carries out the nursing activities necessary to meet Mrs. James' needs; i.e., assist Mrs. James to use her right hand to eat—do not feed her; place bedside table on her right; teach her to stand and move without assistance.	Relates to Mrs. James's behavior in terms of feeding and bathing herself using her right hand. Uses right hand to eat but needs encouragement. Able to get out of bed with assistance; can walk to bathroom; able to dress self with assistance.

(continued)

Table 18-1
(Continued)

Theorist	Assessment	Nursing Diagnosis	Planning	Implementation	Evaluation
Levine	Focus is on using the four conservation principles as a basis for observing and interviewing Mrs. James. Using the principle relative to personal integrity, the nurse questions Mrs. James about her life style before she had the stroke: "What did you usually do each day? How did you get to the garden club?" Analysis of data reflects Mrs. James's balance of strengths and weaknesses in each of the four conservation areas.	Relates to state of illness or altered health reflecting a problem or potential problem with regard to a deficit or threatened deficit; i.e., personal integrity threatened due to increased dependency on others in caring for self.	Focus is on planning therapeutic interventions designed to promote adaptation that contributes to healing and restoration of health; i.e., plan to have Mrs. James ambulate to increase her sense of mobility and independence and conserve energy. Start out slowly—10 minutes twice a day, sitting before walking, and use of the walker.	Carries out the actions necessary based on conservation of energy, and structural, personal, and social integrity; i.e., have Mrs. James sit on the side of the bed for 2 minutes, sit in a chair for 10 minutes, walk to bathroom and back using walker, and increase time of walking as Mrs. James's strength increases.	Relates to Mrs. James's adaptation to changes in her life style that threaten personal integrity, i.e., able to walk with assistance of walker, manipulate walker very well; out of bed all day; has contacted garden club.
Johnson	Focus is on the behavioral subsystems to identify disturbances in struc-	Relates to a description of the behavior that is associated with an actual or	Focus is on identification of short- and long-term goals in the system or sub-	Carries out the necessary activities to assist Mrs. James in modifying, chang-	Relates to the degree of progress in achieving the goals set during planning.

ture and function of subsystems or a discrepancy in behavioral functioning. *Affiliative and dependency subsystems:* Mrs. James has no family for support and affection. Has relied on her outreach through volunteering and her relationship with garden club members for support and assistance. Limited mobility has curtailed outreach. Came to hospital alone.	potential instability in the subsystem. Diminished ability for social behavior due to immobility. Weakening of affiliative subsystem due to limited access to friends.	system by modifying or changing behavior so that the goal of each subsystem will be met. Behavioral objectives are used to show progress toward goal. *Long-range goal:* Diminish the effects of hospitalization and immobilization on Mrs. James. *Short-term goals:* Preserve and strengthen Mrs. James's relationships with friends to encourage and enhance her interest and caring about others.	ing, or regulating behavior so that the goal of each subsystem will be met. Behavioral objectives are used to show progress toward goal. 1. Within two days have Mrs. James contact at least two of her garden club friends. 2. Within four days have Mrs. James, with the use of the walker, visit each client in the room to begin to get to know them.	Mrs. James called her "dearest" friend, Ada Brown, within two days and made plans to call Mrs. Johnson by the next day. Mrs. James also visited each client in the room, using her walker, and decided that she would spend time each day with Mrs. Smith who has no visitors.
Rogers Focus is on collecting data and opinions about the person and the environment relative to principles of integrality, helicy, resonancy; i.e., How is Mrs. James	Relates to rhythms, patterns, and life process and reflects the principles of homeodynamics, i.e., alteration in sleep pattern.	Focuses on promoting dynamic repatterning with regard to alteration in Mrs. James's sleeping pattern. Plans are to provide an environment conducive to sleeping;	Carries out the strategies necessary to strengthen the the individual-environment relationship. Ask Mrs. James to tend plants on unit, thus increasing walking	Relates to optimum state of health; i.e., What is Mrs. James's pattern of sleeping by the third day following nursing implementation? How long is she sleeping? How

(continued)

331

Table 18-1
(Continued)

Theorist	Assessment	Nursing Diagnosis	Planning	Implementation	Evaluation
	interacting with the hospital environment? Mrs. James reports difficulty in sleeping in the hospital. Until she was hospitalized, she slept 6–7 hours a night. Was very active, gardened. How has the life process of Mrs. James progressed to date? What kind of patterns characterize Mrs. James?		increase activity during the day based on Mrs. James's previous life style; use relaxation techniques to promote readiness for sleep.	and providing a purpose. Air and smooth her bed; use appropriate pillows; flex her knees to reduce any pulling on her back muscles.	well is she sleeping? Does she wake at night? Does she need sleep medication? How does Mrs. James feel and look?
King	Focus is on the nurse's and Mrs. James's perception of Mrs. James's health status and her ability to adapt to stresses and to use resources to achieve potential for daily living. Mrs.	Relates to the nurse's understanding and analysis of the data about Mrs. James's social system, perceptions; interpersonal relations, and health; i.e., difficulty coping with feelings of dependency.	Focus is on mutual goal setting with clear communication necessary for setting goals to move Mrs. James toward health. Working with Mrs. James, the nurse and Mrs. James	Carries out the activities necessary for Mrs. James to achieve increased independence; i.e., teach Mrs. James to eat with right hand. Prepare food so she can do so. Stay with Mrs.	Relates to how well the interpersonal process of nursing assisted Mrs. James in meeting the basic activities of daily living and to cope with health and illness; i.e., feels less de-

Neuman	James is viewed as a reacting being, a time-oriented being, and a social being; i.e., being dependent on others to feed and dress me, even to go to the bathroom." Left-handed, no strength in left hand, left-sided weakness.	Relates to stressors identified in each area—intra-, inter-, extra-personal; i.e., immobility due to left-sided weakness; intermittent lack of bladder control; diminished socialization due to immobility.	identify ways to increase Mrs. James's independence in the hospital; i.e., learn to feed self with right hand; learn to walk with walker; progress to using cane; learn to use elevator.	James until she feels confident. Assist Mrs. James to use and manipulate walker in walking and using elevator.	pendent now that she can feed self with right hand; ambulation allows Mrs. James to move out of four-bed room and relate to others; using elevator decreases feelings of dependency. "I feel so much better now that I can go to the bathroom by myself and feed myself."
	Focus is on Mrs. James's reaction to known or possible stressors—intra-, inter-, extra-personal. Also looks at lines of defense and resistance. *Intrapersonal:* Mrs. James is left-handed with muscle weakness of left arm and hand and left leg. Incontinent		Focus is on setting priorities to facilitate Mrs. James's adaptive behaviors to stress. Teach Mrs. James to feed herself with right hand. Teach Mrs. James to use walker to become more mobile. Begin exercises for bladder control. Encourage Mrs. James to use	Carries out the necessary actions to achieve highest level of reconstitution. Focus is on primary, secondary, and tertiary prevention; i.e., primary prevention—reduce the possibility of Mrs. James becoming depressed by increasing independence and as-	Relates to the degree of reconstitution achieved. Mrs. James is able to feed self with right hand with little assistance. Needs help to cut meat. Able to use the walker to use the bathroom. Incontinence is occurring less frequently. Mrs. James

(continued)

Table 18-1
(Continued)

Theorist	Assessment	Nursing Diagnosis	Planning	Implementation	Evaluation
	at times. *Interpersonal:* Separated from friends. *Extrapersonal:* Unable to engage in gardening or do volunteer work. Nurse asks Mrs. James, "What are you doing and what can you do to help yourself?" "I'm being fed, but I think I can feed myself. I want to walk to the bathroom."		walker to get to bathroom.	sisting her to feed herself immediately. Get Mrs. James out of bed and using walker to go to the bathroom. Introduce her to others in the room. Tell her how much she has accomplished. Praise her for her accomplishments.	tries hard to improve the strength of her right side. She is determined to go home as quickly as possible. She tries to cheer the other people in the room.
Paterson and Zderad	Focus is on describing what is and confirming it with Mrs. James. This begins the interdependent relationship between the nurse and the nursed. Mrs. James is a	Based on assessment and relates to comfort-discomfort level. Bruised self-image due to change in body function. Limited support system due to lack of family.	Identification of ways to reduce discomfort and increase comfort to help nursed become all she can be. Assist Mrs. James to become more independent by teaching	The nurse becomes truly present to Mrs. James and behaves in ways to reduce discomfort and relieve tension. Have Mrs. James call at least two of her garden club friends.	The nurse examines how effective her relationship and action with Mrs. James have been in reducing discomfort and alleviating tension. *Increased inde-*

strong, independent woman who has weakness in the left side of her body. She is left-handed, cannot feed or dress herself, cannot walk without help. Depends on garden club friends, has no family.

"Mrs. James, I'm Sue Ryan, your nurse. Can you tell me what is happening with you?"

"Well, I've had a stroke and I can't do anything without help. My friends don't know where I am—I'm a mess."

her how to feed self with right hand and how to use walker to become more mobile. This will give her more control over her life and will increase her comfort. Encourage contact with her garden club friends for needed support system.

Be there for Mrs. James. Feed her when necessary. Share feelings with her. Teach her to use right hand. Encourage Mrs. James to use walker to increase her mobility and independence. Discuss her plans for the future.

pendence: Mrs. James learned to eat with her right hand within two days. Now uses walker with ease. Visits people in room with her. Uses bathroom without assistance. *Decreased discomfort and relieved tension:* Now has more control over her situation. Has decided to return home. Sharing her plans for the next few months. Mrs. James and nurse have been truly present with each other. Mrs. James's self-confidence has been bolstered, and she has learned ways to become independent and in control. She has dis-

(continued)

Table 18-1
(Continued)

Theorist	Assessment	Nursing Diagnosis	Planning	Implementation	Evaluation
					cussed care after discharge. Mrs. James and nurse have planned contact after her discharge.
Roy	*First level:* Focus is on collecting data related to each adaptation mode. Physiological mode: Mrs. James's behavior related to rest and sleep. "I'm having trouble sleeping at night. I'm used to 7 hours sleep a night." Nurses during the night note Mrs. James is awake two to three times each night asking for something to sleep.	Relates to the deficits, or excesses, of basic needs leading to ineffective behavior; i.e., Inability to sleep throughout the night due to change in environment.	Focus is on promoting Mrs. James's adaptation in relation to the four modes. Physiologic mode: goal is Mrs. James will sleep if an environment conducive to sleeping is created.	Carries out activities necessary to manipulate the environment by removing, increasing, decreasing, and/or altering stimuli. The resulting behavior should be adaptive; i.e., provide for fresh air, freshen room at bedtime, reduce light and noise, encourage Mrs. James to fall asleep before others to reduce disturbance from	Relates to Mrs. James's goal achievement. After two nights, check with Mrs. James about restful sleep. Has sleeping improved? Does she look and feel rested in the morning? Review the night nurses' notes relating to Mrs. James's wakefulness.

Second level:
Focal stimuli—Mrs.
James is in a new
environment. Con-
textual stimuli—
other three people
in room snore.
Residual stimuli—
Mrs. James's inter-
nal response to all
the recent changes
in her life.

others' snoring.
Introduce Mrs.
James to relaxation
techniques before
sleeping.

GLOSSARY

Achievement subsystem (Johnson)* The behavioral subsystem relating to behaviors that attempt to control the environment and lead to personal accomplishment.

Adaptation (Levine) Process of adjusting or modifying behavior or functioning to fit the situation.

Adaptation (Rogers) Change resulting from the integration of human beings and their environment. The change occurs as an ongoing evolving process that can never return to the original state.

Adaptation (Roy) Positive response to internal or external stimuli using biopsychosocial mechanisms to promote personal integrity.

Adaptation level (Roy) Condition of the person, or the individual's range of coping ability.

Adaptive responses (Roy) Behaviors that positively affect health through promotion of the integrity of the person in terms of survival, growth, reproduction, and mastery.

Agent (Wiedenbach) The practicing nurse, or the nurse's delegate, who serves as the propelling force in goal-directed behavior.

---

*When a term relates specifically to a theorist, the name of the theorist appears in parentheses after the term.

338

Aggressive subsystem (Johnson)   The behavioral subsystem that relates to behaviors concerned with protection and self-preservation.

Assumption   Statement or view that is widely accepted as true.

Assumption (Wiedenbach)   The meaning a nurse attaches to an interpretation of a sensory impression.

Attachment or affiliative subsystem (Johnson)   The behavioral subsystem that is the first formed and provides for a strong social bond.

Authority (King)   An active, reciprocal relationship that involves values, experience, and perceptions in defining, validating, and accepting the right of an individual to act within an organization.

Automatic activities (Orlando)   Nursing actions decided on for reasons other than the patient's immediate need.

Body image (King)   Individuals' perceptions of their own bodies, influenced by the reactions of others.

Care (Hall)   The exclusive aspect of nursing that provides the patient bodily comfort through "laying on of hands" and provides an opportunity for closeness.

Central purpose (Wiedenbach)   The commitment of the individual nurse, based on a personal philosophy, that defines the desired quality of health and specifies the nurse's special responsibility in providing care to assist others in achieving or sustaining that quality.

Clustering of data   The grouping of data pieces that fit together and show relationships.

Cognator mechanism (Roy)   Coping mechanism or control subsystem that relates to the higher brain functions of perception/information processing, learning, judgment, and emotion.

Communication (King)   A direct or indirect process in which one person gives information to another.

Community (Paterson and Zderad)   Two or more persons striving together, living-dying all at once.

Concept   An abstract notion; a vehicle of thought that involves images.

Conceptual framework   Group of interrelated concepts.

Conservation (Levine)   Keeping together or maintaining a proper balance.

Conservation of energy (Levine)   Balancing energy output with energy input to avoid excessive fatigue.

Conservation of personal integrity (Levine)   Maintaining or restoring the patient's sense of identity and self-worth.

Conservation of social integrity (Levine)   Acknowledging the patient as a social being.

Conservation of structural integrity (Levine)　Maintaining or restoring the structure of the body.

Contextual stimuli (Roy)　Stimuli of the person's internal or external world, other than those immediately confronting the person, that influence the situation and are observable, measurable, or subjectively reported by the person.

Core (Hall)　The shared aspect with any health professional who therapeutically uses a freely offered closeness to help the patient discover who he is.

Covert problem　Hidden or concealed condition.

Culture (Rogers)　The integrated pattern of human behavior that includes thought, speech, action, and artifacts, and depends on man's capacity for learning and transmitting knowledge to succeeding generations.

Cure (Hall)　An aspect with medical personnel in which the nurse helps the patient and family through medical, surgical, and/or rehabilitative care.

Decision making in organizations (King)　An active process in which choice, directed by goals, is made and acted upon.

Deliberative actions (Orlando)　Nursing actions that ascertain or meet the patient's immediate need.

Dependency subsystem (Johnson)　The behavioral subsystem whose behaviors evoke nurturing behaviors in others.

Developmental self-care requisites (Orem)　Maintaining conditions to support life and development or to provide preventive care for adverse conditions that affect development.

Dialogue (Paterson and Zderad)　An intersubjective experience in which individuals relate creatively and have a real sharing.

Discrepancy (Johnson)　Action that does not achieve the goal intended.

Dominance (Johnson)　Primary use of one behavioral subsystem to the detriment of the other subsystems and regardless of the situation.

Eliminative subsystem (Johnson)　The behavioral subsystem that relates to socially acceptable behaviors surrounding the excretion of waste products from the body.

Empirical testing　Measurement or observation of real world events.

Environment (Neuman)　Those internal and external forces that surround humans at any given point in time.

Environment (Nightingale)　External conditions and influences that affect life and development.

Environment (Rogers)   Four-dimensional, negentropic energy field identified by pattern and encompassing all that is outside any given human field.

Environment (Roy)   All conditions, circumstances, and influences surrounding and affecting the development and behavior of persons or groups.

Equifinality   An open system that may attain a time-independent state independent of initial conditions and determined only by the system parameters.

Exploitation phase (Peplau)   The third phase of Peplau's nurse-patient relationship. The patient takes full advantage of all available services while feeling an integral part of the helping environment. Goals are met through a collaborative effort as the patient becomes independent during convalescence.

Extrapersonal stressors (Neuman)   Forces occurring outside the system that generate a reaction or response from the system.

First level assessment (Roy)   Behavioral assessment; the gathering of output behaviors of the person in relation to the four adaptive modes.

Flexible line of defense (Neuman)   Variable and constantly changing ability to respond to stressors.

Focal stimuli (Roy)   Stimuli of the person's internal or external world that immediately confront the person.

Framework (Wiedenbach)   The human, environmental, professional, and organizational facilities that make up the context in which nursing is practiced and constitute its currently existing limits.

General system theory   A general science of wholeness.

Goal   The end stated in broad terms to identify effective criteria for evaluating nursing action.

Goal (Wiedenbach)   Desired outcome the nurse seeks to achieve.

Growth and development (King)   The process in the lives of individuals that involves changes at the cellular, molecular, and behavioral levels and helps them move from potential to achievement.

Health deviation self-care (Orem)   Care needed by individuals who are ill or injured; may result from medical measures required to correct illness or injury.

Health problem

Actual   Client need that currently exists.

Potential   Client need that may occur in the future and which may be averted with appropriate action.

Helicy (Rogers)   The nature and direction of human and environmental change; change that is continuously innovative, probabilistic, and characterized by increasing diversity of the human field and environmental field pattern emerging out of the continuous, mutual, simultaneous interaction between the human and environmental fields and manifesting nonrepeating rhythmicities.

Holism   A theory that the universe and especially living nature are correctly seen in terms of interacting wholes that are more than the mere sum of the individual parts.

Homeodynamics (Rogers)   A way of viewing man in his wholeness. Changes in the life process of human beings are irreversible, nonrepeatable, rhythmical in nature, and evidence growing complexity of pattern. Change proceeds by continuous repatterning of both human beings and environment by resonating waves, and reflects the mutual simultaneous interaction between the two at any given point in space-time.

Humanism (Rogers)   A doctrine, attitude, or way of life centered on human interests or values. A philosophy that asserts the dignity and worth of human beings and their capacity of becoming through choices.

Identification phase (Peplau)   The second phase of Peplau's nurse-patient relationship. The perceptions and expectations of the patient and nurse become more involved while building a working relationship of further identifying the problem and deciding on appropriate plans for improved health maintenance.

Illness (Levine)   State of altered health.

Illness (Neuman)   State of insufficiency in which needs are yet to be satisfied.

Incompatibility (Johnson)   Two behavioral subsystems in the same situation being in conflict with each other.

Ineffective responses (Roy)   Behaviors that do not promote the integrity of the person in terms of survival, growth, reproduction, and mastery.

Ingestive subsystem (Johnson)   The behavioral subsystem that relates to the meanings and structures of social events surrounding the occasions when food is eaten.

Insufficiency (Johnson)   A behavioral subsystem that is not functioning adequately.

Integrality (Rogers)   The continuous, mutual, simultaneous integration process between human and environmental fields.

Interactions (King)   The observable, goal-directed, behaviors of two or more persons in mutual presence.

Interpersonal stressors (Neuman)   Forces that occur between two or more individuals and evoke a reaction or response.

Intrapersonal stressors (Neuman)   Forces occurring within a person that result in a reaction or response.

Lines of resistance (Neuman)   The internal set of factors that seek to stabilize the person when stressors break through the normal line of defense.

Means (Wiedenbach)   The activities and devices that enable the nurse to attain the desired goal.

Meeting (Paterson and Zderad)   The coming together of human beings characterized by the expectation that there will be a nurse and a nursed.

More-being (Paterson and Zderad)   The process of becoming all that is humanly possible.

Need for help (Orlando)   A requirement for assistance in decreasing or eliminating immediate distress or in improving the sense of adequacy.

Negentropy   The open system growth process of becoming more complex and efficient.

Normal line of defense (Neuman)   The biological-psychological-sociocultural-developmental skills developed over a lifetime to achieve stability and deal with stressors.

Nursing agency (Orem)   The specialized abilities that enable nurses to provide nursing care.

Nursing problem (Abdellah)   A condition faced by the client or client's family with which the nurse can assist through the performance of professional functions.

Nursing process   A deliberate, intellectual activity whereby the practice of nursing is approached in an orderly, systematic manner. It includes the following components:

Assessment   The process of data collection that results in a conclusion or nursing diagnosis.

Diagnosis   A behavioral statement that identifies the client's actual or potential health problem, deficit, or concern that can be affected by nursing actions.

Planning   The determination of what can be done to assist the client, including setting goals, judging priorities, and designing methods to resolve problems.

Implementation   Action initiated to accomplish defined goals.

Evaluation   The appraisal of the client's behavioral changes due to the action of the nurse.

Outcome evaluation   Evaluation based on behavioral changes.

Structure evaluation   Evaluation relating to the availability of appropriate equipment.

Process evaluation   Evaluation that focuses on the activities of the nurse.

Reassessment   The process of collecting additional data during the planning, implementing, and/or evaluation phases of the nursing process that may lead to immediate changes in those phases, or a change in the nursing diagnosis.

Nurturer (Hall)   A fosterer of learning, growing, and healing.

Objective   A specific means by which one proposes to accomplish or attain the goal.

Organismic response (Levine)   Changes in behavior or in the level of bodily functioning exhibited by a person adapting or attempting to adapt to the environment.

Organization (King)   An entity made up of individuals who have prescribed roles and positions and who use resources to achieve goals.

Orientation phase (Peplau)   The first phase of Peplau's nurse-patient relationship. Through assessment, the patient's health needs, expectations, and goals are explored and a care plan is devised. Concurrently, the roles of nurse and patient are being identified and clarified.

Overt problem   Apparent or obvious condition.

Parsimonious theory   Theory that is both simple and generalizable.

Partly compensatory system (Orem)   A situation where both nurse and patient perform care measures or other actions involving manipulative tasks or ambulation.

Perception (King)   An individual's view of reality that gives meaning to personal experience and involves the organization, interpretation, and transformation of information from sensory data and memory.

Potential comforter (Hall)   The role of the nurse seen by the patient during the care aspect of nursing.

Potential painer (Hall)   The role of the nurse seen by the patient during the cure aspect of nursing.

Power (King)   A social force and ability to use resources to influence people to achieve goals.

Prescription (Wiedenbach)   A directive for activity that specifies both the nature of the action and the necessary thought process.

Prescriptive theory (Wiedenbach)   A theory that conceptualizes both the desired situation and the activities to be used to bring about that desired situation.

Presence (Paterson and Zderad) The quality of being open, receptive, ready, and available to another in a reciprocal manner.

Primary prevention (Neuman) The application of general knowledge in a client situation to try to identify stressors before they occur.

Problem-solving process Identifying the problem, selecting pertinent data, formulating hypotheses, testing hypotheses through the collection of data, and revising hypotheses.

Professional nursing action (Orlando) What the nurse says or does for the benefit of the patient.

Realities in the immediate situation (Wiedenbach) At any given moment, all factors at play in the situation in which nursing actions occur; realities include the agent, the recipient, the goal, the means, and the framework.

Recipient (Wiedenbach) The vulnerable and dependent patient who is characterized by personal attributes, problems, and capabilities, including the ability to cope.

Reflective technique (Hall) The process of helping the patient see who he is by mirroring what the person's behavior says, both verbally and nonverbally.

Regulator mechanism (Roy) Coping mechanism subsystem that includes chemical, neural, and endocrine transmitters and autonomic and psychomotor responses.

Relating (Paterson and Zderad) The process of nurse-nursed "doing" with each other, being with each other.

Residual stimuli (Roy) Characteristics of the individual that are relevant to the situation but are difficult to measure objectively.

Resolution phase (Peplau) The fourth and final phase of Peplau's nurse-patient relationship. This phase evolves from the successful completion of the previous phases. The patient and nurse terminate their therapeutic relationship as the patient's needs are met and movement is made toward new goals.

Resonancy (Rogers) The identification of the human field and the environmental field by wave pattern manifesting continuous change from lower frequency longer waves to higher frequency shorter waves.

Role (King) The set of behaviors and rules that relate to an individual in a position in a social system.

Secondary prevention (Neuman) Treatment of symptoms of stress reaction to lead to reconstitution.

Second level assessment (Roy) The collection of data about focal, contextual, and residual stimuli impinging on the person.

Self-care (Orem)   Practice of activities that individuals personally initiate and perform on their own behalf to maintain life, health, and well-being.

Self-care agency (Orem)   The human ability to enage in self-care.

Self-care deficit (Orem)   The inability of an individual to carry out all necessary self-care activities.

Set (Johnson)   An individual's predisposition to behave in a certain way.

Sexual subsystem (Johnson)   The behavioral subsystem that reflects socially acceptable behaviors related to procreation.

Space (King)   A universal area, known also as *territory*, that is defined in part by the behavior of those who occupy it.

Status (King)   The relationship of an individual to a group, or a group to other groups, including identified duties, obligations, and privileges.

Stress (King)   A positive or negative energy response to interactions with the environment in an effort to maintain balance in living.

Supportive-educative system (Orem)   A situation where the patient is able to perform, or can and should learn to perform, required measures of externally or internally orientated therapeutic self-care but cannot do so without assistance.

Supportive intervention (Levine)   Action that maintains the patient's present state of altered health and prevents further health deterioration.

Synergistic wholeness (Rogers)   Cooperative action of discrete agencies such that the total effect is greater than the sum of the effects taken independently.

Tertiary prevention (Neuman)   Activities that seek to strengthen the lines of resistance after reconstitution has occurred.

Theory   A set of interrelated concepts that are testable and provide direction or prediction.

Therapeutic interpersonal relationship (Peplau)   A relationship between patient and nurse in which their collaborative effort is directed toward identifying, exploring, and resolving the patient's need productively. The relationship progresses along a continuum as each experiences growth through an increasing understanding of one another's roles, attitudes, and perceptions.

Therapeutic intervention (Levine)   Action that promotes healing and restoration of health.

Time (King)   The relation of one event to another, uniquely experienced by each individual.

Transactions (King)   Observable behaviors between individuals and their environment that lead to the attainment of valued goals.

Unitary humans (Rogers)   Four-dimensional, negentropic energy fields identified by pattern and manifesting characteristics and behaviors different from those of the parts, and which cannot be predicted from knowledge of the parts.

Universal self-care requisites (Orem)   Those requisites, common to all human beings throughout life, associated with life processes and the integrity of human structure and function.

Well-being (Paterson and Zderad)   A steady state.

Wholly compensatory nursing system (Orem)   A situation in which the patient has no active role in the performance of self-care.

INDEX